Basaglia's International Legacy

Basaglia's International Legacy

From Asylum to Community

Edited by

Tom Burns

Department of Psychiatry,
University of Oxford, Warneford Hospital,
Oxford, UK

John Foot

Department of Italian, School of Modern Languages,
University of Bristol, Bristol, UK

OXFORD
UNIVERSITY PRESS

OXFORD
UNIVERSITY PRESS

Great Clarendon Street, Oxford, OX2 6DP,
United Kingdom

Oxford University Press is a department of the University of Oxford.
It furthers the University's objective of excellence in research, scholarship,
and education by publishing worldwide. Oxford is a registered trade mark of
Oxford University Press in the UK and in certain other countries

First Edition published in 2020

Impression: 1

Published in the United States of America by Oxford University Press
198 Madison Avenue, New York, NY 10016, United States of America

British Library Cataloguing in Publication Data

Data available

Library of Congress Control Number: 2020935856

ISBN 978–0–19–884101–2

Printed and bound by
CPI Group (UK) Ltd, Croydon, CR0 4YY

Acknowledgements

The editors would like to thank all the authors for their hard work and remarkable punctuality, and for those who contributed to two days of friendly and stimulating discussion in Oxford in September 2018, and who travelled from as far afield as Brazil. The preparation and running of the seminar would not have been possible without the superb and generous work of Ksenija Yeeles and Mio Shimazaki. Jocelyn Catty took notes from the discussions which were invaluable in the revisions of chapters for publication. The symposium was funded from sources within the Department of Psychiatry at the University of Oxford with a contribution from the Association of Modern Italy. St Anne's College provided hospitality and a perfect venue for our discussions, which continued into the pubs of Oxford. Excellent photos from Trieste were generously provided by Claudio Erné. Peter Stephenson, Lauren Tiley, and Rachel Goldsworthy from Oxford University Press provided excellent support and encouragement throughout.

Tom Burns
John Foot

Contents

Abbreviations ix
Contributors xi
Introduction xiii

1. Franco Basaglia: a man, a movement, institutions, and outcomes 1
2. Basaglia and the British anti-psychiatrists, 1960–70 23
3. Basaglia after Basaglia: recovery, human rights, and Trieste today 43
4. Basaglia's legacy and Italian mental healthcare today 69
5. Basaglia's international influence 79
6. The impact in Latin America of Basaglia and Italian psychiatric reform 95
7. The optimism of practice: the impact of Basaglia's thoughts on Brazil 113
8. From the asylum to community mental health services: the path to human rights 129
9. Spain: the critical movements and the influence of Franco Basaglia and 'Democratic Psychiatry' 147
10. Franco Basaglia's influence on the Greek mental health system 161
11. The United Kingdom's rejection of Basaglia 175
12. Franco Basaglia: another conspicuous non-event in the history of psychiatry in Ireland? 191
13. *Asylum*: a magazine for democratic psychiatry in England 205
14. 'Visions of another world': Franco Basaglia and German reform 227
15. Has the spirit of Basaglia affected Polish psychiatry? 245
16. A spectre for some, a Mecca for others: the impact of Basaglia in the Netherlands 257
17. Basaglia in France: the marginality of exemplarity 275

18. Borderline deinstitutionalization: Yugoslav resonance and dissonance with Basaglia 295

19. The Trieste model: obstacles to replication in San Francisco 317

20. Deinstitutionalization, the welfare state, and social engineering: Basaglia in the Swedish context 333

21. Making sense of Basaglia: cross-cutting themes and unresolved issues 347

Index 361

Abbreviations

ABRASME	Brazilian Association of Mental Health
ACT	assertive community treatment
AMP	Psychiatry Association of Minas Gerais
AO	aziende ospedaliere
APO	Ausserparlamentarische Opposition
ASEPSI	Association pour l'Etude et la Promotion des Structures Intermédiaires
BR	Brigate Rosse
CAPO	Campaign against Psychiatric Oppression
CAPS	centres for psychosocial care
CELS	Centro Estudios Legales y Sociales
CEO	Chief Executive Officer
CIM	centri di igieni mentali
CMH	community mental health
COPERSAMM	Permanent Conference for Mental Health in the World
CRPD	Convention on the Rights of Persons with Disabilities
DGPN	Deutsche Gesellschaft für Psychiatrie und Nervenheilkunde
DGSP	Deutsche Gesellschaft für Soziale Psychiatrie
DI	deinstitutionalization
DMH	Department of Mental Health
EBM	evidence-based medicine
ECT	electroconvulsive therapy
EU	European Union
GDP	gross domestic product
GIA	Groupe d'Information sur les Asiles
IBRAPSI	Brazilian Institute of Group and Institutional Psychology and Psychoanalysis
IMHCN	International Mental Health Collaborating Network
LHT	local hospital/health trust
MDRI	Mental Disability Rights International
MHC	mental health centre
MK	Mannheimer Kreis
MTSM	Mental Health Workers' Movement
NBSA	National Board of Social Affairs
NGO	non-governmental organization
NHS	National Health System/Service
NICE	National Institute of Health and Care Excellence
NIMH	National Institute of Mental Health
PAHO	Pan American Health Organization
PHA	Psychiatric Hospital of Attaca

PNASH	Valuation and Restructuring Programme of the Psychiatric Assistance in Hospitals [Brazil]
PROMPT	Protection of the Rights of Mental Patients in Treatment
PT	Workers' Party [Brazil]
RAF	Rote Armee Fraktion
RENILA	Anti-Asylum Fight Centres' Network
RMPC	Royal Medico-Psychological Association
SIEP	Italian Society of Psychiatric Epidemiology
SOU	Statens Offentliga Utredningar
SPDC	social psychiatric service centre
SPK	Sozialistisches Patientenkollektiv
SRO	single-room occupancy
SSI	Supplemental Security Income
SUS	Unified Health System [Brazil]
TAPS	Team for the Assessment of Psychiatric Services
UN	United Nations
USSL	Unità Socio-Sanitaria Locale
WHO	World Health Organization

Contributors

Paulo Amarante The Oswaldo Cruz Foundation (FIOCRUZ), Brazilian Ministry of Health, Rio de Janeiro, Brazil

Alejandra Barcala National University of Lanús, Buenos Aires, Argentina

Victor Aparicio Basauri Central University Hospital of Asturias, Principality of Asturias, Spain

Thomas Becker Department of Psychiatry II, Ulm University, Günzburg, Germany

Gemma Blok Open University of the Netherlands, Heerlen, The Netherlands

Maria Stella Brandão Goulart Federal University of Minas Gerais, Belo Horizonte, Brazil

Tom Burns Department of Psychiatry, University of Oxford, Warneford Hospital, Oxford, UK

José Miguel Caldas de Almeida Lisbon Institute of Global Mental Health, Lisbon, Portugal

Nataša Cvetković Jović International Aid Network (IAN), Belgrade, Serbia

Heiner Fangerau Heinrich Heine University Düsseldorf, Düsseldorf, Germany

Angelo Fioritti Department of Mental Health, AUSL Bologna, Bologna, Italy

Vito Flaker Faculty of Social Work, University of Ljubljana, Ljubljana, Slovenia

John Foot Department of Italian, School of Modern Languages, University of Bristol, Bristol, UK

Nicolas Henckes Center for Research Medicine, Sciences, Health, Mental Health and Society, Paris, France

Grażyna Herczyńska Public Health Department, Institute of Psychiatry and Neurology, Warsaw, Poland

Vladimir Jović Center for Rehabilitation of Torture Victims, International Aid Network (IAN), Belgrade, Serbia

Brendan D. Kelly Department of Psychiatry, Trinity College Dublin, Trinity Centre for Health Sciences, Tallaght University Hospital, Dublin, Ireland

Anne M. Lovell Center for Research Medicine, Sciences, Health, Mental Health and Society, Paris, France

Chantal Marazia Heinrich Heine University Düsseldorf, Düsseldorf, Germany

Diana Mauri University of Milan-Bicocca, Milan, Italy

Theodoros Megaloeconomou Former Director of the Ninth Department of Psychiatry, Psychiatric Hospital, Athens, Greece

Roberto Mezzina WHO Collaborating Centre for Research and Training in Mental Health, Trieste, Italy

Jacek Moskalewicz Department of Studies on Alcoholism and Drug Dependence, Institute of Psychiatry and Neurology, Warsaw, Poland

Robert Okin Professor Emeritus Psychiatry, UCSF School of Medicine, San Francisco, California

Katarzyna Prot-Klinger Institute of Psychology, Maria Grzegorzewska University Academy of Special Education, Warsaw, Poland

Andreja Rafaelič Faculty for Social Work, University of Ljubljana and Social Protection Institute of the Republic of Slovenija, Ljubljana, Slovenia

Benedetto Saraceno Lisbon Institute of Global Mental Health, Lisbon, Portugal

Sashi P. Sashidharan Institute of Health and Wellbeing, University of Glasgow, Glasgow, UK

Felicitas Söhner Heinrich Heine University Düsseldorf, Düsseldorf, Germany

Helen Spandler School of Social Work, University of Central Lancashire, Preston, UK

Alain Topor Department of Psychosocial Health University of Agder, Norway

Ernesto Venturini University of the Republic of San Marino, San Marino

Oisín Wall School of History, University College Dublin, Dublin, Ireland

Introduction

The closure of mental hospitals is the dominant feature of mental healthcare in the second half of the twentieth century. These enormous institutions, offspring of the lunatic asylum building programme of the nineteenth and twentieth centuries in many countries across the world, had come to symbolize all that was fearful about mental illness and psychiatry. They often housed thousands of souls—the largest ever built Pilgrim State Hospital in New York had an inpatient population of over 13,000 at its height. Their fearsome reputation—that once admitted you never emerged again—earned them a place in local folklore, used as a threat to frighten naughty children. By the 1950s, there were 150,000 patients in such institutions in the UK, 100,000 in Italy, and 500,000 in the USA, many having been there decades. Morale was dreadful and reports of scandalous abuses began to filter out to a shocked public. Their time was undoubtedly up and the process of reforming or closing them began.

A name that dominates the literature of this process is that of the Italian psychiatrist Franco Basaglia (1924–1980). Basaglia rose to international fame in the 1970s as the reforming director of two obscure mental hospitals in northern Italy—the first in Gorizia, the other in Trieste. Basaglia turned his back on the international consensus of reforming and reducing the size of mental hospitals and insisted that they simply had to be closed. He viewed them as irremediably destructive and was impatient to liberate patients from them. This movement, which came to be called Psichiatria Democratica (Democratic Psychiatry), caught the public imagination with its slogan 'libertà è terapeutica' ('freedom heals'). Basaglia was one of the main protagonists of this movement in Italy, but was by no means the only reforming voice to emerge from that system. Energetic and charismatic, Basaglia was outward looking, and politically and culturally well connected. The crowning achievement of this Psichiatria Democratica was the passing in 1978 of Italian Law 180 (which became known in common parlance as 'Basaglia's Law'). This is considered the most radical mental health legislation ever passed in any country. It prohibited the admission of any new patients to mental hospitals throughout Italy from that day forward. With a limited three-year transition period for established patients, it restricted all admissions to small, separate units, with stringent control over the use of compulsion. No new asylums were allowed to be built.

Of course, it was not that simple. Its application throughout Italy was patchy and it met pockets of resistance. It was extremely difficult to move thousands of patients out into the community, and to create new institutions to help those who had significant mental health problems but had never been inside what were called 'total institutions'. But Trieste and other centres (such as Arezzo and Perugia) flourished and became centres for both visiting psychiatrists wanting to learn and many young people, from across the world, wanting to volunteer. Basaglia's dramatic success in opening what were once appallingly repressive and abusive institutions met with acclaim in Italy and abroad, although opinion was always divided. His influence in Latin America and several Mediterranean countries has been decisive in shaping not just their practice but also their mental health policy and law. Trieste has been strongly promoted as a model by the World Health Organization (WHO) and remains a designated centre for teaching and research. This book was originally conceived to mark the fortieth anniversary of Law 180 and to reflect on Basaglia's international impact.

Much has been written about Basaglia and the Italian mental health reforms and practice of the 1960s and 1970s, but very little research or reflection has taken place with relation to the global influence of these experiences, writings, and legislation. This book aims to fill this gap, and to open up a number of questions for further discussion.

There were many different roads to deinstitutionalization, and some countries never embarked on this route at all. Italy was proud of its lack of psychiatric beds; other countries saw the lack of beds as a problem to be resolved. Italian solutions were sometimes praised, occasionally adopted, and often dismissed as utopian. Knowledge about what had actually happened in Italy was often sketchy, or based on brief visits to centres of excellence. Moreover, Italian mental healthcare varied widely from region to region. This was not just a classic north/south, rich/poor divide, but also depended on a series of other factors and varied over time—including the strength (or weakness) of the movement, individual initiatives, historical and political structures, the role of local universities, and social change, such as the arrival of new groups of immigrants. Many Italian mental health employees and psychiatrists rejected the more radical aspects of Psichiatria Democratica in terms of practice *and* theory. In any case, Psichiatria Democratica was itself highly divided. There was no single Italian model, and this book is also about different forms of translation, understanding, and misunderstanding across international borders.

The book is timely but, more importantly, we believe it is also unique in bringing Basaglians and non-Basaglians together. It not only explores what happened in countries where Basaglia's teachings were warmly received and implemented and interpreted in various ways, but also in those where they were either ignored or even actively rejected. Basaglian writers and practitioners have often disregarded these rejections, or simply dismissed them as medical or social conservatism. We believe this is a mistake. There is much to be learned from understanding the content and origin of this resistance. It can sharpen our focus on the cultural fit of Basaglia's ideas in different contexts. It can also help tease out what were the essential features of the Basaglian movement—distinguish its unique character and separate it out from the wider, global deinstitutionalization movement or simply the inevitable closure of large-scale mental health institutions across much of the world. This is not only important for contrasting, for example, Germany and Italy, but also for understanding Basaglia's relevance to Italy now—a very different place to Italy in the 1970s.

Psychiatry now has to operate in a radically different world to 40 years ago. Globalization, mass migration, the move of women into the workplace, smaller, more mobile and fragmented families, and an ageing population all demand a different mental health service. Being able to illuminate the Basaglian approach from different angles yields a deeper, nuanced understanding of its strengths and weaknesses. Moving beyond the often acrimonious polemic, and acknowledging shades of grey, should improve our understanding of Basaglia and Psichiatria Democratica and the Italian movement as a whole, both before and after the 1978 Law, and its global reach and translation. Through this process, we can come to a more balanced and focused appraisal of what Basaglia has to offer modern mental healthcare and its reform.

Structure of this book

Countries represented

Choosing who to invite to the two-day symposium in Oxford in September 2018 (the genesis of this book) was not straightforward. There is no simple catalogue of Basaglia experts or exponents. Inevitably, the process was organic. We contacted those who had written about the Italian experience, and then obtained leads from them. Although the focus of this book is on Basaglia's international impact, it made sense to capture the Italian experience comprehensively. Our three 'Italian' authors detailed the implementation of Psichiatria Democratica both in Italy (in Trieste and also in its varied forms across the country) and also, with a WHO overview, more internationally.

Many parts of the world are not covered in this book. Edited books which seek to be absolutely comprehensive, with chapters commissioned to fulfil a matrix, are not uncommon. We did not think there was anything served by replicating non-stories simply for the sake of completeness. There is no real evidence of a Basaglian influence in Asia, the Middle East, nor Africa (other than in Mozambique). During the symposium, Ernesto Venturini provided the following description of the Basaglian interlude in Mozambique. However, it may well be that there are experiences which are not covered in this book, and we hope its publication will stimulate further interest, bring such experiences to light, and fuel discussion.

In Geneva, at a meeting of Ministers of Health, Basaglia met Hélder Martins, Minister of Health of Mozambique. Martins asked Basaglia for help in building a psychiatric organization in his country, similar to the model of Italian reform. At the time of independence, most of the former Portuguese settlers, who operated the state apparatus, had fled to South Africa. The psychiatric system was based on four psychiatric hospitals (three in Maputo and one in Nampula) and on three psychiatric services in general hospitals (Maputo, Beira, Chissui). Only one Mozambican psychiatrist had remained in the country. Three South American psychiatrists (who had escaped from military dictatorships) were subsequently recruited, along with three Cuban psychiatrists and some nurses. Cuba, at that time, supported all sectors of the fraternal socialist country with such resources. The Italian State also supported Mozambique, and the Italian ambassador organized Basaglia's trip to Mozambique.

In 1978, Basaglia visited the psychiatric services and held a seminar in Maputo. A lively debate ensued between Basaglia and the Cuban psychiatrists who favoured a model centred on the psychiatric hospital. Upon returning to Italy, Basaglia enlisted the support of the Trieste team to co-operate with Mozambique. Venturini went, as an expert from the Italian Foreign Ministry, in September 1979. His aim was to prepare for the arrival of a group of Italian doctors. He remained for two years. A few months after the group's arrival, the minister was dismissed, the Italian ambassador was transferred, and Basaglia died suddenly. Venturini, however, remained and contributed to the closure of two psychiatric hospitals. In one hospital, he organized the first public meeting with traditional healers in the region, who had been persecuted by the Mozambican state, being considered charlatans and supporters of superstition. However, traditional healers had continued to be, clandestinely, the point of first health contact for the population. This initiative encouraged the integration of traditional medicine, as recommended by the WHO. However, the largest hospital in the city—Infulene—run by Cuban psychiatrists, did not adopt any deinstitutionalization project.

So, the first government of the Republic of Mozambique adopted ideas from Franco Basaglia and the Italian movement for reform. Although limited, important traces of his impact have remained. Twenty years later, the Trieste team was again involved in study visits, internships, and training seminars in Mozambique.

Both Australia and Japan have writers who have been personally very influenced by Basaglia and contact with Trieste. Active advocates for the Italian message in their countries, they are not however included here since there appears to be no substantive story to tell beyond their personal engagement: no story either of implementation or of a wider rejection by the psychiatric establishment. Clearly, if we are wrong in our judgement, we hope this book will stimulate others to tell these forgotten or less well-known stories.

The chapters in this book cover three main areas: Basaglia and his life, Italy and Basaglia's widening influence, and individual national responses. A final concluding chapter focuses on cross-cutting issues from the symposium discussions.

Basaglia and his life

While we write and speak of Basaglia, it is important to keep in mind that Basaglia worked and wrote jointly with a team of creative and forceful individuals—his équipe (which changed over time). His published statements and his approach often demonstrate an inconsistency that reflect this constant vibrant interaction. Despite this, he emerges as the clear leader and figurehead of Psichiatria Democratica and a symbol of the reforms. It is meaningful to speak of 'Basaglian psychiatry'. So who was Franco Basaglia, and what were the key moments in his life?

The first chapter in this book, 'Franco Basaglia: a man, a movement, institutions, and outcomes', is by John Foot. He has written a history of the Italian movement with a focus on the biography of Basaglia, but with a wider reach to many other areas of experimentation and reform. Foot's work gives a picture of this charismatic personality and how he moved, precipitously, from a sheltered university post to take charge of a run-down asylum in Gorizia on the former Yugoslav border. The chapter charts his struggles to implement his vision, the importance of his wife Franca Ongaro in the process, and the growth of a strong team around him. It follows his departure from Gorizia (via New York and Parma) to Trieste, where his developing community services and Law 180 bring him to international fame before his untimely death at the age of just 56 years. Foot tackles head on the problems of understanding a man whose history has been largely written by his followers, and how one gets beyond the mythology to the complex individual behind. He calls for an approach that does not just concentrate on Basaglia's career and practice, but also takes into account the experience in other cities and asylums in Italy. He also calls for exploration of the contradictions of the movement, and the various forces behind Law 180. This includes opposition to the ideas of Psichiatria Democratica, the divisions within the movement itself, and the role of more moderate or reformist psychiatry.

Early on, Basaglia was dismissed by his detractors as 'just another anti-psychiatrist'. This accusation—often based on a simplistic reading of both anti-psychiatry and the Basaglian movement itself—is still common today. Basaglia and many of his companions in the psychiatric reform movement were undoubtedly swept up in the radical movements of the time—cultural, political, and psychiatric. The UK anti-psychiatrists, and in particular R.D. Laing, had an important influence on Basaglia and many others in Italy. In Chapter 2, 'Basaglia and the British anti-psychiatrists', Oisín Wall outlines and explores the central similarities of much of their thinking. However, he also notes the crucial differences imposed by their wider political influences and aims.

Italy and Basaglia's widening influence

Chapters 3 to 5 take their origin from Basaglia's homeland, Italy. In Chapter 3, 'Basaglia after Basaglia: recovery, human rights, and Trieste today', Roberto Mezzina, the current director of Trieste mental health services (the most important place in terms of 'Basaglian' practice today within Italy), outlines the model service and how it has changed over time. Mezzina also considers how Basaglian ideas play out in many of the central concepts in current mental health thinking such as recovery and the struggle for civil rights.

In Chapter 4, 'Basaglia's legacy and Italian mental healthcare today', Angelo Fioritti (head of mental health services in the city of Bologna) analyses the practical implementation of the Basaglia reforms across Italy since 1978. Fioritti does not shy away from cataloguing the difficulties of applying the lessons of Trieste to larger cities and to the south of Italy with its greater poverty, stronger families, and relative lack of civic cohesion. He addresses the changes over time as Italy has come more to reflect the rest of Europe, particularly in its family structure. Fioritti also notes how Basaglia's successes, reflecting the spirit of the age, moved beyond mental health to influence other social organizations.

In Chapter 5, 'Basaglia's international influence', Benedetto Saraceno and Sashi Sashidharan outline how Basaglia's ideas and practice, and those of the movement, influenced international mental health policy initiatives. Saraceno had worked in Trieste and was WHO Director of Mental Health from 2000 to 2010. The authors explore how Basaglia's ideas might be applied within a public health framework. They also observe the failure of Basaglia's ideas to be taken up in much of the English-speaking world (the dominant language of science) and how reservations about his motivation may have inhibited that spread.

Individual national responses

The remaining bulk of the book is a series of reports outlining the reception and implementation of Basaglia's reforms in a number of different countries. These chapters were first presented in an intense and unique two-day workshop in Oxford, in the summer of 2018, which included researchers from 14 different countries. A wide-ranging and complicated debate took place over the legacy and meaning of the Italian story and Basaglia's ideas. Before briefly describing these individual contributions, they can be broadly assigned to three rough categories.

Chapters 6 to 10 describe the rapid uptake and profound influence of the Italian experience and 'model' in Spain and Latin America, and the limited but iconic impact in Greece. The next four chapters then report clear rejections of Basaglia. These differing national responses were based on examination of his proposals and decisions, in some countries, that they were not either useful or applicable. However, in some cases, Basaglia's ideas simply failed to circulate beyond a small or relatively insignificant number of psychiatrists and thinkers. In many chapters, issues are raised connected to questions of translation, understanding, and the practical issues related to rapid deinstitutionalization.

Of those countries that rejected the Basaglia experience, the UK was the most high-profile case and the most resented by the Italians (although the rejection by Germany was probably more acrimonious). France experienced a conflict with its own highly developed, radical, and idiosyncratic approach to mental hospital reform. The country's radical psychiatrists decided to work within the institutional framework of the asylum rather than close it down and construct alternative institutions. In Poland, meanwhile, a strongly entrenched and institution-based profession simply saw no need to change. In all these 'rejecting' countries, Basaglia's influence on the 'counterculture' was evident and often vigorous. A minority of clinicians and thinkers did embrace the ideas and practice emerging from Italy. Despite rejection by established psychiatry, visits to Trieste persisted and cordial relationships were maintained.

However, the local development of psychiatric reforms in these areas did not draw on Basaglia's approach, apart from in a few isolated cases.

The remaining chapters in this volume present a mixed picture. In the Netherlands and in Yugoslavia (before and after the war), Basaglia's practice and the Italian example received a warm reception in cultural and radical mental health circles. Some of his ideas achieved local implementation but not wholescale adoption. Similarly, in California, a spirited attempt to introduce Basaglian principles into San Franciscan mental health services foundered on the brutal reality of a grotesquely unequal society with impoverished or absent social provision. Sweden stands out as a country that took a radically different approach. It was initially welcoming of Basaglia's message and achieved the early abolition of all mental hospitals. However, in the end, it followed a diametrically opposite approach by sharply limiting, rather than softening and expanding, psychiatry's remit. Reform of the system and closure of the asylum did not have to be 'Basaglian'. There were (and are) many possible routes towards deinstitutionalization.

These groupings are simply an aide to thinking through the pattern of Basaglia's influence. They are in no way absolute. In those countries where Basaglia triumphed, there are still critics and alternatives. Similarly, in those that rejected the message, pockets of enthusiasm developed and survived. In Germany, Basaglian ideas were eagerly taken up and championed by some alternative service providers alongside mainstream psychiatry. In the UK, despite the establishment's rejection, relationships and visits have persisted. Chapter 13, '*Asylum*: a magazine for democratic psychiatry in England', by Helen Spandler, describes Basaglia's influence in one British city, Sheffield. It also outlines the legacy of the Italian movement amongst groups who worked, or are still working, within the mental health system.

In Chapter 6, 'The impact in Latin America of Basaglia and Italian psychiatric reform', José Miguel Caldas de Almeida focuses on high-level international processes to foster mental health reforms in the area. Starting with the Basaglian influence on the Caracas Declaration in 1990, Basaglian psychiatrists worked, through the Pan American Health Organization (PAHO), to support humane service development throughout the region. Basaglia's emphasis on civil rights was central to these initiatives and solidarity was leveraged to great benefit. Basaglia's impact in Brazil is probably his most spectacular achievement. Chapter 7, 'The optimism of practice: the impact of Basaglia's thoughts in Brazil', by Ernesto Venturini, Stella Goulart, and Paulo Amarante confirms the electrifying consequences of Basaglia's tour of the country in 1978 and 1979. The books based on his contributions during the lectures and debates in which he took part were published in a number of languages. The thorough reforming of Brazil's mental health services, resulting in the 2001 Mental Health Reform Law, all bear the stamp of his thinking. The Brazilian celebration of Basaglia outdid even that in Italy, with its sense of theatre and public engagement and in its political militancy and anti-fascist thinking (key components of the Italian movement).

The receptivity of Brazil to Basaglia's message is, in no small measure, a consequence of this being a country just emerging from the oppression of military dictatorship. The same dynamic is evident in Spain and Argentina and, to a lesser extent, in Italy itself after the decades of fascism. Chapter 8, 'From the asylum to community mental health services', by Diana Mauri and Alejandra Barcala, describes a similar though less dramatic impact. As in Brazil, ideas and lessons of the Italian experience were a major influence on the revisions of the Mental Health Act and on national policy. In Argentina, the military dictatorship persisted longer. Basaglia's ideas also had to compete with a very powerful and well-established psychoanalytical establishment. However, a permanent Basaglia Institute was successfully established in Buenos Aires. A downside of the arrival of Basaglia's ideas in Argentina, however, was that many of the newly enthused young doctors left to take jobs in Europe.

Basaglia's ideas, and those of Psichiatria Democratica, took root in Spain during, and despite, the Franco regime. Victor Aparicio Basauri, in Chapter 9, 'Spain: the critical movements and the influence of Franco Basaglia and 'Democratic Psychiatry'', provides a thrilling description of an illegal underground network of Spanish psychiatrists working for radical reform. Many of these lost their jobs. Links were close with Italy, and the seminal Basaglia text *L'Istituzione Negata* (*The Institution Denied*—which was never translated into English, but did appear in many other languages) was already available in Spain in 1972. Young Spanish psychiatrists shifted their allegiance from the French *secteur* approach to Basaglia and, after years of conflict, took over the lead of the very powerful Spanish Association of Neuro-Psychiatry in 1977. Basaglia's thinking became central to the ministerial document underlying the reform of mental health policy in 1985.

Young psychiatrists in Greece also welcomed Basaglia's ideas, but this was not echoed in their professional bodies. Theodore Megaloeconomou describes, in Chapter 10, 'Franco Basaglia's influence on the Greek mental health system', how the scandal of Leros brought practitioners and ideas from Trieste to Greece. The dreadful conditions of the neglected mentally ill in this island colony became an international scandal. Money poured in from the European Union to reform it and rehabilitate its residents. The Greek psychiatric establishment took little interest, and so teams from the Netherlands and Trieste worked alongside some individual Greek psychiatrists. Basaglian ideas took root and influenced the development of community services in a handful of areas across the country, but they failed to be generalizable. Could it be that the memory of Leros became, paradoxically, an impediment to reform? Was it so shameful that the memory had to be suppressed?

The UK in the 1970s considered itself in the vanguard of social psychiatry and deinstitutionalization. In Chapter 11, 'The United Kingdom's rejection of Basaglia', Tom Burns describes how the Italian claims were initially treated with some scepticism and then utterly rejected. Their fate was sealed by two damning articles in the *British Journal of Psychiatry* in 1985 and 1986. Kathleen Jones, a professor of social policy at York University, was interested in mental health implementation, not theory. She reported from her visits to Italy that, contrary to claims, the mental hospitals were simply not closed. Despite the furore generated by these articles in Italy, no productive dialogue was established to explore or contradict them. The UK (with some notable exceptions, as outlined in Helen Spandler's contribution) simply turned its back on Basaglia. Nonetheless, the large hospitals were scaled down here as well, and alternative services were created. In Chapter 12, 'Franco Basaglia: another conspicuous non-event in the history of psychiatry in Ireland', Brendan Kelly reports that Ireland took its lead from this debate in the UK, and rejected Basaglia. As Kelly demonstrates, however, the reasons for the Irish rejection were more complex and rooted in its unique social history, not simply a concern with data and figures. Ireland's status as the country with most psychiatric beds per head of population was a reflection of very specific social pressures rather than medical opinion. Similarly, its reforms were driven from outside the profession, such that now it has half the rate of compulsion in mental health as its UK neighbour.

Such rejections were never absolutely comprehensive. In Chapter 13, '*Asylum*: a magazine for democratic psychiatry in England', Helen Spandler describes an enduring radical mental health journal for practitioners and users. This was established in 1986 by the professor of psychiatry in Sheffield, Alec Jenner, after a visit from Trieste staff. Initially, it made many references to Basaglian psychiatry. Later issues have focused more on the survivor movement. However, it still retains its title as a 'magazine for democratic psychiatry' from its Basaglian origins. Similarly, Ireland produced some of the central figures of the 'critical' or 'post-psychiatry' movement who acknowledge their debt to Basaglia.

Basaglia was energetically discussed in German anti-psychiatry circles and stimulated some alternative provision, but the Italian movement was forcefully rejected by the established professional organizations. In Chapter 14, "Visions of another world': Franco Basaglia and German reform', Chantal Marazia and colleagues describe a very blunt dismissal of the Italian message. Much of this relates to the very strained relationships between the two countries during the 1970s, when both were racked by home-grown urban terrorism. However, the main source of the rejection (as in the UK) arose from the well-established and sophisticated planning for deinstitutionalization that was outlined in the German Enquète. The Italian plans seemed rough and ready by comparison, and their claims exaggerated. They were also seen as excessively politicized, and were often dismissed as utopian and dangerous. In later years, Basaglia and the Italian experience has been written about in much more positive terms. However, the move from the asylum is still seen essentially as a consequence of the international zeitgeist, rather than stemming from one individual or one set of ideas.

The language used (on both sides) in the German rejection of Basaglia is more personal and barbed than that between the UK and Italy. Despite this, the UK's rejection is more keenly felt by the Italians. This is in part due to the perceived power of English as the premier language of scientific journals. It is also a reflection of the compromised position of German psychiatry after its behaviour in the Second World War. It seems that Germany could be ignored in a way that the UK could not.

Basaglia's ideas were initially very warmly received in Poland in the context of an internationalized debate on radical psychiatry and anti-psychiatry. In Chapter 15,

'Has the spirit of Basaglia affected Polish psychiatry?', Jacek Moskalewicz and colleagues describe Polish engagement in these issues in the 1960s and 1970s. Several pilot projects were initiated across the country, with an emphasis on deinstitutionalization. These included a Basaglia-inspired model in a hospital just outside Warsaw in the 1970s. However, the 1980s and 1990s saw a retrenchment and a remedicalization of psychiatry. The Polish experience also portrays the 'colonization' of emergent East European states by the international pharmaceutical industry for drug trials. The dominance of large mental hospitals (which in practice had not gone away) became reasserted in Polish psychiatric life. Not every country closed its asylums, and in many places the 'old' system is alive and well. Many countries still have mental hospitals, albeit on a smaller scale. These are often transformed on the inside, compared to those of the 1950s and 1960s. Italy, meanwhile, has also recently closed its criminal asylums.

In several countries, Basaglia generated intense intellectual interest and admiration for what he had achieved in Trieste and elsewhere in Italy, but which failed to translate into reforms in established psychiatry. The Netherlands is a very clear example of this process. In Chapter 16, 'A spectre for some, a Mecca for others: the impact of Basaglia in the Netherlands', Gemma Blok outlines how Basaglia's work was translated for the Dutch arena in the mid-1970s. Basaglia's ideas were prominently discussed, and 'pilgrimages' to Trieste became common. Law 180, however, divided opinion and generated increased caution during an already timid reform process. Despite all the discussion, deinstitutionalization was remarkably slow. The Italian reforms, as often as not, were held up as the 'Italian mistake'.

The relationship between Basaglia's thinking and psychiatric reform in France is even more paradoxical. In Chapter 17, 'Basaglia in France: the marginality of exemplarity', Nicolas Henckes and Anne Lovell describe a meeting of two highly intellectual, politicized, and self-confident—but fundamentally different—approaches. Basaglia's ideas were warmly welcomed, and figured prominently in cultural and policy debates. Personal relationships were also close, with a lively interchange and high-profile debates in both countries. However, the French *secteur* system saw community provision run from within reformed mental hospitals. The French aim was not to close the asylum. Apart from some isolated services, such as that in Lille, Basaglia's approach failed to take root.

If the relationship with France is considered complex, what can one say of that with the former Yugoslavia? In Chapter 18, 'Borderline deinstitutionalization: Yugoslav resonance and dissonance with Basaglia', Vito Flaker and colleagues describe how impressions and ideas from Gorizia and Trieste (both within sight of the former Yugoslavia) were received and impacted by the upheavals in that country. Basaglia's ideas were initially welcomed, but then rejected as they clashed with local high-status social psychiatry. They then became overshadowed by the political fallout of the demise of Yugoslavia. During the 1980s, there were vigorous contacts with the Italian movement during the period of political liberalization. However, rivalries with local deinstitionalization movements became prominent. The relationship between liberalism and Yugoslav (anti-Stalinist) socialism led to endless complexities. These became overwhelmed by the wars in the 1990s and transition to more stable nation states, each of which had its own style of mental health development. The devastation from the wars has left impoverished mental health services still reliant on poor-quality asylums. Flaker and colleagues vividly describe what they term 'hiccups' in deinstitutionalization, a consequence of the vulnerability of the process to major political upheavals.

Basaglia and other Italian reformers developed their ideas and approach in a public healthcare system with access (at that time) to relatively generous social supports and in a community richly endowed with social capital. Could these ideas transfer to the USA with its highly commercialized medical care system and impoverished social welfare network? Robert Okin, in Chapter 19, 'The Trieste model: obstacles to replication in San Francisco', describes a spirited and persistent attempt to apply Basaglia's thinking in San Francisco. Not surprisingly, this would be a challenge in one of the most economically divided cities in the world. The USA has only rudimentary healthcare provision for the poor, and minimal welfare provision that effectively traps them in poverty. California had recently enacted one of the most savage retrenchments of mental healthcare in the developed world, so it was no surprise that such a radical and humane approach was doomed.

The last of these regional case histories, and in many ways one of the most remarkable, is that of Sweden. In Chapter 20, 'Deinstitutionalization, the welfare state, and social engineering: Basaglia in the Swedish context', Alain Topor describes how Sweden was probably the first country, after Italy, to totally close all its mental hospitals. However, their approach was embedded in a social democratic welfare state long used to 'social engineering' and diametrically opposite to Basaglia's. Rather than 'putting the diagnosis in brackets' and expanding psychiatry's reach to the whole person, Sweden actively decided to consolidate psychiatry into its medical roots. In a culture where the state had long accepted its responsibilities for the welfare of its citizens, the long-term care of the mentally ill was split off from medicine. It was taken over by local authorities who saw the provision of comprehensive support to the mentally ill as simply the same as that owed to any other group of vulnerable citizens. Psychiatry was left with a restricted role in treating acute episodes.

Conclusions and cross-cutting themes

Most of the authors of these chapters met for a two-day symposium in Oxford (St Anne's College, 14 and 15 September 2018). Each paper presented was followed by intense discussion. This was a unique experience, in many ways, as it brought committed Basaglians together with dispassionate historians and even critics. The meeting was not without its measure of conflict! The last chapter in this book reports on the emergent ideas from this symposium. Not surprisingly, there were no simple 'final answers'. The range and style of interpretations reflected the range and style of contributors and their cultures. 'Style'—cultural, political, philosophical—was clearly very important in how Basaglia and the Italian reforms were perceived and received in different countries. Such differences in national styles are apparent in the chapters in this book. These differences determine what they focus on, what they emphasize as important, and *how* they are described. We have made no attempt to homogenize the chapters or to impose a strict editorial format, so allowing these crucial differences to be reflected and taken up in Chapter 21.

Three types of issue emerged from the symposium. The first was a growing awareness of what is *not* dealt with in Basaglian literature and practice. There is nothing about gender, nothing about primary care, and nothing about specialist teams. The second focus was on a number of key matters where symposium members had differing, often strongly differing, perspectives. Some of these were about Basaglia himself and the movement which emerged in Italy in the 1960s and 1970s. Was Basaglia an anti-psychiatrist? Was he a Marxist? Was the movement ideological or simply pragmatic? In exploring the response to the reforms, the issue of the source of resistance, and in particular the role of professional hegemony, was hotly debated. Similarly, so too was the role of social capital in the patchy implementation in Italy and its impossibility in the USA. Lastly, the discussion flushed out ambiguities in our use of language and forced us to consider the meaning of the terms 'therapeutic community' and 'mental hospital'.

The book that follows does not give simple answers. As Basaglia himself would have wanted, it informs and challenges. There are common threads, but there are also contradictions and ambiguities. Language is used by different authors in very different ways, and this variation in language may explain some of the misunderstandings and conflicts. Experiencing this variation across a range of settings and authors gives us the possibility of reflecting on Basaglia without retreating to point scoring or a reductive insistence on 'either . . . or'.

1
Franco Basaglia
A man, a movement, institutions, and outcomes

John Foot

Reflections on sources and Franco Basaglia's life

Franco Basaglia has been the subject of a number of biographies, numerous newspaper articles, a feature film, a graphic novel, a two-part nationally transmitted semi-fictional TV play, a series of documentaries, a memoir by his daughter, academic studies of all kinds, histories, studies of his political thought, exhibitions, sculptures, art works, plays, contemporary accounts, and photographic collections (Foot, 2014a, b, c, 2015a, b, 2016; Pivetta, 2012). He has schools, squares, and other public spaces named after him, as well as cafés and shops. His collected works were published in Italian in 1982, in two volumes totalling over 900 pages, and have recently been re-published (Basaglia, 2017). A critical edition of a translated selection of his writings came out in English in 1987 (Figure 1.1), and some of his and Franca Ongaro's (his wife, collaborator, and often co-writer) work has been translated into Spanish, Portuguese, Dutch, German, French, Japanese, and other languages (Scheper-Hughes and Lovell, 1987) (Figure 1.2). The extensive archive of Basaglia and Ongaro has been exhaustively catalogued, but is difficult to access—and includes numerous letters and other materials.

Basaglia also gave a number of interviews and wrote extensively for the press and other publications (much of this material is not collected, or relatively hard to find) and gave frequent TV interviews between the 1960s and his death in 1980. He wrote no autobiography, but during lecture and 'Q and A' tours to Brazil in 1978–1979 he made a number of autobiographical reflections which were later collected and included in the highly influential publication, *Conferenze Brasiliane*, which appeared in various editions in Portuguese and Italian (Basaglia, 2000/2018). In 1976, Basaglia's former friend and by then rival, Giovanni Jervis, published an autobiographical essay which made extensive reference to Basaglia's work and personal life (Jervis, 1977). Recently, some other accounts have begun to appear, such as that by Basaglia's colleague in Gorizia, Antonio Slavich (Slavich, 2018).

In general, the story of Franco Basaglia's life has largely been written by his own 'supporters', or by those sympathetic to his work within and outside psychiatry and his (contested) legacy. Some of this work verges on the hagiographical. There is a key

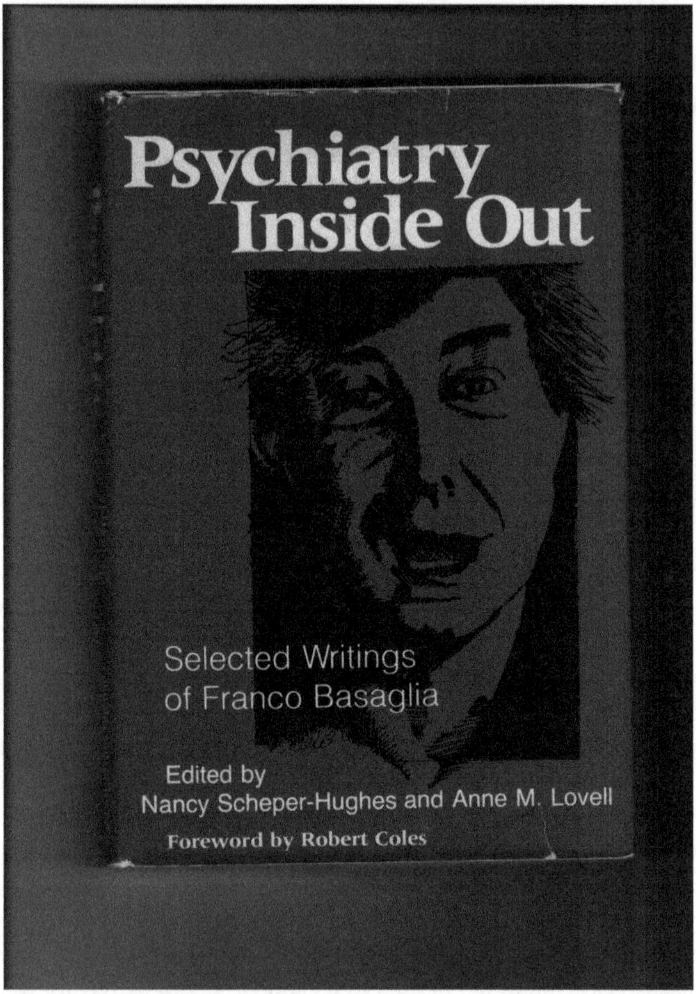

Figure 1.1 Front cover of *Psychiatry Inside Out: Selected Writings of Franco Basaglia.*
Reproduced with permission from N. Scheper-Hughes and A. Lovell, *Psychiatry Inside Out: Selected Writings of Franco Basaglia*. Copyright (1987) Columbia University Press.

problem here of *sources and circularity*. Basaglia's *own account* of his life and work—usually taken from *Conferenze Brasiliane*—is often used uncritically, without the checking of sources or attempt to carry out *independent* research into his statements or claims. *Basaglia himself is often the key source for Basaglia's life and work.* This has provided us with an oft-repeated, standard, and largely linear story of militancy and reform.

In reality, I would argue, although there were continuities, Basaglia's theory and practice were often in flux, not always coherent, often experimental, and adaptable to changing circumstances, times, and institutions. The same could be said of the

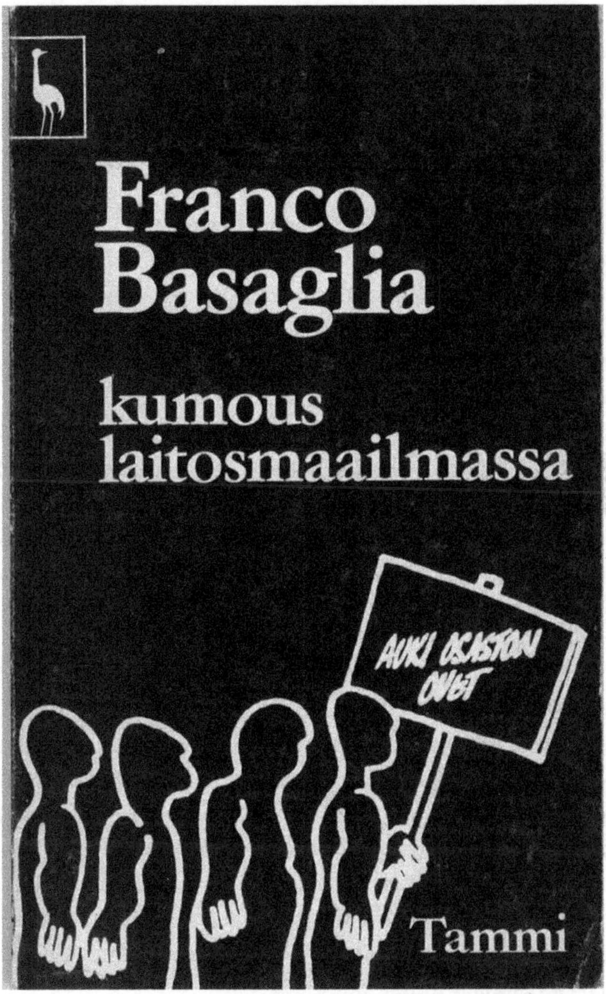

Figure 1.2 Front cover of *Kumous Laitosmaailmassa* [*Negated Institutions*], Finnish edition of Franco Basaglia's *L'istituzione negata*. Translated by Pirkko Peltonen. Helsinki: Tammi, 1972.
Courtesy of Archive of the Mental Health Service, Trieste and Tammi Publishers.

work by psychiatrists who came after Basaglia, either in Italy or elsewhere. I have argued that this 'incoherence' was a virtue, not a flaw, although Basaglia's supporters have attempted to invent or construct a kind of coherence which was not there at the time. Disputes, in addition, tend to be read backwards. Thus, Basaglia's friendship and florid working relationship with Giovanni Jervis and the psychologist Letizia Comba in 1966–1968, in particular, is eliminated from the history books, given the bitter dispute between the two men in the 1970s. Jervis was (and sometimes still is) seen as a traitor, and as such his contribution to the movement was to be downplayed or simply excised from the record. Two separate historiographies have emerged—a Basaglian one and a Jervisian one—and the two do not come into contact with each other. The relative lack of access to the Basaglia archive is crucial here, as the letters held there often tell a very different story—of splits, depression, disputes, jealousies, controversies, but also of long friendships and kindness and fruitful working relationships.

A further (connected) issue here is the tendency to tell the story of psychiatric reform and critical psychiatry in Italy in a *Basagliacentric* way. The classic biographical, geographical, and psychiatric pathway—Basaglia in Gorizia (1961–1968), Basaglia in Colorno (1970–1971), and Basaglia in Trieste (1971–1979)—is usually simply repeated, and dominates the accounts we have. It is too linear, and too personally centred on the life and work of Basaglia himself. This approach also, inevitably, downplays or excludes altogether the role of Franca Ongaro, who is sometimes labelled as a 'secretary', despite the Ongaro–Basaglia co-authorship of much of the work that appeared in the 1960s and 1970s, and her central role in the movement itself from 1961 onwards. Moreover, Basaglia almost always worked with allies and as a part of teams—with psychiatrists, politicians, publishers, intellectuals, volunteers, and others. A Basagliacentric approach is profoundly 'unBasaglian'.

A further repercussion of this standard way of telling the story is that other key Italian experiences—from Perugia to Varese to Nocera Inferiore to Naples to Colorno itself—(with and without Basaglia) have often been ignored, or simply reduced to a footnote. This is also true, to an extent, of the fate of the Basaglian diaspora. Slavich's activities in Ferrara have led to very little research, for example, as has Lucio Schittar's work in Pordenone. There is more available on Agostino Pirella's time in Arezzo and Jervis's period in Reggio Emilia, but it is the Gorizia–Trieste–Basaglia story that dominates. Paradoxically, one of the results of some recent work about Franco Basaglia has been the repositioning of Basaglia's own role in the movement. In any case, the only way to understand this movement is to write its history as a movement, not as a cohesive group led by a visionary individual.

What we do and do not know about Franco Basaglia

There are many parts of Basaglia's life we know little or nothing about—above all the first 37 years. We also know little or nothing about how Basaglia dealt with clinical issues. It appears that he kept minimal or non-existent medical records on patients, and that this was a deliberate policy. But how did he actually communicate with patients, and discuss their problems? We know almost nothing about his university years—beyond his few academic publications (which are rarely read or cited), the fact that he became interested in phenomenology, his participation in courses organized by Pier Francesco Galli in Milan, plus some accounts of encounters with other like-minded young psychiatrists and others. Going back further, little or nothing has been written about his family life, his family background in Venice, his school years, his siblings, and his coterie of friends.

We know little or nothing about Basaglia's brief experience as a university lecturer in the early 1970s in Parma (teaching 'mental hygiene'). Nobody has studied the documentation relating to the competitions for jobs which Basaglia took part in. It is often claimed, for example, that Basaglia was 'expelled' from the university system in 1961. However, he continued to gravitate around the university sector and taught for a time in Parma. It is also said that he wanted to create a new university department inside the asylum in Parma. He was not 'anti-university' per se.

Basaglia's networks

Basaglia and Ongaro travelled frequently—to conferences, to visit other asylums, to stay with colleagues (Figure 1.3). They lived for six months in New York in 1969, and Basaglia spent another six months travelling around central and Latin America and the Caribbean. But these journeys and encounters have rarely been studied, especially those on a global scale. He was part of a global *network* of psychiatrists and

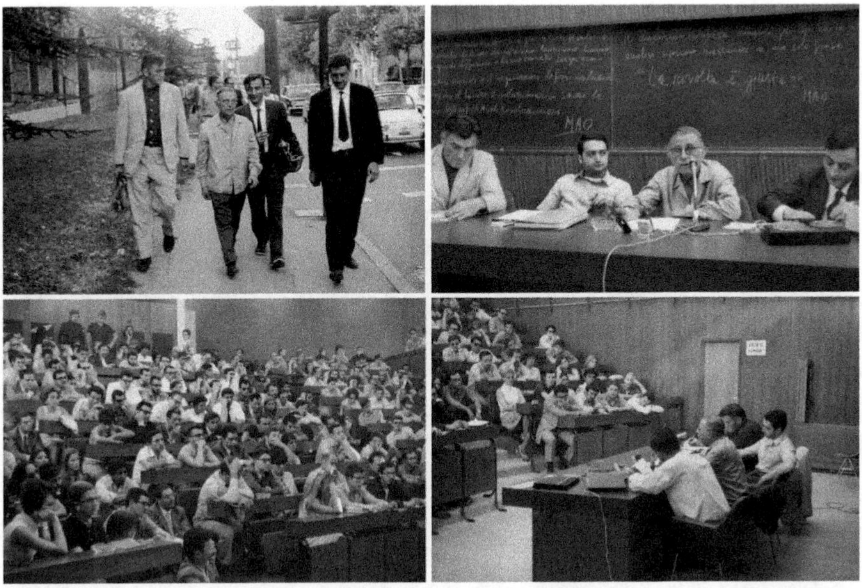

Figure 1.3 Left to right: the historian Vladimir Dedijer, Jean-Paul Sartre, the psychiatrists Gian Franco Minguzzi and Franco Basaglia. Bologna, 1968.
Courtesy of Luciano Nicolini (Archivio Storico Alma Mater Studiorum Universita' di Bologna).

others interested in psychiatry and social change. However, the way this global network worked has not been the object of research—until now, with the Oxford symposium in September 2018 and this volume. Basaglia also entered into correspondence with numerous psychiatrists and others across the world, such as Henry Ey and Maxwell Jones.

These unknown areas are important, because they leave us with gaps as to an understanding of Basaglia's 'conversion' to the anti-asylum cause in the early 1960s. From a fairly standard (if innovative) researcher in the 1950s, Basaglia moved towards a more radical position after his encounter with the asylum in Gorizia in 1961–1964, writing his famous paper, presented in London in 1964, which called for the *destruction* of the asylum. We can extrapolate and draw conclusions, as historians, as to *why* this conversion took place. This would include Basaglia's anti-fascism, his experiences in prison, the state of the asylum system in Italy in 1961, the appearance of a number of texts around that time—by Laing, Foucault, Goffman, Fanon, and others. But many other psychiatrists were also shocked by the state of the asylum system, and many thought the system was useless. Basaglia was amongst very few (along with Laing and Cooper) who thought the system itself was defunct and damaging—and that *it could not be saved.* As the 1960s wore on, Basaglia would be joined by many others in this position. Why did he take up such a position on the asylum so early on in his career, and so abruptly? The encounter with the asylum itself in Gorizia is certainly one part of the answer, but is it the only one (Figure 1.4)?

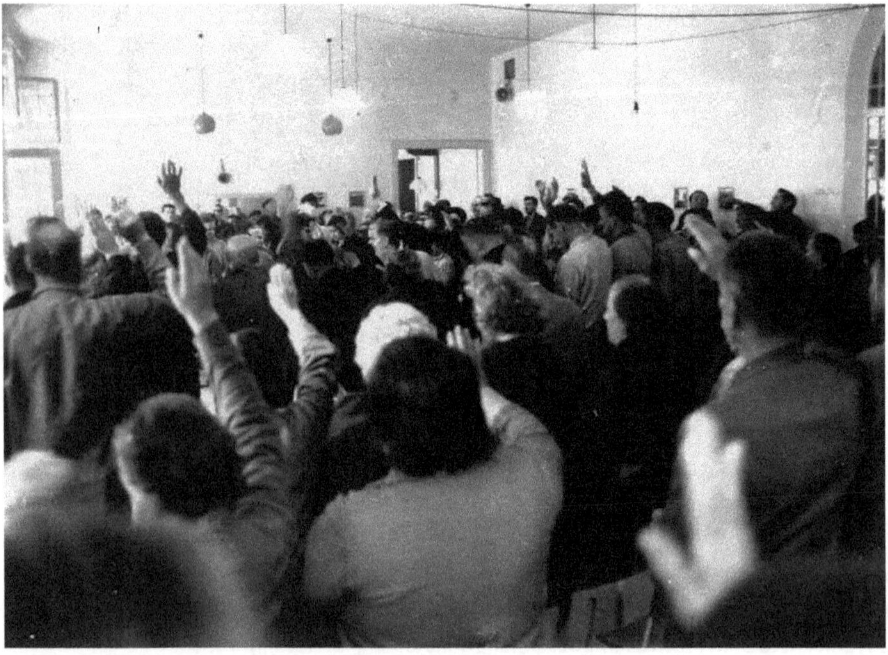

Figure 1.4 Voting by the General Assembly (of patients).
Gorizia Psychiatric Hospital, 1960s (private collection).

Contradictions

Like most people, Basaglia was a contradictory personality: ambitious, but also willingly destructive of his own (psychiatric and academic) career; a strong leader who worked almost exclusively in a collective way; a revolutionary who was fond of the trappings of bourgeois society (there is no particular contradiction here). He understood many of these contradictions. After the (self-edited) collective volume *L'istituzione negata* appeared in 1968, Basaglia embarked on a popular book tour and spoke to big audiences. But he found some of this distasteful. He compared himself to a 'travelling salesman'. He hated the thought of being misinterpreted, although this happened frequently. He often bent the stick for propaganda purposes—in order to make his point—but this was also something he occasionally found unpleasant, or dishonest. He invited people to Gorizia to see what had taken place there, but then denied that Gorizia was 'a model' of any kind—although it clearly became precisely that for many people. These contradictions were not always resolvable. At the height of his fame, he left Italy for more than a year, disappearing from the national scene altogether and leaving others to take up his legacy in Gorizia and elsewhere.

His life

Anti-fascism

Basaglia had a comfortable upbringing. His father, Enrico, managed a lucrative tax collection company. Franco grew up in the Venetian neighbourhood of San Polo. His family were loyal to the fascist state, but Franco became involved in the anti-fascist movement in the city as a teenage student. One of his teachers at the Liceo Classico Foscarini was Agostino Zanon Dal Bo, who recruited a number of students to the anti-fascist cause. Dal Bo helped to set up the anti-fascist Partito d'Azione in the Veneto in 1942. His influence led to a whole group of anti-fascists emerging from the Foscarini school. However, Lucio Rubini, another student of Zanon Dal Bo's, later claimed that Basaglia 'was *always* anti-fascist'.

In the spring of 1944, Franco Basaglia and a colleague crept into a classroom in the Liceo Marco Polo at night and covered the walls with anti-fascist slogans and leaflets. Basaglia became part of the anti-fascist milieu in the city. He was arrested, probably after a tip-off, on the 11 December 1944. After five days (and nights) of police interrogations he was sent to prison in Venice. Dozens of other anti-fascists were arrested at the same time. The authorities had discovered the key anti-fascist base in a tailor's shop and this had given them a link to a whole network of activists. The time in the police station was terrifying, and the young men arrested were subjected to violence and threats. It is said that Basaglia's wealthy father used his influence to prevent his son from being deported, and that Basaglia would spend the next six months in a series of large group cells in Venice's forbidding central prison. This experience is often linked, known largely through a few passages in the *Conferenze Brasiliane*, to Basaglia's decision, between 1961–1964, to reject the entire asylum system.

On 26 April 1945, the city's prison was the spark for the uprising that would see the Nazis kicked out of Venice. The guards and political prisoners took control of the institution. For a time, there was a serious danger of violent clashes inside the prison between ordinary prisoners and political internees. Then, after a struggle, armed political prisoners and guards defended the prison from Nazis and fascists who were attempting to break in. A pitched battle followed. Then the fascists withdrew, and the prisoners (including Basaglia) broke out into the city itself. Basaglia presumably played a part in this uprising, although he would never write a word about it in the years to come. An armed insurrection followed right across the city.

The Nazis finally left Venice on the 28 April 1945 and the Allies arrived the very next day. The war was over. If this moment was formative in Basaglia's political consciousness, he kept very quiet about it. His time in prison seemed to have had a deep impact on him, although he rarely if ever spoke about his experiences there, even with friends or family. He would, however, sometimes sing songs that he had learned inside the cells. His intense, almost visceral reaction to the asylum system in Gorizia in 1961 has often been traced to his memories of time behind bars as a young man. As he later stated, in an oft-cited passage:

> The first time that I went to prison I was a medical student. I was an active anti-fascist and I was imprisoned as a result. I remember the terrible situations which I found myself in. It was the time of slopping out. There was a terrible smell, the smell of death. I remember that it felt like being in an anatomy theatre where the bodies were dissected. Thirteen years after I graduated, I became the director of an asylum and when I entered the building for the first time, it took me straight back to the war and the prison. It didn't smell of shit, but there was the symbolic smell of shit. I was convinced that that institution was completely absurd, that its function was only to pay the psychiatrists who worked there. In the face of this absurd, disgraceful logic of the asylum—we said 'no'.
>
> **(Basaglia, 2000/2018, p. 49).**

His anti-institutionalism was, it seems, intimately connected to his own time as a prisoner, and what he had seen around him at that time. He was also deeply affected, later on, by his first reading of the work of Primo Levi, and in particular *If This is a Man*. (The excellent work of Bucciantini (2011) is one of the few studies to look deeply at this aspect of Basaglia's intellectual journey.) But this account is also a little flimsy, based entirely on this single passage from the *Conferenze* (read backwards, as a cause of an earlier event). No other evidence is provided. The circularity of the account is plain to see here.

The resistance would appear to have patterned Basaglia's life in other ways. Alberto Ongaro, a school friend of Franco's, was a key participant in the Venetian movement, a semi-mythical figure as one of the first students to openly oppose the regime. Arrested before Basaglia, after his release back to the army he deserted to join the partisans in the mountains. Alberto introduced Franco to his sister Franca Ongaro. The couple would marry in 1953, and they remained together right up to Basaglia's death in 1980. The relationship between Franca Ongaro and Franco Basaglia has rarely been studied, but is central to any understanding not just of their respective biographies, but also of the vast quantity of published writings and practical activities carried out by Basaglia, Franca Ongaro, and others after 1961. It was a complicated relationship, with ups and downs and difficult aspects connected to power, fame, and work–life balances.

Psychiatry and university

In 1943, Basaglia had signed up to study 'medicine and surgery' in Padua. He would later claim that he had chosen his degree subject completely at random. Nonetheless, it seems he was a brilliant student. He graduated in 1949 (despite the war years and his time in prison) and spent the entire next decade studying philosophy and psychiatry. We know, as I have stated, little or nothing about these long years within the university system, and most of what we 'know' comes from Basaglia himself, and in particular the *Conferenze*. In 1952, Basaglia specialized in the field of *Malattie nervose e mentali*, qualifying in 1958 as a doctor in that area. Basaglia's 'failure' to obtain a university post has often been attributed (including in my work) to his 'unorthodox' approach to psychiatry. But once again, the evidence here is flimsy—and contested. Some, looking back on Basaglia's life, have compared the university itself to an asylum, as another kind of 'total institution'. Basaglia himself made this point in an 'interview' book published in the 1970s:

> When I went to Gorizia as director of the provincial asylum, I had worked for ten years in an institution as a university assistant. I had learnt (in a personal way) about the workings of institutions, and how power can destroy people and how you can become ill with a kind of 'university sickness'. It was as if someone's entire existence came down to one thing only: a university career. I couldn't stand it anymore and I applied for a job in an asylum.
>
> **(Basaglia, 1978, pp. 94–5)**

In this version—the only one we have—the decision to leave the university system is attributed, by Basaglia, to Basaglia himself: he 'couldn't take it any more' and he 'applied for the job in the asylum'. This is, without doubt, a key moment in Basaglia's life. From a dedicated researcher, specializing in academic articles, he became something different—very different—after 1961. November 1961 was clearly a turning point in his life, his career, and his psychiatric practice. If he had obtained a university post, what would he have become? Would we have even heard of him? His practical impact on the asylum, and the power he had as a Director, provided a potent mix of anger and opportunity which Basaglia then applied to his ideas and to his practice.

Basaglia appears to have been frustrated in Padua, and when he went (briefly) back into the university system, in Parma in the early 1970s, it seems his promotion was again blocked from above, at least twice. Yet, it was in the 1950s that Basaglia began to define himself as a phenomenologist. Soon, his professor began to refer to him, a little disapprovingly, as 'the philosopher'. Was it these ideas, above all, that were important in the 'leap' of 1961, as some have argued? Jervis later wrote, interestingly, that 'he thought of himself, correctly, as an *outsider*' (Jervis, 1977, p. 20). But what made him an outsider, precisely? Was it his rejection of traditional psychiatry (which he seems to have embraced to some extent at Padua)? Was it his decisive activities after 1961 in Gorizia and then in Trieste?

The time in Padua was certainly crucial in terms of friendships and acquaintances. Basaglia studied with Antonio Slavich, who would become the second member of the Gorizian équipe in 1962, and would share the whole Gorizian experience, as well as that in Colorno. Links were also forged with psychiatrists such as Agostino Pirella and others through the academic world of conferences and workshops. Moreover, Basaglia developed a close friendship with a powerful academic neurologist of Armenian descent, Hryay Terzian, who had been born in Addis Ababa in 1925 and educated at the Armenian College in Venice. Terzian would later prove to be an important ally of the movement, and turned up (not by chance) on various appointment commissions.

Basaglia had friends in high places (so was he really an outsider?) and he knew how to build alliances and work with those who had power. He also tended to work within institutions, and after Padua he would take up positions of authority. Moreover, the philosophical and political ideas he developed in Padua appear to be crucial to his approach to running an asylum after 1961. His life and his career would be marked by radical breaks and strong continuities.

Personality

Tall, charismatic, and good looking, Basaglia was something of a workaholic. Michele Risso (his friend, and a psychoanalyst and an ally in the movement) compared him to a 'big cat'. It has often been said that Basaglia had a particular skill at communicating with those in distress (something which is also often said of R.D. Laing)—and there are many anecdotes which testify to this. He could be both decisive and indecisive. After the Miklus murder in 1968 (when a patient murdered his wife while on day release, causing a national scandal and leading to a court case), Basaglia wanted to give up the struggle altogether, and close down the hospital again. He was persuaded not to do so by the other members of the équipe.

Basaglia liked to talk (both in person and on the phone) and to discuss everything, and could be very persuasive. He was certainly extremely charismatic: people have told me, in detail, their stories of a single meeting with him, or just a coffee. But he was not a particularly charismatic public speaker, and he could be very impatient with his 'followers'. He nurtured a deep hatred of parts of the psychiatric establishment, for whom he held deep contempt (which was often mutual). However, he knew how to use power structures and institutions in order to get his way. His writing was disorderly; he often used sayings and little stories to make his point. It often needed editing and was not immediately accessible to a wider audience. He was deeply affected by a varied range of texts (apart from Primo Levi's aforementioned *If This is a Man*): works by Sartre, Pirandello, Goffman, and Minkowski. He was a kind of intellectual magpie, in this sense, drawing on different texts in order to make his points. Basaglia was extremely well-read, with a vast and eclectic library and set of interests. He had no time for psychoanalysis. He had private patients, although he never discussed this contradiction. He (liberally) prescribed antipsychotic medication—but rarely if ever discussed its use.

Once he had power, Basaglia fought hard to get his way. He loved to argue things out, but could also be intolerant of criticism or take it personally. A stubborn man, he could occasionally act in an authoritarian manner, although he also worked collectively and was aware of the importance of building a team. He was both authoritarian *and* an extreme democrat (contradictions of which he was aware). Basaglia understood his position as both inside and outside of 'the system'. As he later wrote (in a collective resignation letter, sent in 1972):

> Fanon was able to choose the revolution. But we, for obvious objective reasons, cannot do so. Our situation is that we are forced to live through the contradictions of a system which creates us, managing an institution we deny/negate, carrying out therapy which we refuse to acknowledge as useful, denying the fact that our institution—which has become, thanks to us, an institution where violence is hidden and masked—does not continue to be functional to the system, trying to resist the temptations provided by new scientific solutions which tend to crush the contradictions which our work makes explicit; well aware that we are attempting the impossible in trying to uphold values while non-rights, equality and the daily death of man are part of the very legal system itself.
>
> **(Basaglia, 1968, pp. 377–80)**

Basaglia was ambitious, and enjoyed fame and authority, but was completely uninterested in money. He would usually wake early and work until very late, fuelled by chain-smoking, bottles of coca cola, and occasional glasses of whisky. For Jervis,

> Basaglia asked his collaborators for unconditional support, and wouldn't tolerate theoretical dissent, which he tended to see, in a dramatic way, as personal attacks on him . . . Basaglia's leadership was above all authoritarian . . . Basaglia wasn't very happy with the idea of a 'Gorizia without Basaglia'.
>
> **(Jervis, 1977, p. 26)**

Basaglia's roots were very much in Venice, and he tried to return to the city every weekend after leaving Gorizia in 1969. His daughter talks about him feeling 'the lure of water'. Basaglia rarely took holidays, and when he did go away with the family his time would often be taken up with discussions over work and future strategies. He was anti-establishment in terms of his psychiatric practice and political activity, but his trappings were bourgeois. He rarely went out of the house without a tie, especially in the 1960s. In Gorizia, lunch and dinner would be served by a maid, at set times, with all the family present. He was a strict father. The clash between the generations was also something that took place within the Basaglia family itself.

Many were seduced by his intellect and his personality (including those who had never met him). Some saw him, at the time and later, as a hero, or a saint, or a revolutionary, or a combination of all three. Charismatic and charming, he inspired not only love and admiration, but also fear, jealousy, and sometimes hatred. He became a hero to many, but also an anti-hero for those who were opposed to the movements linked to 1968 (as well as for some who were key figures in '1968' itself). In 1968 he became a symbol for a whole epoch overnight, a household name. A key law was later (unofficially) named after him—a rare honour in Italy, especially for a non-politician. He was often seen as a 'good man', but was also criticized for what was seen as extreme irresponsibility. He had a strong empathy with his patients, but was blamed by many within society for abandoning them to their fate. He suffered from depression, but he never discussed this publicly.

His life was sometimes chaotic, but he never missed an appointment. Work was at the centre of his life. He dedicated himself totally, for nearly 20 years, to 'the struggle', and he paid a heavy personal price for this commitment. Various epithets were applied to him over time, some linked to his well-to-do background and Venetian upbringing: 'natural leader', 'aristocrat', 'patrician'. These were labels used, in the main, by those who did not know him. Jervis, however, did know him, and wrote that 'from his aristocratic and bourgeois origins he derived a sense of taste, culture, a ruthless streak and leadership qualities, as well as a dislike of euphemisms and for the petty features of everyday life' (Jervis, 1977, p. 20). He embraced creativity—some have compared him to a surrealist. For example, this was the case with the illustrator Hugo Pratt, the theatre director Giuliano Scabia, the artist (and his cousin) Vittorio Basaglia, and numerous film-makers and photographers. He had an eye for the visual and the aesthetic.

He was a member of the Socialist Party in his youth, but held no party card in the 1960s and 1970s. He believed in political organization, helping to set up Psichiatria Democratica in the 1970s, but never himself played a direct role in its organizational committees. He was strongly attracted to the ideas and slogans of Maoism (although this was later played down in most accounts). Franca Ongaro visited China, as did Giovanni Jervis. He was able to work closely with politicians of all colours and parties on the left and centre left—Christian Democrats, Communists, Socialists, and others. In Gorizia, he lived in a flat provided by the Province in the town centre. In Parma, he stayed in a hotel in the town centre. In Trieste, he lived within the asylum itself. He lived his life within and across these boundaries, inside and outside of the asylum, his own family, and the system itself.

Friendships: personal and political

Basaglia struck up strong and often lifelong friendships with a number of people. These friendships crossed over from his personal into his political life (and vice versa). Key figures included Terzian (from childhood), Giulio Bollati (from the Einaudi publishing house, who he met in 1967), and the politician Mario Tommasini. Some friendships disintegrated or were placed under extreme pressure by the stresses and strains of the movement—as with Giovanni Jervis, where friendship became a kind of 'enemyship' (the men eventually stopped talking to each other). Basaglia also had public debates/polemics with a number of figures—most famously Mario Tobino, the writer and psychiatrist who attacked Law 180.

In 1979, in Brazil, Basaglia looked back on his past life and his own family. He was extremely auto-critical:

> In those years [the 1960s and 1970s] the feminist struggle began. And it was difficult, because you couldn't lie any more. You couldn't say to your wife that you were a revolutionary and still act like an oppressor. *So—bad father, terrible husband, good revolutionary.* And here the real struggle began, an internal struggle, a real dialogue where a militant looks at their own individuality and relationships with others and their own individuality.
>
> **(Basaglia, 2000/2018, pp. 192–3)**

But here, the challenge of feminism is denied any sense of agency (Franca Ongaro but also the movement in general), and the struggle to 'not lie' anymore is presented as a *male* challenge.

In a later passage, Basaglia referred directly to contradictions between political pronouncements and the private sphere:

> When I began to fight against psychiatric oppression, I was much less mature than I am now. I wanted to destroy an oppressive world, but I also wanted to preserve my own privileges as a psychiatrist and a member of the middle classes. As time passed, and in line with the struggle itself, I noticed that I began to be transformed as well—and this was difficult because I began to lose my privileged position, and when we lose something personal we either regress or mature. *I'm sorry if I am talking about myself, but I am doing so in order to highlight the meaning of the structures we are fighting against . . . For example, I remember that in 1968 . . . when the rebellion of the younger generation began . . . I was a symbol of that rebellion, one of its leaders . . . well, one day I went home, and I found that my 16-year-old son had run*

> *away. It was an incredible surprise for me,* something that caused me great pain. It was also clearly something that helped me grow … because I understood that I was a terrible father—perhaps *I was a good revolutionary but a bad father.* It is a huge contradiction, something that is very difficult and painful.
>
> **(Basaglia, 2000/2018, p. 192)**

However, this combination of the personal and political was not always seen as legitimate. Basaglia stated, for example, that some of Jervis's contested statements and writings were his 'personal way of seeing things' (Basaglia, 1978). Personal divisions were also often explained through politics, and vice versa. Here, more explicitly, the tension between the 'good revolutionary' and the 'bad father' is expressed as something painful for Basaglia himself—and not particularly for his family, his wife, or his son. It is *his* (Basaglia's) problem, and he sees it essentially in that way and that way alone. Basaglia continued:

> What are our relationships with our children? … They are clearly … to do with power. I, as a father, educate my children through a logic of rewards and punishment. How do relationships within couples work? … In public, in the political world, we are all important political figures, we want freedom for everyone. In private, within the family, we are oppressors. We oppress our children, our wives. This is not an evangelical or Catholic position—it is a realistic one. I think that our world—and therefore also psychiatry itself—will not work if selfishness and injustice are at the heart of our existence. *I don't think we can resolve psychiatric problems if we don't resolve our own problems.* And this is a difficult and complicated issue.
>
> **(Basaglia, 2000/2018, p. 191)**

Franca Ongaro left even less autobiographical material than her husband, and wrote almost nothing about her marriage. There is, however, this well-known passage in an article written just after Franco's death in 1980:

> Now that my long struggle with and against the man who I loved has ended, I know that every word that was written in this period was the result of an endless discussion with him—to understand, to make myself understood. Sometimes it was a dialogue. Sometimes, the other person vanished, and I remained alone.
>
> **(Basaglia Ongaro, 1982, p. 59)**

There is a certain bitterness here, and signs that the marriage was not as perfect as it has often been painted. She writes of a 'long struggle *with and against*' her husband, and of an 'endless discussion'. There is also a sense of abandonment. But, of course, this piece was written at a moment of deep grief and pain.

Some reflections on Gorizia (1961–1972)

> The actual history of the anti-institutional movement he led is not to be found in Basaglia's own writings ... It must be reconstructed from numerous books and articles.
>
> **(Scheper-Hughes and Lovell, 1987, p. 5)**

Gorizia was where it all began, and where it all went wrong. Basaglia was Director in the asylum there from 1961–1968, and the experiment continued until the mass resignation of the Basaglian équipe in 1972. But all of those involved found Gorizia difficult in terms of explanation and narration. In her introduction to the new edition of *L'istituzione negata*, published in 1998, Franca Ongaro told the story of a failure—of her own, personal failure. In the beginning of the 1990s, she had decided to look back at the Gorizian period in order to demonstrate that many of the later accusations against the Basaglia law were wrong. In doing so, she had come to realize that

> the deeper meaning of that 'institutional overturning' had, over the years, disappeared and had been reduced to a sterile if necessary debate between those who were for and those who were against a reform which appeared detached from the services it was designed to produce, and this meant that nothing was done in a practical sense.
>
> **(Basaglia Ongaro, 1998, pp. 1–2)**

'I didn't want to tell the story in the first person', she wrote (and the reader can only wonder why, since what a fascinating account that would have been). Instead, she collected a series of writings which, 'chronologically, laid out what had happened'. However,:

> When the work was finished, I found myself faced with something that seemed dead: works, debates, judgements, speeches which were disconnected from the reality of those years, from the tiny things which changed bit by bit and the meaning they had. Something was missing. It was an account of an experience—critical and self-critical—which was lacking in the vitality, the physicality, the effort, the concrete contradictions, the anxiety, the problems, the emotions and the sense of relationships and connections ... what was missing was the reality of life as it was lived in those years in Gorizia.
>
> **(Basaglia Ongaro, 1998, p. 2)**

Ongaro was not looking for reflection, therefore, but immersion in the Gorizian experience.

For Franca Ongaro, the here and now was what mattered. She wanted to (re) examine the past in order to inform the present; to finish what Franco Basaglia had started (something which became her mission in life after he died). Ongaro argued that there had been a series of mistaken or willful misinterpretations of that past. But she gave up her attempt to recreate that past. She simply waited for the books from that time to come out again. She wrote that those books, 'born during the time of struggle … and which registered, as it happened, discussions, judgements, reflections about those tiny, real things which were a sign of change … were alive' (Basaglia Ongaro, 1998, p. 3). The history of Gorizia was difficult to tell, in part because it had already been told (but only partially) at the time.

It was not easy, therefore, to write about Gorizia, even (or perhaps especially) for someone who was there. Let us take another protagonist from the time, Agostino Pirella. In 1982, in a special issue of the periodical *Sapere* dedicated to Franco Basaglia, he wrote that 'it is so difficult to write about Franco Basaglia' (Pirella, 1982, p. 4). Later in the same piece, he seemed to contradict himself. First, he argued that 'the experience of Gorizia is too well known to be described', but then he went on to correct his own statement: 'Perhaps [Gorizia] has not been sufficiently debated'. Pirella concluded that 'this history has not been written, and we are all partly responsible for this state of affairs' (Pirella, 1982, p. 8). But *why* was Gorizia so difficult to talk about? Were there too many tensions, bad memories, silences, or lies? Was it the ending itself, and the 'abandonment' of the patients there, which hurt so deeply? Had the experience been too emotional, too all-encompassing? Had it failed? Was it better to simply forget what had happened there, and move on?

As with Basaglia's life in general, most of the accounts we have of Gorizia from 1961–1972 are those of the équipe themselves, either thanks to memoirs and accounts written later, or those from the time. Once again, the circularity of sources returns. The Gorizians told their own stories, although these stories were not always in agreement with each other. They also self-identified as a group, or a series of groups, and excluded some from that self-defined group. The secondary studies written by journalists, historians, sociologists and others are largely based on these internal narratives. Central to all this are the two collective books published by the Gorizian équipe in the late 1960s: *What is Psychiatry?* (1967) and *The Negated Institution* (1968). In addition, numerous journalists visited and wrote about Gorizia, especially during and after 1968, and their accounts were almost always sympathetic.

By 1968, Basaglian ideas were reaching out to a wide readership, across left-intellectual and the radical chic milieu in the press, and even within the television and radio services. Visitors and others quickly became converted to the Basaglian cause, carrying the word out to the world. An accepted version of the Basaglia story took hold. It was the version the Basaglians wished to portray, and it has largely held sway in the literature up to the present day. Beyond the first-hand accounts and images, much of the research on Basaglia and Gorizia has concentrated on his theories, philosophy, and ideas. This has meant that many of the accounts of Gorizia tend to be circular and repetitive. This circularity of internal sources has also meant that there is a standard 'Gorizia' story, which has then been told and retold in various formats.

In 1977, Giovanni Jervis provided a different account of Gorizia, setting himself up at the same time as an alternative (perhaps *the* alternative) critical historian/narrator of the movement. This version has usually been excluded from 'official' or Basaglia accounts, and is rarely even cited. The concentration on Basaglia's ideas and writings in order to tell the 'Basaglia story' has also meant that the historical details about Gorizia are rather vague. Nobody has written a history of what happened there. The 'Gorizia story' is well known, but critical and new approaches towards this story have been rare. There are also lots of gaps in this story.

In truth, we know very little about Gorizia beyond what the 'Gorizians' have told us. Moreover, most of the accounts we have are *Basagliacentric*. Generally, the story is told in this way: Franco Basaglia had some original ideas, he applied them, and then he moved on and applied them somewhere else. (There is also very little material on Gorizia itself after 1969: this story tends to follow Basaglia.) Contemporary accounts play down the collective aspects of the Gorizia story (and often exclude Franca Ongaro) and tend to ignore the other members of the équipe, the patients, and the nurses. Exceptions to this are two works not translated into Italian: a Brazilian doctoral thesis and a fascinating Belgian study.

Most of the accounts we have from Gorizia are therefore circular, limited, insular, and top down. They rarely tell the story from the point of view of the citizens of Gorizia at the time and afterwards, the patients, the nurses, the non-Basaglian doctors, the local politicians, or the administrators. The Basaglians wrote the history of their movement, and this history has been taken forward in a subjective and partial way. It is a 'standard story', which has rarely deviated from that laid down in the late 1960s.

These accounts thus became the main sources for what happened and how to analyse it, and were often simply cited or translated into other media—film, journalism, documentaries. This is not to say that the Basaglian account was acritical on its own terms. One of the main features of Basaglian thought was the sense that everything was up for grabs and fair game, but even this critical approach was quite tightly controlled. What we do not have are the details, a sense of the story that goes beyond the canonical texts, a view from outside the core group. Gorizia has not been subjected to any kind of serious historical research, so much so that even the key facts (when people arrived, when they left, the numbers of patients, the arrival and departure of nurses) are difficult to ascertain and often contradictory. The way the story has been told has also affected the story that has been told.

Trieste: 1971 to the present day

> I want to start something completely different from Gorizia, as I realized that revolutionary situations are immediately consumated (sic.) from

> 'power' as a new solution of its own contradictions, and I don't want to be functional to its social system which I don't like.
>
> **(Basaglia archive, letter, 1968)**

Trieste represents the most famous and celebrated period of Basaglia's work within the psychiatric system. It also coincided with the peak period of the national movement, with reformist psychiatrists taking charge of asylums all over Italy and experimenting with change along the lines seen in Gorizia—meetings, humanization, new forms of psychiatry, the discharge of patients (made possible by the 1968 reforms, which allowed for voluntary admissions and provided funding for external services), and a series of creative activities. Thus, crucial centres of change developed in Arezzo, Ferrara, Naples, and many other places, to add to those seen in Gorizia and, without Basaglia's influence, Perugia.

Trieste saw the dismantling of much of the asylum,—quickly, and without the creation of a therapeutic community (which was seen as unnecessary). It also provided evidence of Basaglia's ability to change tack and adapt his tactics and ideas. Sectoral reformist techniques were also used in Trieste. Mental health centres were opened. Many patients were discharged and rehoused. Cooperatives came into play to help with this process. The envelope was pushed. The province pumped money into the reformed asylum in order to close it down, effectively and humanely, allowing for a large staff and social care for those who left the asylum.

The 1978 law, Basaglia's death, and the movement's afterlife

The law of May 1978—Law 180—was passed just in time for it to be enfolded into the creation of an Italian national health service. It did three things. First, it called for the closing down of all asylums (apart from the criminal asylums). Second, it banned the building of new asylums and the placing of new patients within the old asylums (although amnesties extended this for a period of time). Third, it codified forms of forced treatment. Once the law was passed, it needed to be implemented, and this occurred with great regional variations, as healthcare was decentralized to regional governments. Closure, accompanied by new, external institutions and emergency clinics within general hospitals was often complicated and politically difficult. It required resources, manpower, will, and commitment. The uneven nature of the movement itself affected the patchy levels of closure and development of alternative mental healthcare services. Some areas saw the speedy closure of asylums, and effective and innovative use of decentralized services, cooperatives, and housing. Other areas did very little: closure was merely technical; patients were transferred, en masse, to old people's homes, or simply left to rot in crumbling asylums which people thought had already 'closed'.

A comprehensive study of these closures, their histories, their politics, and their legacies has not been written, but there are numerous local studies, many of them partisan or justificatory. Basaglia had died too young, in 1980: he was just 56. He had no time to implement his own law, or even to really contemplate its implementation. The 'Basaglia' law was thus implemented by many others, with great difficulty, over a long period of time, in the face of opposition from psychiatrists, politicians, locals, nurses, and occasionally patients. Most of these 'implementers' were not 'Basaglians'. The global legacy of the movement and the reform was equally uneven, contradictory, and complicated.

But what is/was 'Basaglianism' and the '180 model' (and perhaps these are not the same thing at all—perhaps they represent movement, activity and outcome), and what were/are the lessons of the Italian experience? First, there is the idea that the asylum system was to be destroyed, not reformed. This is a crucial red line for Basaglians (and the Italian experience in general) in comparison with other systems, where the asylum has survived in most cases in one form or another. Basaglianism thus advocated a form of radical deinstitutionalization, moving from one system to another. In many countries, whilst asylums were scaled down and replaced with more modern/humane hospitals, the psychiatric hospital itself survived. Not in Italy. Thus, Basaglianism not only said that asylums *had to be closed*, it said that *all* asylums were to be closed, and it showed a *way* for this closure to happen. Trieste revealed to the world how an asylum could be closed. The World Health Organization adopted it as a model. Basaglians, and those who came after them, became to be seen as experts in closing down outdated psychiatric systems. The use of cooperatives and shared houses was particularly important and influential in Trieste.

Yet the replacement institutions were not always particularly innovative, or specific to Italy. Most countries adopted decentralized systems of care and closed down large-scale psychiatric hospitals. Most countries modernized treatment and used open-door policies. Some did this *before* it happened in Italy. A further key feature of the Basaglian worldview was that linked to the demedicalization of psychiatric diagnosis, with the 'suspension' of diagnosis. (Indeed, has this survived in any form?) It is not clear if this survived the 'heroic' period of the movement in the 1970s. Moreover, the Basaglians worked within the system, unlike, for example, many of the anti-psychiatrists in the 1960s and 1970s in the UK. Basaglia argued that there was no such thing as 'an outside of the system'. Did, and do, the Basaglians practice new or different forms of psychiatry? Was there a counter-revolution in the 1980s and 1990s? Basaglia and his legacy is seen in very different ways within different psychiatric cultures (and in divided ways even within those cultures—where the translation of the Basaglian experience often produces different forms of psychiatric care). In addition, what about the role of patients, nurses, and administrators?

Constant and long-term accusations have been made against Basaglia and Law 180. It is often said that Basaglia 'abandoned the patients', that no structures were set up to replace the asylum, and that families have had to take up a huge burden. Over the years, there have also been other accusations, such as the idea that the asylums were not actually closed at all, or that Basaglia was a 'Marxist' exploiting patients for political ends. Others have accused the movement, especially in the early period, of ignoring gender considerations and patient/survivor rights.

What did the Basaglian experience and the 'Basaglia' law mean in other psychiatric and political cultures? This depended to a large extent on two factors. The first was the attitude to the asylum. Was it a place which could be reformed, humanized, transformed into a place of care and refuge in the true sense of the word? Or was it an abomination, a place which caused more harm than good? This debate raged on within global psychiatric cultures, leading to divisions between 'Basaglians' and non-Basaglians. In France, the reformers and revolutionaries tended, in the main, to want to preserve a radically reformed psychiatric hospital, especially with the development of institutional psychotherapy. (For the current situation, see Raymond Depardon's extraordinary 2017 film, *12 days*.)

Everywhere, Basaglia's ideas caused debate and division, although there was often confusion about *what had happened* in Italy (and the differences within Italy itself). Many people visited—and continue to visit—the 'concrete utopia' of Trieste, but have they also visited areas where reform was less successful, or less extensive? Trieste was never Italy, and Italy was never Trieste. Closure of the asylums was contradictory, painful, and often politically explosive, especially at a local, street by street level. That it happened at all was due to the hard work and commitment of thousands of psychiatrists and other care workers in the sector, and also to the resources committed to the process by politicians.

References and further reading

Babini, V. (2009). *Liberi tutti. Manicomi e psichiatri in Italia: una storia del Novecento*. Bologna: Il Mulino.

Balconi, S. (1997–1998). *L'esperienza goriziana dal '61 al '72. Un percorso paradigmatico di valorizzazione della professionalità in ambito psichiatrico*, Unpublished thesis, Università degli studi di Torino.

Basaglia, A. (2014). *Le nuvole di Picasso*. Milan: Feltrinelli.

Basaglia, F. (1968). *L'istituzione negata. Rapporto da un ospedale psichiatrico*. Turin: Einaudi.

Basaglia, F. (1997). *Che cos'è la psichiatria?* Milan: Baldini & Castoldi.

Basaglia, F. (2000) (new edn 2018). Ongaro Basaglia, F. and Giannichedda, M. (eds). *Franco Basaglia. Conferenze Brasiliane*. Milan: Raffaello Cortina Editore.

Basaglia, F. (2017). *Scritti 1953–1980*. Milan: Il Saggiatore.

Basaglia, F., et al. (1978). *La nave che affonda. Psichiatria e antipsichiatria a dieci anni da 'L'istituzione negata'. Un dibattito*. Rome: Savelli.

Basaglia Ongaro, F. (1982). *Una voce. Riflessioni sulla donna*. Milan: Il Saggiatore.

Basaglia Ongaro, F. (1998). Nota introduttiva alla nuova edizione. In: F. Basaglia (ed.), *L'istituzione negata*. Milan: Baldini & Castoldi, pp. 1–2.

Brandão Goulart, M.S. (2004). *De profissionais a militantes: a Luta Antimanicomial dos psiquiatras italianos nos anos 60 e 70*. Universidade Federal de Minas Gerais, Tese de Doutorado, Belo Horizonte.

Bucciantini, M. (2011). *Esperimento Auschwitz*. Turin: Einaudi.

Cipriano, P. (2018). *Basaglia e le metamorfosi della psichiatria*. Milan: Eleuthera.

Colucci, M. and Di Vittorio, P. (2001). *Franco Basaglia*. Milan: Bruno Mondadori.
Crossley, N. (2006). *Contesting Psychiatry. Social Movements in Mental Health*. London: Routledge.
De Salvia, D and Rolle, A. (eds) (1984). Franco Basaglia. Conferenze Brasiliane. *Fogli d'informazione*, 100.
Donnelly, M. (1992). *The Politics of Mental Health in Italy*. London: Tavistock.
Foot, J. (2014a). Franco Basaglia and the radical psychiatry movement in Italy, 1961–78. *Critical and Radical Social Work* 2(2):235–49.
Foot, J. (2014b). Gli esperimenti di Kingsley Hall e Villa 21 a Londra negli anni Sessanta. Mito, memoria e storia. In: M. Carli and V. Fiorino (eds), *Spazi manicomiali nel Novecento, Memoria e Storia*, volume 47, pp 65–82.
Foot, J. (2015a). *The Man Who Closed the Asylums. Franco Basaglia and the Revolution in Mental Health Care*. London: Verso.
Foot, J. (2015b). Photography and radical psychiatry in Italy in the 1960s: the case of the photobook *Morire di Classe* (1969). *History of Psychiatry* 26(1):19–35.
Foot, J. (2016). *La repubblica dei matti. Franco Basaglia e la psichiatria radicale in Italia*. Milan: Feltrinelli.
Foot, J. (2017). Franco Basaglia and the radical psychiatry movement in Italy 1961–1978. In: D. Mangano and M. van Rooy (eds), *Homestead of Dilution*. The Netherlands: Onomatopee, pp. 53–69.
Foot, J. (2018). Franco Basaglia. In: G. Stanghellini, et al. (eds), *The Oxford Handbook of Phenomenological Psychopathology*. Oxford: Oxford University Press.
Forgacs, D. (2016). *Italy's Margins. Social Exclusion and Nation Formation since 1861*. Cambridge: Cambridge University Press.
Jervis, G. (1977). *Il buon rieducatore. Scritti sugli usi della psichiatria e della psicanalisi*. Milan: Feltrinelli.
Jones, K. and Poletti, A. (1985). Understanding the Italian experience. *British Journal of Psychiatry* 146:341–7.
Legrand, M. (1988). *La psichiatrie alternative italienne*. Toulouse: Editions Private.
Manacorda, A. and Montella, V. (1977). *La nuova psichiatria in Italia. Esperienze e prospettive*. Milan: Feltrinelli.
Ongaro Basaglia, F. (ed.) (2005). *Franco Basaglia. L'utopia della realtà*. Turin: Einaudi.
Pirella, A. (1982). Il giovane Basaglia e la critica della scienza. *Sapere* 851:4–7.
Pitrelli, N. (2004). *L'uomo che restituì la parola ai matti. Franco Basaglia, la comunicazione e la fine dei manicomi*. Rome: Riuniti.
Pivetta, O. (2012). *Franco Basaglia. Il dottore dei matti*. Milan: Dalai Editore.
Ramon, S. (1985). The Italian psychiatric reform. In: S.P. Mangen (ed.), *Mental Health Care in the European Community*. London: Croom Helm, pp. 170–203.
Ramon, S. (ed.) (1988). *Psychiatry in Transition. The British and Italian Experiences*. London: Pluto.
Scheper-Hughes, N. and Lovell, A. (eds) (1987). *Psychiatry Inside-Out. Selected Writings of Franco Basaglia*. New York: Columbia University Press.
Slavich, A. (2003). *La scopa meravigliante. Preparativi per la legge 180 a Ferrara e dintorni 1971–1978*. Rome: Riuniti.
Slavich, A. (2018). *All'ombra dei ciliegi giapponesi. Gorizia 1961*. Merano: Edizioni Alphabeta.
Venturini, E. (1979). *Il giardino dei gelsi. Dieci anni di antispsichiatria Italiana*. Turin: Einaudi.

2
Basaglia and the British anti-psychiatrists, 1960–70

Oisín Wall

Introduction

The London-based psychiatrists, R.D. Laing, Aaron Esterson, and David Cooper were some of Basaglia's best known contemporaries. They attended the same conferences as Basaglia; they drew on similar influences from the therapeutic community movement and existential philosophy; and their experimental communities in the 1960s, Villa 21 and Kingsley Hall, are often mentioned in the same breath as Basaglia's experiments at Gorizia and Trieste. Indeed, many writers have referred to Basaglia, Laing, Cooper, and others collectively as 'the anti-psychiatrists', a term coined by Cooper in the mid 1960s (Cooper, 1967). However, this chapter will argue that, in spite of their similarities, the British anti-psychiatric project was fundamentally different to that of Basaglia and Democratic Psychiatry, focusing more on affecting political revolution than changes in the care of psychiatric patients.

Who were the British anti-psychiatrists?

Laing, Esterson, and Cooper, studied, practiced, and came to prominence at the same time as Basaglia. Their 1950s were not unlike those of many ambitious young psychiatrists—they graduated, found their first jobs, and drifted closer to London. Laing graduated with a medical degree from the University of Glasgow in 1950. After his degree, and a stint in the Royal Army Medical Corp for National Service, Laing worked in Scotland until 1957 when he moved to London, in what his son referred to as 'a complete and courageous break from the past' (Laing, 1996, p. 60). Here he began his psychoanalytic training, started working at the Tavistock Institute for Human Relations, established a private practice, and worked on his first book, *The Divided Self* (1960), before becoming director of the Langham Clinic in 1962. Esterson graduated from Glasgow a year after Laing and went to Israel to practice medicine on a kibbutz before returning to Britain, where he moved between different institutions before settling at Napsbury Hospital on the Northern fringe of London, where he stayed until 1962. Cooper was South African by birth and graduated from the University of

Cape Town in 1955, moving to London immediately after his degree. It would later be rumoured that he had left under pressure from the South African security services and that he was a member of the Communist Party, and that he had trained with a revolutionary cadre in Poland and China. Like Esterson, Cooper moved between several hospitals in the 1950s, including two years at Belmont Hospital where Maxwell Jones was running his large-scale therapeutic community. In 1960, Cooper was appointed as a Senior Registrar at Shenley Hospital, just outside London, four miles from Napsbury (see Figure 2.1).

Unlike Basaglia, whose youth was marked by his imprisonment for resistance activities during the war, there is not much in their early history that would distinguish the three from the countless other ambitious young psychiatrists of their generation, apart from Cooper's rumoured political affiliations. This began to change in 1960 when Laing published his first book, *The Divided Self*. The book laid out an existential–phenomenological approach to analysis for psychotic and schizoid patients. It argued that schizoid symptoms were presentations of a radical ontological insecurity in which a person might

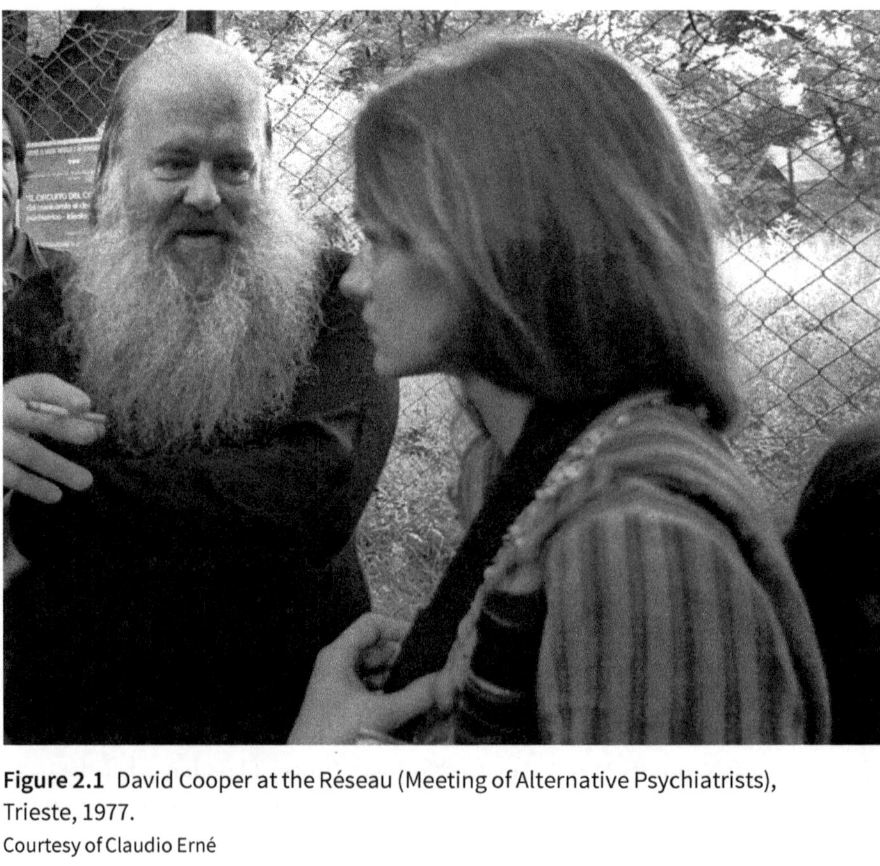

Figure 2.1 David Cooper at the Réseau (Meeting of Alternative Psychiatrists), Trieste, 1977.
Courtesy of Claudio Erné

> feel more unreal than real; in a literal sense, more dead than alive; precariously differentiated from the rest of the world, so that his identity and autonomy are always in question. He may lack the experience of his own temporal continuity. He may not possess an over-riding sense of personal consistency or cohesiveness. He may feel more insubstantial than substantial, and unable to assume that the stuff he is made of is genuine, good valuable. And he may feel his self as partially divorced from his body.
>
> **(Laing, 1960, p. 93)**

To an ontologically insecure person, Laing posited, every action or interaction in the course of everyday life poses a threat to the self's existence. The argument of *The Divided Self* is a seductive one, both easy to grasp and a complex reflection of both clinical experience and theoretical writing. However, the initial reception of the book was cold, the reviews were few and unflattering. One, in *The Annals of the American Academy* (1961), concluded that the book was 'simply rehashing old cases and concepts and trying to make them sound like new and stimulating notions', finishing with damning praise: 'There is an extensive Bibliography' (Lonsdorf, 1961, p. 190). Laing himself thought that the book had 'bombed', and yet in spite of this, *The Divided Self* has been translated into more than 30 languages and has been described as 'one of the most influential books of the sixties' (Laing, 1996, p. 40; Burston, 2000, p. 7; Maitland, 1988, p. 215).

There were two keys to the book's success: the first was the sense, which the book cultivated, that it was a challenge to old established authority; and the second was the empathy and understanding which is so evident in its pages. Both of these features are exemplified early in the book when Laing reinterprets an incident described half a century earlier by Emil Kraepelin, who is often cited as one of the founders of modern psychiatry. In this example, Laing sets up an old, out-dated authority to be challenged by telling the reader that 'the classical clinical psychiatric attitude has not changed in principle since Kraepelin' and that similar exercises could be done with contemporary textbooks. He then includes a long quotation from Kraepelin's magnum opus *Lectures on Clinical Psychiatry* (1905) in which a patient 'showing signs of catatonic excitement' is brought into a lecture theatre to be exhibited to medical students (Laing, 1960, p. 29). Kraepelin describes how the patient has to be almost carried into the room and immediately starts exhibiting bizarre behaviour, kicking off his shoes, singing a hymn, and shutting his eyes to ignore his surroundings. When asked where he is, he responds in an increasingly loud and apparently incoherent speech which Kraepelin interprets symptomatically. Laing, however, sees this outburst as an internally coherent conversation with the patient's 'parodied version of Kraepelin':

> Kraepelin asks him his name. The patient replies by an exasperated outburst in which he is saying what he feels is the attitude implicit in Kraepelin's approach to him: What is your name? What does he shut? He shuts his eyes ... Why do you give me no answer? Are you getting impudent again? You don't whore for me? (i.e. he

> feels Kraepelin is objecting because he is not prepared to prostitute himself before the whole classroom of students).
>
> **(Laing, 1960, p. 31)**

Laing concludes that this externalized internal dialogue is, far from being incoherent, an assertion of the patient's existence. Through it he is objecting to being objectified by Kraepelin. He 'wants to be heard' but knows that his voice, that of the patient-object, is never heard, so he is expressing his 'tormented and desperate' experience in Kraepelin's voice, the voice of the doctor-subject, the voice that is always heard.

It is this empathetic and challenging approach that gave *The Divided Self* such weight. Its primary impact was not on Laing's fellow psychiatrists: instead, it found favour with the emergent counterculture in the early 1960s. This would set a pattern which would repeat, and indeed shape, the work done by the British anti-psychiatrists throughout the 1960s. They began by writing and working, firmly set in a psychiatric context, but found that their work was more enthusiastically received by the counterculture. Over the decade they began to focus on working within a countercultural milieu, and, indeed, their work eventually became generative of that milieu (Wall, 2018).

The group's therapeutic communities

As well as writing books, Laing, Cooper, and Esterson established two therapeutic communities in the 1960s that garnered international interest. The first was established by David Cooper in Shenley Hospital and lasted from January 1962, only two months after Basaglia became the Director of Gorizia, until Cooper left the hospital to focus on his private practice in April 1966 (RMPA, 1969, p. 46). Shenley, most of which had been built in the 1920s, had struggled with decades of overcrowding and underfunding, and most of the hospital's buildings were old-fashioned and in need of care. However, in the early 1960s, under the increasingly progressive stewardship of doctors like S.T. Hayward, the hospital was beginning to modernize its practices. A patient's social club, called the Alpha Club, had been established following the model of therapeutic community adherents like T.P. Rees and Joshua Bierer. The railings that surrounded the hospital had been removed (although they would later be re-erected after complaints from the inhabitants of a nearby village), and the practice of locking all wards had been discontinued in all but a few cases. As part of this modernization, Hayward, who was in charge of the men's section of the hospital, allowed Cooper to establish an experimental 'ultra liberal' therapeutic community in one of the hospital's outlying villas, the former insulin coma ward, Villa 21 (Cooper, 1965, p. 14, 1967, p. 83).

At Villa 21, Cooper was primarily concerned with how patients and staff became 'institutionally deformed' by hospitals, either through treatment, hospital discipline, or association with people who had internalized their roles as patients or staff (Cooper, 1967, p. 84). In many ways, the Villa was a radical version of what other therapeutic communities were doing. Staff and patients were put on an equal footing: both wore civilian clothes, rather than white coats; they ate with the same crockery and ware; and the only institutional authority that the staff maintained was their handling of the administrative contact between the Villa and the rest of the hospital, and holding the key to the medicine cabinet, which was a legal requirement (Cooper, 1965, p. 13; Conran, 1971, p. 30). The practical tasks normally done, or assigned to patients, by staff, like tidying and maintaining the building, were allocated at regular community meetings where staff and patients had equally weighted votes, similar to those held at Gorizia. In the initial phase of the experiment all of the hospital rules were removed until everything, except public nudity and masturbation, was permitted. This phase lasted one year, reaching a crisis while Cooper was away on holiday in Eastern Europe. Rubbish had been piling up in the corridors, windows had been broken and not repaired, and the garden around the villa was unkempt and rubbish-strewn. In a foreshadowing of later debates in Kingsley Hall about 'smellspace', an emergency community meeting was called and some rules about hygiene were established (interview between OW and Adam, 2010). After this, the Villa's community was not dissimilar to many other therapeutic communities, albeit more extreme in some of its practices. However, it had developed a bad reputation within the hospital, and Cooper remarked that there was a 'fantasy existing in the minds of many staff outside the unit that rape, sexual orgies and murder [were] daily occurrences in the unit' (Cooper, 1965, p. 16).

Just like the government of the Villa, therapy also became a group activity. Cooper's Villa 21 relied primarily on group therapy, and the therapeutic atmosphere was not unusual and had been an established feature of the therapeutic community movement since Bion and Rickman's Northfield experiment in 1943; Cooper's work, however, went even further (Harrison and Clarke, 1992, p. 705). While most patients at the Villa did not receive any medication unless they specifically requested it, there were instances where the community meeting collectively decided on a course of medication for one of their number. For instance, one former resident described how an 'inmate was found dabbling with a couple of electric wires and a basin full of water' and, because of the danger that this posed to himself and the rest of the community, and because of his acute state at the time, the community agreed that he should be medicated (interview between OW and Adam, 2010).

The controversy that surrounded Villa 21 may have dashed Cooper's hopes for promotion and, throughout 1965 and 1966, he applied for consultancies in Shenley and elsewhere, but to no avail. He felt increasingly trapped at Shenley Hospital, which Laing referred to as the 'straight-jacket he's got himself into' (Briskin, 1966). Eventually, he decided to resign from the hospital and concentrate on his private practice on Harley Street. After he left the hospital, he wrote an account of the experiment in *Psychiatry and Anti-Psychiatry* (1967), in which he claimed that the experiment was a 'prototype for a small autonomous unit which could function in a large house in the community, outside the psychiatric institutional context'—an allusion to Kingsley Hall, which was, at that stage, already operational (Cooper, 1967b, p. 84).

During the first half of the 1960s, the group had been growing, accruing friends, followers, and hangers-on. In 1965, 'the inner group' (what Laing called the group of friends at the heart of the movement) formalized their relationship as the Philadelphia Association Ltd. Their primary aim was to 'relieve mental illness of all descriptions' and, in doing so, to establish communities and clinics, and to organize training (a first step towards the school of existential analysis that Laing and Esterson had been planning) (Philadelphia Association, 1965; Berke, 1964). The signatories of the articles of association were Laing, Cooper, Esterson, and four of their patients (Sid Briskin, Clancy Sigal, R.K. Wilkinson, and Joan Cunnold). However, the Association soon began to grow (Philadelphia Association, 1965).

Not long after they formed the Philadelphia Association, they signed a peppercorn lease on Kingsley Hall, a former community centre in the working-class area of Bow in East London (Kingsley Hall Repair Fund, 1970). By the time the anti-psychiatrists moved in, the Hall had already seen its fair share of radical politics, having provided a base for suffragettes and pacifists during the First World War, as well as lodgings for the Jarrow Marchers and for Mahatma Gandhi during his negotiations with the British (Koven, 2012). The Hall was a red and grey brick building with two large halls, a kitchen, various smaller meeting rooms, and accommodation for 14 people, including eight 'cells' on the building's roof. In the five years between 1965 (when the Association moved in) and 1970 (when they left the Hall), 119 people lived there. Many of these stays were brief, but others, like the celebrated artist Mary Barnes, spent months or even years living in the Hall (Itten, 2005, p. 4).

Like Villa 21, Kingsley Hall was focused on demystifying interactions so that residents could learn new, 'authentic' ways of relating to each other. In many ways, the Hall was able to go further than Villa 21, particularly in relation to the flattening of staff–patient boundaries. The biggest difference in this respect was that while at the Villa, the boundaries were reduced, the staff were still paid to be there and could go home at night. At the Hall, every resident paid a rent to be there, and nobody was financially obliged to care for anyone else. As a result, they believed, the therapeutic relationships that formed were entirely voluntary and not mystified by the power dynamic that exchanging money creates. Another approach to creating 'authentic' relationships was to strip away the unspoken social rules. In Villa 21, this was attempted by removing the hospital rules and allowing the patients to set their own; in Kingsley Hall, the axiom was 'everything that is not forbidden is allowed' (Huxley, 1989). This may seem tautological, but it enforced the principle that there were no unwritten rules and that no behaviour should be curtailed unless it was explicitly banned by the community.

The extent of their attempt to demystify relationships and rules can be seen particularly clearly in the case of Mary Barnes, the community's most famous patient, whose experience at the Hall was the subject both of a book which she co-wrote with Joseph Berke (Berke and Barnes, 1971), and a play written by David Edgar (Edgar 1997). Barnes entered the Hall in 1965, after several years of analysis with Laing.

During her time at the Hall she regressed for long periods to childhood and infancy, and even lived for a time *in utero*, in a womb built for her in the basement by the artist John Latham. At several times, the extremity of her regression tested the limits of the community's commitment to abolishing staff–patient boundaries. For instance, when she had regressed *in utero* she stopped eating, demanding instead to be tube fed, sparking a heated argument. On the one hand this kind of behaviour was not forbidden, but on the other hand it imposed a significant burden on the medically trained residents, forcing them to act as doctors with responsibility for Barnes' health. In the end, it was decided that if she wanted to pursue tube feeding she would have to move out of the Hall to a place that could facilitate it safely, and she began to eat again (Berke and Barnes, 1971, p. 219).

This was one of several moments where the medical world almost impinged on the community's life. Indeed, this was the subject of a long-running power struggle between different factions within the Association, with Esterson arguing that the Association needed a medical officer and Laing arguing that this would medicalize the community and defeat its anti-authoritarian purpose. Indeed, in spite of the community's commitment to demystifying social relations, it seems to have been riven by unspoken tensions. As early as 1968, Sid Briskin wrote to Laing that 'the network @ Kingsley hall . . . [needs to look] @ ourselves ie. what we have done, are doing + may wish to do with special focus on the fragmentation of our endeavour + the personal feuds which are rarely brought out in the open' (Briskin, 1968). That same year, Esterson split from the group, citing Laing's 'mental instability' (Laing, 1996, p. 175). The community struggled on until 1970 but, like the anti-psychiatric group, it did not fare well. When they finally left the Hall, it was in a severe state of disrepair, so much so that the landlords, in spite of their sympathy with the Association's cause, issued a bill for £5,000 worth of repairs to the building (Kingsley Hall Repair Fund, 1970).

In reality, the dissolution of the Kingsley Hall community was also the end of British anti-psychiatry. Laing had begun to withdraw from public life in 1969 and, in 1971, a few months after they left the Hall, he departed for an ashram in Ceylon. When he came back, his interests had shifted away from the cultural politics that had been so important in his work throughout the 1960s. Cooper resigned from the Association in 1971, citing its growing authoritarian and hierarchical structure, and the following year he left London for South America to find a more active revolutionary scene. In 1970, Joseph Berke refused to show Laing the manuscript for *Mary Barnes: Two Accounts of a Journey Through Madness*, indicating growing hostilities. The following year, Berke and Morton Schatzman resigned from the Association to form their own therapeutic community group, the Arbours Association. By the end of 1973, the newly depoliticized Laing was the only remaining member of the original Philadelphia Association, and although he was still a prominent face of the Association, he was increasingly sidelined.

Basaglia and the British anti-psychiatrists

Laing had always sought relationships with prominent figures: as an undergraduate, he had corresponded with Bertrand Russell; as a medical student, he had arranged a studentship with Karl Jaspers; and when beginning his analytical training, he had tried to have D.W. Winnicott appointed as his training analyst. This pattern continued throughout the 1960s, and the British anti-psychiatric group were in correspondence with many of the best-known and most influential scholars, psychiatrists, and analysts of their period. These included the philosophers Jean-Paul Sartre and Michel Foucault, the anthropologist Gregory Bateson, and the psychoanalysts Erich Fromm and John Bowlby. Indeed, in its early years, the Philadelphia Association's fellowship programme included two weekly analytical sessions with another Fellow, conducted by R.D. Laing and Marion Milner; fortnightly seminars, held by the Philadelphia Association and the Institute of Phenomenological Studies; and a monthly group session with all three Fellows, conducted by D.W. Winnicott (Philadelphia Association, *c.*1967). By this stage, Milner and Winnicott were the two leading members of the Independent Group at the British Psychoanalytical Society, and, indeed, Winnicott was a household name in Britain having been a regular broadcaster on, among other programmes, *Women's Hour* from 1939 to 1962.

We can be reasonably confident that Laing had known of Basaglia since the First International Congress of Social Psychiatry in London in 1964. Both Laing and Basaglia presented on the same day, in the Community Treatment and Part Time Services section organized by Joshua Bierer. Laing presented the paper 'Is Schizophrenia a Disease?' and Basaglia presented the paper 'The Destruction of the Mental Hospital as a Place of Institutionalisation', a title that Laing could hardly have resisted (World Association of Social Psychiatry, 1964, pp. 11, 31). In spite of this early convergence, the group's international connections, and the growing prominence of both the British group and Basaglia, there is far less evidence of interaction between them than we might conceivably expect. Basaglia is not referenced in any of their published works, and the Laing Archive at the Library of the University of Glasgow contains only four letters between Laing and Basaglia, written between 1972 and 1977, inviting Laing to contribute to a collection that would become *Crimini di Pace* (*Crimes of Peace*), and two invitations to be involved in research forums, all of which were after the disintegration of the British group (Basaglia, 1972–77).

There is only one recorded meeting between Basaglia and his British counterparts during their 'anti-psychiatric' period, and that was during Basaglia's visit to the UK in September 1969. En route to the Congress of the International Multi-Disciplinary Federation of Social Psychiatry, Basaglia and a documentary film crew, led by Paolo Tranchina, stopped briefly in London where they interviewed Laing, Cooper, Sid Briskin, Leon Redler, and Mary Barnes, and visited the community at Kingsley Hall. The interviews were intense but friendly and, according to Tranchina, there was the sense that they were 'on the same side of the barricades' (Tranchina, 2008, p. 52).

Basaglia and Tranchina's experience of Kingsley Hall contrasts sharply with that of other visitors at the time:

> The entire situation was very simple, modest, at the edge of poverty, but it was never slovenly. The house simply reminded one of all the comfortable apartments which are a little decayed, in which the Berlin students live, and of other great European cities ... Nothwithstanding the modest appearance, one breathed at Kingsley Hall an intense sense of peace, of acceptance, like a place where one could remain in peace, rediscovering peace with oneself. Truly a place 'to go to recover oneself, in case of need', exactly as Cooper described it to us.
>
> **(Tranchina, 2008, p. 53)**

This is one of the few descriptions of Kingsley Hall at this time that emphasize the modesty, peace, and acceptance of the community. The descriptions of Sedgwick and Adrian Laing paint a very different picture of a 'roller coaster' of performance, parties, paranoia, and even violence (Laing, 1996, pp. 107, 110, 149; Pickering, 2015, pp. 59–61; Sedgwick, 1987, p. 117). Indeed, as I have mentioned earlier, by 1969 the inner group was riven with interpersonal tensions; it had already lost Esterson, and would disintegrate entirely over the next two years. It may be that Basaglia visited the Hall on a quiet day or, perhaps more likely, it is an example of the residents playing up to the particular needs or fantasies of visitors.The latter is certainly a practice that the anti-psychiatrists had used in the past. For instance, Adam, a former patient of Villa 21 and regular visitor to Kingsley Hall, explained:

> Cooper used to use me as a kind of star patient really, because ... when there were visitors and that sort of thing, you know, I'd be called in to speak to them and stuff like that ... because I was, perhaps, more coherent than ... because I never really went completely nutty. And he said to me 'you realise you're being used' ... which I didn't actually. (Adam, 2010b)

If this is what the residents were doing when Basaglia visited, it was successful. Basaglia was impressed by the community and, Tranchina recalled, enthusiastically discussing the therapeutic and political potential of this kind of community.

There are many parallels to be drawn between the rise of Basaglia and the British anti-psychiatrists. They were all born within seven years of each other, they graduated from medical school within five years of each other, and they began to be recognized internationally in the early 1960s for their critique of psychiatry. Indeed, they are often mentioned together as part of a more or less coherent movement. The standard for this seems to have been set by Peter Sedgwick in *Psycho Politics* (1982), when he identified an international movement built around Erving Goffman, R.D. Laing, Michel Foucault, and Thomas Szasz, with, in his view, less significant people like Franco Basaglia, David Cooper, and the Socialist Patients' Collective following on (Sedgwick, 1987, pp. 197–9). This pattern has been followed by more recent books like Burtson's *The Wing of Madness* (1996) in which Cooper, Guatarri, and Basaglia are characterized as 'weaker and more ideological theorists' than Laing (Burston, 1998, p. 94). Others did not make such assertions about talent or fame, and variations of the list can be found in, for instance, Edward Shorter's *A Historical Dictionary of Psychiatry* (2005) and Michael Staub's *Madness is Civilization* (2011). Some even invert the hierarchy to a degree: Zbigniew Kotowicz in *R.D. Laing and the Paths of Anti-Psychiatry*, for instance, argues that Basaglia's work at Gorizia is 'the greatest experiment in alternative psychiatry' (Kotowicz, 2005, p. 82). This constellation of anti-psychiatrists has become so hegemonic that it is difficult to address this period without addressing a form of this list, even for people critical of the characterization of the movement, like Adrian Laing, who argued that David Cooper had been the only real anti-psychiatrist, and Thomas Szasz, who tried to show that he was not an anti-psychiatrist in *Antipsychiatry: Quackery Squared* (Laing, 1996, p. 187; Szasz, 2009, pp. 27–30).

This chapter contends that the British 'inner group' can legitimately be identified as anti-psychiatrists, in spite of Laing's retrospective denials. In 1977, Laing wrote to Joseph Berke, who was then preparing an article refuting Thomas Szasz's *Anti-Psychiatry: The Paradigm of a Plundered Mind* (Laing, 1977; Szasz, 1976). Laing told Berke that he had never used the term 'anti-psychiatry' and had always been opposed to it. Berke then claimed that the use of the term 'anti-psychiatry' was the main cause of the split between Cooper and Laing (Berke, 1977a, pp. 1–2). Privately, however, Berke was surprised, writing that he had not known how strongly Laing had felt about the word (Berke, 1977b).

It seems that Laing was content to be seen as an 'anti-psychiatrist' when it suited his purposes: that is, when his fame was tied to the success of the group and the promotion of its radical image. In 1967, when the term 'anti-psychiatry' became current, Laing was working, and continued to work, closely with its advocates. In light of this, he was publicly identified as an 'anti-psychiatrist', and although I have not been able to find any place where he explicitly refers to himself as such, neither can I find any evidence that he made any attempt to publically refute this identification before the 1970s. Indeed, Laing was repeatedly identified as an anti-psychiatrist by organizations of which he was a leading member. For instance, when the Institute of Phenomenological Studies brought out recordings of the Congress on the Dialectics of Liberation (which we will discuss later), one third of them, including Laing's lecture, were advertised as being about 'anti-psychiatry'. Similarly, his friends and close collaborators often referred to him as such. In 1971, for instance, Salmagundi published a collection entitled *Laing and Anti-Psychiatry* which included contributions about Laing from Morton Schatzman, who had worked closely with Laing at Kingsley Hall and had trained at the Philadelphia Association (Boyers and Orrill, 1973). Laing seems to have raised no objection to this very public association of his name with anti-psychiatry. What is more, variations of the term had been current within the group from as early as 1964. In a letter to Laing that year, Sid Briskin referred to his being 'anti-psychology', and in 1965, in *The Politics of the Family*, Laing himself praised

Cooper's Villa 21 community, referring to it as the 'anti-hospital' (Briskin, 1966; Laing, 1976).

While I contend that the British group can be rightly called anti-psychiatrists, at least from the mid 1960s to the beginning of the 1970s, I maintain, as I have argued in *The British Anti-Psychiatrists*, that Sedgwick's characterization of an international anti-psychiatry movement is flawed. Each figure that he identified on the international stage had such varied critiques and practices, and worked in such disparate historical circumstances, that trying to retrospectively unite them as one movement adds nothing to our critical framework and actively obscures their diversity. Not only this, but some of the people that Sedgwick identified rejected the sobriquet. For instance, Basaglia rejected his categorization as such, referring to his work in 1968, the year after the term anti-psychiatry was popularized by Cooper's *Psychiatry and Anti-Psychiatry* (1967), as 'non-psychiatry' (Laing, 1996, p. 187). In the late 1970s, Basaglia summed up the fundamental difference between his project and that of the British anti-psychiatrists:

> I would like to say that this child, anti-psychiatry which is ten years old, does not exist—or rather exists only in the heads of people because it has had great success from the ideological more than the practical point of view. We have never been anti-psychiatrists—we are simply employees . . . we worked in the real world within psychiatric institutions in order to give people who were suffering an alternative to the violence and repression of the asylum.
>
> **(Foot, 2015, p. 30)**

Basaglia's sentiment had in fact been foreshadowed almost a decade earlier by Tranchina, after they had interviewed the British anti-psychiatrists and visited Kingsley Hall. In a passing remark, Tranchino described the anti-psychiatrists as 'persone molto colte, appassionate, che credevano in quello che facevano, pur avendo rinunciato ad intervenire nelle istituzioni' ('very cultivated people, passionate, who believed in what they were doing, properly renouncing the interventions of the institutions')— implicitly querying the anti-psychiatrists' renunciation of interventions in psychiatric institutions (Tranchina, 2008, p. 51). One of the distinguishing aspects between the British and Italian groups,was that while Basaglia and Democratic Psychiatry were focused on reforming the psychiatric system and relieving the immediate suffering of institutionalized people, the British anti-psychiatrists, in the late 1960s, were focused on remaking the world through a project that was influenced more by Alexander Trocchi's *Invisible Insurrection of a Million Minds* than by Maxwell Jones' *Social Psychiatry in Practice* (Trocchi, *c.*1963; Jones, 1968).

As we have already noted, there were clear parallels to be drawn between Villa 21 and Basaglia's work in Gorizia, through the democratization of the institution and partial flattening of staff–patient hierarchies, and these similarities have been discussed at greater length by Foot in *The Man who Closed the Asylums* (Foot, 2015, p. 139). The projects were very much about deinstitutionalizing the institution, challenging the power structures of the hospital as a way of giving patients agency both therapeutically and politically. Kingsley Hall was different. Basaglia saw in it a model for community households and intermediate facilities that might eventually supplant the psychiatric hospital, but by the time he visited in 1969 it had become far more than that. It had become, in Schatzman's words, 'a link in a chain of counter-cultural centres' (Boyers and Orrill, 1973, p. 194).

Anti-psychiatry beyond psychiatry

From the early 1960s onwards, the British anti-psychiatrists became increasingly disengaged from psychiatry and increasingly significant members of the international counterculture. This is clearly evident in three events that they organized in the mid 1960s: the conference at Braziers Park (1964), the Congress on the Dialectics of Liberation (1967), and the Anti-University of London (1968). Each event demonstrated the growing countercultural credibility of the anti-psychiatrists, but they also inform our understanding of the function of the anti-psychiatric communities, particularly Kingsley Hall, and how their project diverged from that of Basaglia.

In 1964, the anti-psychiatrists organized a conference in a neo-Gothic country house called Braziers Park. The meeting was attended by the inner group, then beginning to call itself the Philadelphia Institute or Association, and some of their followers, including at least one patient from Villa 21. They were joined by a very loosely-knit group of people who had come together around Alexander Trocchi's 'Project Sigma', including Trocchi himself, Jeff Nuttall, John Latham, and Tom McGrath. Project Sigma was a template, as Trocchi saw it, for an 'invisible insurrection' in which the revolutionaries would seize control of 'centres of consciousness', rather than television stations, rail networks, or government buildings (Trocchi, 1963). They would create an international network of spontaneous universities and communities that would eventually supplant the repressive institutions of capitalism and the state, which would promptly wither away. Mick Farren later reflected:

> Sigma was impossibly romantic, wildly utopian and fundamentally unworkable. Sure, if Trocchi's Invisible Insurrection had been attained and put into practice, we would all have died of either starvation or cholera in the first eighteen months. Okay, so it was the pipe dream of an opiate-dependant poet. Back in those days of golden haze, though, it was also exactly what many of us wanted, and within a year or so a great many of us would be playing variations on Trocchi's initial themes and embracing them as our own.
>
> **(Farren, 2001, p. 35)**

The two groups met because they shared similar goals, although they approached them in very different ways. Both groups sought a cultural revolution rooted in a shift in consciousness that would make repressive institutions redundant. Indeed, by this time it was beginning to become apparent that the psychiatric hospital was not the only institution that the anti-psychiatrists were interested in overturning.

The meeting was initially wildly optimistic, but it rapidly degenerated into a drunken and drug-fuelled shambles, leading Jeff Nuttall to speculate that 'with co-operation we could all actually win. Do we really want to win?' (Nuttall, 1970, p. 219). On the first day of the conference, Trocchi had a minor overdose of heroin, which delayed the beginning. After that there were some meetings and discussions, but most of their time seems to have been spent drinking. In spite of its objective failure to bring the two groups together, the conference seems to have spurred the anti-psychiatrists on. Very soon after the meeting, the Philadelphia Association started looking for spaces for their first community, eventually settling on Kingsley Hall. Moreover, Adam, a patient at Villa 21 who attended the Braziers Park conference and who used to visit Kingsley Hall, speculated that the Braziers Park conference may also have been the first step towards the Congress on the Dialectics of Liberation (interview between OW and Adam, 2010).

The Congress on the Dialectics of Liberation was held in the Roundhouse in Chalk Farm, London, between 15 and 30 July 1967. Eamonn McCann, a Northern Irish civil rights activist who attended the Congress, recalled that 'everybody who was anybody on the left was there'– from hippies to black liberationsists, feminists to phenomenologists (interview between OW and McCann, 2008). Each day was structured around a plenary address at 10.30 a.m. from a well-known speaker, after which the audience of several hundred broke up into as many as 20 seminar groups. The plenary speakers ranged from Herbert Marcuse, who had come to countercultural prominence in 1964 with the publication of *One Dimensional Man*, to Stokely Carmichael, the black power activist and then Chair of the radical Student Non-Violent Coordination Committee, who had been released from jail only a few days before coming to London. While the primary speakers were well known, the seminars could be proposed by anyone and, although a full list does not exist, the diversity can be seen in the proposals in the Institute of Phenomenological Studies Archive. Some of these were formal and highly developed proposals like 'Fragility and dictatorship: socio-pathology of political behaviour'; others were scribbled on torn notepaper, like Danny Schechter's proposal which read:

> Are hippies a force for change
> I
> think.
> So.
> And can talk about why—(or read a paper about these possibilities)
>
> **(Schechter, 1967)**

One clinical psychologist from Amherst Massachusetts, Joseph Havers, summed up much of the Congress' content in the rather wordy title of his seminar proposal: 'Methods of changing consciousness and the relation of such changes to a new, non-violent social order: meditation, new forms of worship, group therapy, group dynamics, psychedelic drugs, etc' (Havers, 1967).

The Congress sought to strengthen the sense of a diverse, but shared, international project. Throughout the Congress, the anti-psychiatrists took every opportunity to promote this sense, beginning with the poster which advertised the Congress' aim to 'demystify human violence in all its forms, the social systems from which it emanates, and to explore new forms of action'. This unifying tendency can also be seen in the questionnaire about 'communes/communiversities' that was circulated among the audience, which asked about respondents' interest or participation in communes or communities, and how they imagined an ideal community. The questionnaire aimed 'to establish preliminary contact between individuals and/or groups of persons who recognise the need of re-creating society now not only at the macro-level but also at the inter-personal and micro-communal levels' (Sprengen, 1967).

Above all, the intention to unify can be seen in the opening and closing addresses of the Congress. It opened with a paper by Laing entitled 'Mediations between the individual and society', and closed with a paper by Cooper called 'Beyond words'. At their core, both papers articulated the same argument —the revolutionary imperative to mediate between the micro-social and the macro-political. Drawing together the ideas of the theorists and the activists who attended the Congress, they argued that revolutionary action would have to take place in the institutional mediations that hold bourgeois society together. They argued that the authority of institutions like hospitals, schools, universities, factories, and the state came from an internalized power structure instilled by bourgeois family relations and, as a result, a political revolution, in the traditional sense, would never really change the world, because we would inevitably continue to project and realize these internalized structures of violence. What was needed, they argued, was an 'inner revolution' that would enable people to create new ways of being together (Cooper, 1968, p. 197).

Cooper used this framework to bring together the ideas of most of the speakers into one, more or less coherent, project, describing them as 'a transactional network of expertise ... [which] can transform each institution—family, school, university, mental hospital, factory—each art form, into a revolutionary centre for a transforming consciousness' (Cooper, 1968, p. 197). Cooper posited the anti-institution, which would disrupt the mediations between the micro-social and the macro-political, as the form of action that would facilitate this transformation.

After the Congress, the Institute for Phenomenological Studies finally had the momentum to establish the Anti-University of London. It was an idea that they had been developing since late 1965, when Joseph Berke tried to establish the Free University of London, modelled on the Free University of New York with which he had been involved before leaving America (Berke, 1965, p. 8). On 12 February 1968, the campus of the Anti-University opened its doors at 49 Rivington Street, a building belonging to the Bertrand Russell Peace Foundation which had been the former home of the Vietnam Solidarity Campaign. They offered 42 courses, on a wide array of subjects, including *Experimental Music*, taught by the composer Cornelius Cardew; *Black Power*, taught by the Nigerian-born activist Obi Egbuna; *Communications*, taught by the cultural theorist Stuart Hall; *Dragons*, taught by the anthropologist Francis Huxley; and, of course, *The Invisible Insurrection*, taught by Alex Trocchi (Anti-University, 1968a). However, the Anti-University was more than just an educational experiment: it was a social space, with regular parties and even a 'kip-in' (an all-night party to which members were asked to 'bring drink, music, joss-sticks … sleeping bags and food') (Anti-University, 1967). There were also weekly 'counteruniversity meetings' at which members were encouraged to interrogate the ideological and intellectual underpinnings of the whole organization. For instance, in June 1968, it was agreed that they would abolish the system of quarters, which had previously structured the year at the Anti-University, and that

> the formal distinction between student and teacher embodied in the present money relationships be dissolved by abolishing set student fees and relying instead on a yearly membership fee plus voluntary contributions and abolishing payment to faculty.
>
> **(Anti-University, 1968b)**

The Anti-University, however, was short-lived. In spite of accruing more than 300 students, by May (four months into its existence), the Anti-University was two and half months behind on its rent, and Stuart Montgomery, then in charge of the finances, had stopped accepting phone calls or answering letters (Farley, 1968). In July, the Anti-University officially decamped from Rivington Street and moved into the Drury Lane Arts Lab. After that, they began to meet in local pubs and members' flats. As the organization became less formal, it created less paperwork, and I have been unable to identify when it officially ceased to be. However, it certainly seems to have disappeared by the end of 1968.

The Anti-University was an attempt at an anti-institution of the type described by Cooper in his closing address to the Congress on the Dialectics of Liberation. There were three aspects to this. The first took place on an individual level, in the classes where students were encouraged to examine their own consciousness and experience of power and society. The second happened at the 'micro-social' level, where members collectively interrogated and 'destructured' the power structures within the Anti-University. Finally, on the 'macro-political' level, the Anti-University attempted to contribute to an international movement of 'revolutionary experiments in universities', to the 'communities, communes and direct action … taking place in Europe and America' (Anti-University, 1968c).

Conclusion

It is striking that Basaglia does not feature in any of the British anti-psychiatrists' work in the 1960s, especially given that he has so often been mentioned in the same sentence as Laing and Cooper, and that the British group would have been familiar with his work, at least since 1964. However, from 1964 onwards, the British anti-psychiatrists were moving away from psychiatry. There are superficial aspects to this: for instance, we could point to the group resigning from their positions in mainstream psychiatric organizations (Esterson in 1962, Laing in 1964, and Cooper in 1966), or we could point to the declining references to psychiatrists in their writings, particularly those of the most prolific writer, Laing. Laing had always had a broad reference base, but his early work is dominated by psychiatric and psychoanalytic references, interspersed with cultural, political, and philosophical writings. For instance, early works like *The Divided Self* (1960) had an extensive reference list including Wilfred Bion, Harry Stack Sullivan, Theodore Lidz, and Feida Fromm-Reichman; and *Self and Others* (1961), although a much shorter and more psychoanalytically focused book, still made sure to reference a wide range of psychiatric authors including Bion, John Bowlby, Jay Haley, and Harold Searles. His work in the later 1960s clearly shifts away from his psychiatric reference base. While *The Politics of Experience* (1967) still refers to some psychiatrists, like Bion and Haley, the text is dominated by references to cultural and political figures like Jean Cocteau, Franz Fanon, Karl Marx, Herbert Marcuse; and by the time he published *The Politics of the Family* (1969), his references to psychiatrists had been almost completely overshadowed.

While Basaglia and others looked at Villa 21 and Kingsley Hall as potential models for psychiatric practice and reform, the anti-psychiatrists saw them not only as sites of anti-institutional care but as 'revolutionary centres for transforming consciousness'. Basaglia saw them as useful models that could be adapted to further his project, which he had laid out in the paper that Laing likely saw him give in London in 1964:

> through the destruction of the 'loony bin', and then through the gradual reduction of the open-door hospital as the mentally ill patients asylum, we will be able to arrive—through the out-side service—at a psychiatric service which will save the liberty of one who misses it by illness.
>
> **(Basaglia, 1964, p. 5)**

Laing, on the other hand, referred to Villa 21 as an 'anti-hospital', and Cooper called communities like Kingsley Hall 'anti-families'. Both communities aimed to 'destructure' their residents' internalized oppressions; they both attempted, and to a greater or lesser extent failed, to create a demystified, democratic social environment in which residents could discover new, authentic modes of being together; and both attempted to engage the macro-political, albeit in different ways. Villa 21 directly challenged the hospital institution, with Cooper aiming to cause and record 'disintegrative effects on the rest of the hospital' (Cooper, 1965, p. 11). He argued that, to the staff and inmates of the hospital, Villa 21 posed an existential threat because it attempted to destroy the very basis of their livelihood and culture. Indeed, both of the patients of Villa 21 that I interviewed seem to have been aware of this tension on some level, and one of them remembered that this was a source of pride for some of the patients. Kingsley Hall, on the other hand, engaged with the macro-political by becoming a hub for the international counterculture. It became a centre of pilgrimage for every beat writer and hip artist passing through London; while residents like Murray Korngold travelled to distribute 'propaganda' for the Hall in America, and Sid Briskin travelled to communes in Europe, spreading stories about the Hall (Laing, *c.*1965, 1996, p. 108; Crossley, 1999, p. 814; Guattari, 1984, pp. 51–9; Berke, 1966). Kingsley Hall was fighting hard to become a part of the 'international network' of revolutionary cultural centres that Trocchi had called for in *Sigma: A Tactical Blueprint*.

Perhaps the final reason that the anti-psychiatrists did not engage with Basaglia, or others like him, as the 1960s wore on, was hinted at by Cooper in his final address to the Congress on the Dialectics of Liberation:

> If we persist with the theme of transforming our institutions into revolutionary centres of consciousness, we have to be clear about why more has not been achieved by what we have already done in this way. The most immediate answer is that we have become victims of a very old colonizing technique—the technique of divide and rule. Innovators in the fields of education, psychiatry, all the arts and sciences, have been atomized, split off from people doing much the same thing in another area. In this way we lay ourselves open to the strategy of engulfment into the monolithic bourgeois bureaucratic system, with the consequence that we get ourselves invalidated and suppressed if we carry innovation 'too far'.
>
> **(Cooper, 1968, pp. 197–8)**

There are two conclusions to be drawn about this statement. The first is that Cooper seems to have learned, at Villa 21, that presenting too radical a critique to the institution, at too close quarters, could see your project suppressed and ridiculed. This may be why Kingsley Hall had disengaged with conventional psychiatry almost entirely by the end of its five-year life. The second conclusion is that the anti-psychiatrists feared being sucked back into the disciplinary silo of psychiatry and divided from other people who were part of the same revolutionary project as them. Central to both of these conclusions and, more broadly, to grasping why the anti-psychiatrists did not engage with Basaglia, is understanding how they conceptualized their project. At Gorizia, Foot argues, Basaglia came to the radical conclusion that the psychiatric institutions needed to be destroyed. This chapter contends that the anti-psychiatrists came to believe that they were part of a fundamentally different project, that their aim was not to change the psychiatric system, but to remake society through a cultural revolution fostered in anti-institutions.

References

Anti-University (1967). *Kip-In* [flier]. Planned Environmental Therapy Trust Archive, Institute of Phenomenological Studies Archive, PP/JB/IPS 10.7 (1).

Anti-University (1968a). *Catalogue Supplement* [booklet]. University of Glasgow Special Collections, R.D. Laing Collection, MS Laing L229/12.

Anti-University (1968b). *Anti-University of London Newsletter (7 June 1968)*. Planned Environmental Therapy Trust Archive, Institute of Phenomenological Studies Archive, PP/JB/IPS 10.7 (1).

Anti-University (1968c). *'Statement' from Ad Hoc Committee of the Anti-University of London Meeting Minutes (8 January 1968)*. Planned Environmental Therapy Trust Archive, Institute of Phenomenological Studies Archive.

Basaglia, F. (1964). *The destruction of the mental hospital as a place of institutionalisation*. Paper presented at the First International Congress of Social Psychiatry, London.

Basaglia, F. (1972–77). *Four letters from Franco Basaglia to R.D. Laing, 1972–1977*. University of Glasgow Special Collections, R.D. Laing Collection, MS Laing GB2-11.

Berke, J. (1964). *Letter from Joseph Berke to R.D. Laing (2 April 1964)*. University of Glasgow Special Collections, R.D. Laing Collection, MS Laing GB666/16.

Berke, J. (1965). Free University of New York. *Peace News*, 29 October 1965.

Berke, J. (1966). *Catalogue: Paul Kaplan, Gabriel Weissmann, John O'Conner, John Maizels (4 November–2 December 1966)*. University of Glasgow Special Collections, R.D. Laing Collection, MS Laing GT20.

Berke, J. (1977a). *Untitled draft response to anti-psychiatry's 'The Paradigm of the Plundered Mind'* [manuscript]. University of Glasgow Special Collections, R.D. Laing Collection, MS Laing GB 666/51.

Berke, J. (1977b). *Letter From Joseph Berke to R.D. Laing (9 January 1977)*. University of Glasgow Special Collections, R.D. Laing Collection, MS Laing GB 666/53.

Berke, J. and Barnes, M. (1971). *Mary Barnes: Two Accounts of a Journey Through Madness*. London: MacGibbon and Kee.

Boyers, R. and Orrill, R. (eds) (1973). *Laing and Anti-Psychiatry*. Harmondsworth: Penguin Books.

Briskin, S.I. (1966). *Letter from Sidney Briskin to R.D. Laing (14 February 1966)*. University of Glasgow Special Collections, R.D. Laing Collection, MS Laing GB44.

Briskin, S.I. (1968). *Letter from Sidney Briskin to R.D. Laing (10 June 1968)*. University of Glasgow Special Collections, R.D. Laing Collection, MS Laing GB58.

Burston, D. (1998). *The Wing of Madness: The Life and Work of R.D. Laing*. Cambridge, MA: Harvard University Press.

Burston, D. (2000). *The Crucible of Experience: R.D. Laing and the Crisis of Psychotherapy*. Cambridge, MA: Harvard University Press.

Conran, M. (1971). *The family as a model in an application of psychoanalysis to the care and treatment of young male schizophrenics*. Unpublished doctoral thesis. London: University of London.

Cooper, D. (1965). The anti-hospital: an experiment in psychiatry. *New Society*, 3 May 1965, pp. 11–16.

Cooper, D. (1967). *Psychiatry and Anti-Psychiatry*. London: Tavistock Publications.

Cooper, D. (ed.) (1968). *The Dialectics of Liberation*. Harmondsworth: Penguin Books.

Crossley, N. (1999). Working utopias and social movements: an investigation using case study materials from radical mental health movements in Britain. *Sociology* 33:809–30.

Edgar, D. (1997). *'Jail Diary of Albie Sachs'; 'Mary Barnes'; 'Saigon Rose'; 'O Fair Jerusalem'; 'Destiny'* [plays]. London: Methuen Drama.
Farley, C. (1968). *Letter from Chris Farley to Stuart Montgomery (9 July 1968).* Planned Environmental Therapy Trust Archive, Institute of Phenomenological Studies Archive, PP/JB/IPS 10.8 (2).
Farren, M. (2001). *Give the Anarchist a Cigarette.* London: Random House.
Foot, J. (2015). *The Man Who Closed the Asylums: Franco Basaglia and the Revolution in Mental Health Care.* London: Verso.
Guattari, F. (1984). *Molecular Revolution: Psychiatry and Politics.* Harmondsworth: Peregrine Books.
Harrison T. and Clarke D. (1992). The Northfield Experiment. *British Journal of Psychiatry* 160:698–708.
Havers, J. (1967). *Seminar Proposal: Joseph Havers.* Planned Environmental Therapy Trust Archive, Institute of Phenomenological Studies Archive, PP/JB/IPS 5.3.
Huxley, F. (1989). The liberating shamen of Kingsley Hall. *The Guardian,* 25 August 1989.
Itten, T. (2005). *All the lonely people where do they all come from: facts, feelings and experience from the Philadelphia Association, London.* Paper presented at the Association for Community Living Conference, New York.
Jones, M. (1968). *Social Psychiatry in Practice: The Idea of the Therapeutic Community.* Harmondsworth: Penguin Books.
Kingsley Hall Repair Fund (1970). *Kingsley Hall Repair Fund Appeal* [flier]. University of Glasgow Special Collections, R.D. Laing Collection, MS Laing L259/91.
Kotowicz, Z. (2005). *R.D. Laing and the Paths of Anti-Psychiatry.* London: Routledge.
Koven, S. (2012). The 'sticky sediment' of daily life: radical domescticity, revolutionary Christianity, and the problem of wealth in Britain from the 1880s to the 1930s. *Representations* 120:39–82.
Laing, A. (1996). *R.D. Laing: A Biography.* New York: Thunder's Mouth Press.
Laing, R.D. (1960). *The Divided Self: A Study of Sanity and Madness.* Chicago: Quadrangle Books.
Laing, R.D. (*c.*1965). *Letter from R.D. Laing to unknown American psychiatrist (possibly John Thompson).* University of Glasgow Special Collections, R.D. Laing Collection, MS Laing L666/65.
Laing, R.D. (1976). *The Politics of the Family and Other Essays.* Harmondsworth: Penguin Books.
Laing, R.D. (1977). *Letter from R.D. Laing to Joseph Berke (4 January 1977).* University of Glasgow Special Collections, R.D. Laing Collection, MS Laing GB 666/52.
Lonsdorf, R.G. (1961). Reviewed work: 'The Divided Self: An Existential Study in Sanity and Madness' by R.D. Laing. *Annals of the American Academy of Political and Social Science* 338:189–90.
Maitland, S. (1988). *Very Heaven: Looking Back at the 1960s.* London: Virago Press.
Marcuse, H. (1968). *One-Dimensional Man.* London: Routledge & Kegan Paul.
Nuttall, J. (1970). *Bomb Culture.* London: Paladin.
Philadelphia Association (1965). *Articles of association of the Philadelphia Association Limited* [legal document]. University of Glasgow Special Collections, R.D. Laing Collection, MS Laing L 230/2.
Philadelphia Association (*c.*1967). *Philadelphia Association training programme* [memorandum]. University of Glasgow Special Collections, R.D. Laing Collection, MS Laing GS100/8.
Pickering, A. (2015). Laing beyond words. In: M.G. Thompson (ed.), *The Legacy of R.D. Laing.* London: Routledge, pp. 59–69.

Royal Medico-Psychological Association (RMPA) (1969). *Royal Medico-Psychological Association Year Book, 1969*. London: Royal Medico-Psychological Association.

Schechter, D. (1967). *Seminar proposal: Danny Schechter* [manuscript]. Planned Environmental Therapy Trust Archive, Institute of Phenomenological Studies Archive, PP/JB/IPS 5.3.

Sedgwick, P. (1987). *Psycho Politics*. London: Pluto Books.

Shorter, E. (2005). *A Historical Dictionary of Psychiatry*. Oxford: Oxford University Press.

Sprengen, R. (1967). *Response by R. Sprengen to the commune/communiversity survey* [manuscript]. Planned Environmental Therapy Trust Archive, Institute of Phenomenological Studies Archive, PP/JB/IPS 10.7 (1).

Staub, M.E. (2011). *Madness is Civilization: When the Diagnosis was Social, 1948–1980*. London: Chicago University Press.

Szasz, T. (1976). Anti-psychiatry: the paradigm of the plundered mind. *The New Review* 3:3–14.

Szasz, T. (2009). *Antipsychiatry: Quackery Squared*. New York: Syracuse University Press.

Tranchina, P. (2008). Lotte antistituzionali, Legge 180. *Fogli d'Informazione* 5–6. Available at: http://www.psychiatryonline.it/sites/default/files/Libro180-Articolo5.pdf [accessed 2 November 2018]

Trocchi, A. (1963). Technique du coupe du monde. *Internationale Situationniste* 8.

Trocchi, A. (*c*.1963). *The Invisible Insurrection of a Million Minds*. Washington University Archive, Alexander Trocchi Papers (MSS116), Box 43, Folder 36.

Wall, O. (2018). *The British Anti-Psychiatrists: From Institutional Psychiatry to the Counter-Culture, 1960–1971*. London: Routledge.

Wall, O.W., Interview with 'Adam', 2010.

World Association of Social Psychiatry (1964). *First Congress of Social Psychiatry (17–22 August 1964): conference programme*. The National Archives, LAB 20.

3
Basaglia after Basaglia

Recovery, human rights, and Trieste today

Roberto Mezzina

Introduction

Basaglia's main question was 'what is psychiatry?' rather than 'what is mental illness?' (or, more philosophically, 'madness'). Adopting the concept of 'epoché' (that is 'suspending judgement' for the philosopher Edmund Husserl), he would discuss mainly the relationship with the illness in psychiatry, taking into account the implication of the observer's presence, and also the overall context (i.e. the institution).

> If the psychiatrist wishes to understand and, especially, to have some effect upon the mentally ill person, he finds himself in the position of being forced to place the illness, the diagnosis and syndrome with which that person has been labeled between parentheses, given that the person is harmed much more by what the illness is presumed to be and the restrictive measures which have been imposed as the result of such an interpretation, than by the illness itself.
>
> **(Basaglia, 1967a, p. 388)**

> Psychiatry's current task might be that of refusing to seek a solution for mental illness as illness, and instead approach this specific kind of ill person as a problem which—only to the degree to which it is present in our reality—might represent one of the contradictory aspects which will require conceiving and inventing new forms of research and new therapeutic structures.
>
> **(Basaglia, 1967b, p. 392)**

Starting with its critical stance and questioning, we are specifically interested here in the seminal character of Basaglia's work, especially with respect to its anticipation of major questions that have emerged in recent years. Today, the 'recovery' construct challenges medical–biological reductionism in psychiatry, since such reductionism opposes the active role of the person and the importance of factors associated with his/her concrete existence which influence the course of his/her psychopathological condition. Basaglia's action is recognized among the premises of the recovery movement (Davidson et al., 2010a), that seems to be almost as important today as the earlier anti-institutional movement. The players, methods, and philosophies, even the powers involved, appear, however, to be different and completely new. More recently, the disability movement achieved a great victory with the Convention on the Rights of Persons with Disabilities (CRPD) (UN, 2006), to which organizations of people with psychiatric issues significantly contributed.

Basaglia firstly called into question interpretive models of psychiatry and the very biomedical concept of mental illness. He acknowledged the contradiction of objectifying a subjectivity through an operation based on power and specific knowledge. This 'reductionist' view was again revived in recent international reflections (Bracken et al., 2012; Priebe et al., 2013; Mezzina, 2005). The so-called technological paradigm has re-proposed invariances as founding principles of scientific knowledge within a framework exclusively centred on the positivist vision of the sciences of nature. This takes no account of the crisis of scientific models inspired by the knowledge of complexity (as in the works of Von Forster, Prigogyne, and Morin). The Special Rapporteur to the UN Human Rights Council, on the right to enjoy the highest attainable standard of physical and mental health, considered the biomedical model as part of the 'global burden of obstacles' to 'address the grossly unmet need for rights-based mental health services for all'—a problem, rather than a solution (UN, 2017).

Institutionalism: mental illness, its double, and recovery from the institution

According to Basaglia, criticism of the illness that overlaps madness and the person who lives it, as dictated by psychiatry when it imposes itself as an objectifying medical science, is the heart of the matter.

> Just as medicine has been built on a dead body, so psychiatry was built on a dead mind. By analogy, we could define psychiatry as 'mental anatomy'. So, psychiatry has entered the same field of medicine: the behavioural disorder has been included among the disorders of the body, body and behaviour have become the same thing, and similarly body disorders and mind disorders have become the same thing, both within the positivist logic of the cause–effect relationship.
>
> **(Basaglia, 2000, p. 61)**

> The disease has been made to coincide with the behavioural disorder, organic body and social body have been homologated. Both the sick organic body and the sick social body cannot express their sick subjectivity. Instead, they express their objectivity of sick things.
>
> **(Basaglia, 2000, p. 173)**

This disease is not only shaped by the institution, as sociological and psychiatric studies have described (Wing, 1962; Goffman, 1961), but even its 'institutional double' emerges as the effect of the reduction of the human within the imposition of rules and powers.

> The double disease is the transformation of reality (experience) into an ideological reality, that is to say practical–ideological parameters used to destroy the experience and take it to the level of a common behaviour that is, in fact, only its double.
>
> **(Basaglia and Ongaro Basaglia, 1971, p. 178)**

> It is through this process of rationalization and organization of needs that the individual is deprived of the opportunity to possess himself (his own reality, his own body, his own disease) ... but lives his place in the world as a sick entity; which means that he lives the passive role that is imposed on him and that confirms the rift between himself and his own experience. The disease becomes ill behaviour, false relationship that replaces a non-existent relationship: occasion and confirmation of domination.
>
> **(Basaglia and Ongaro Basaglia, 1971, p. 180)**

Also, when the scenario of the asylum was about to be liquidated in Italy by law 180, Basaglia wrote, referring to the new medicalization of psychiatry, that:

> Keeping this connotation of sick person, the individual who suffers from mental disorders is included in the positivist framework of medicine, so that behaviour is homologated to a body, and therefore the notion of disease is confirmed in a new way, recycled.
>
> **(Basaglia, 1980, p. 480)**

There is an extremely deep point here, that Basaglia and the anti-institutional movement had already identified: while the individual fights to get rid of the double institutional identity with all its implications (psychological and relating to deprivation of power), there must be a radical repositioning of psychiatry and medicine with respect to him. A deinstitutionalization of practices, powers, knowledge, roles, players, institutions and healthcare, and legal and social circuits is needed. This could only happen with a change of thinking and practices, not only of services or institutions themselves (IMHCN, 2017).

Basaglia refers to Foucault's analysis of madness. Madness does not appear but as an epiphenomenon which is only 'permitted' to emerge through the language of power (i.e. mental illness). In revealing the nexus between madness and deprivation/misery, it contains and reproduces that deprivation, like Foucault's history of madness reconstructed. The all-pervasive presence of the asylum infects the community like a 'social germ' (Maccacaro, 1978). It rationalizes madness as 'mental illness', in a place conceived around it (Goffman, 1961). The institution creates a 'double' of the illness, as a social role and overlapping behaviour. For Basaglia, deprived of a personal history, and thus without responsibility, the patient finds his new identity in the institution.

Institutionalization is harmful not just because internment/seclusion prevents social reintegration and recovery and therefore favours chronicity (Harding et al., 1987; Ciompi, 1984), but because internment actually generates new forms of illness, such as 'institutional neurosis' (Barton, 1959) or 'institutionalism' (Wing, 1962). Ultimately, Basaglia came to the stark and radical conclusion that the mental hospital had to be phased out and, ultimately, 'destroyed' (Basaglia, 1964, 1965).

Deinstitutionalization of the illness and the movement of subjectivity in the recovery process

Deinstitutionalization means not only shutting down psychiatric hospitals but also establishing procedures, or anti-procedures, which are critical of existing psychiatric practices. It should eventually result in the gradual disappearance of 'illness' and the emergence of the 'person' as a global entity. But has deinstitutionalization made personal suffering more visible, both within and beyond the context of illness (see Figure 3.1)?

For any possible healing to be true, Basaglia urges us to abandon the notion of a total delegation of the body and mind to the 'technicians and the institute' that treat the disease together. This can coincide with the *re-emergence of a 'subjectivity issue'*.

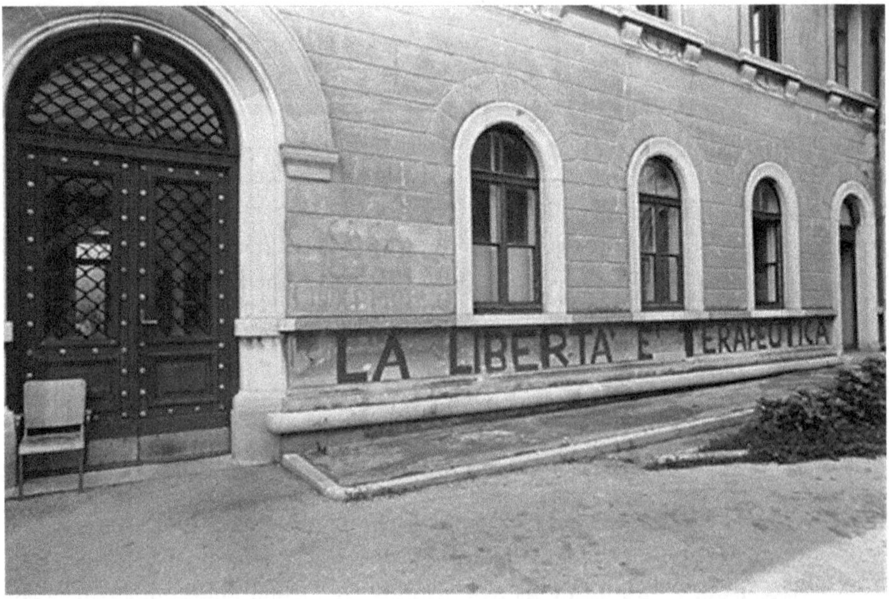

Figure 3.1 'Freedom is therapeutic': graffiti on a wall inside Trieste Psychiatric Hospital, 1970s.
Courtesy of Emilio Tremolada

The treated individual could set himself free from the uncertainty of the dominating relationship (Basaglia, 1979). During a series of conferences in Brazil, just a few months before he died, Basaglia said:

> We want to change the pattern that makes the patient a dead body and strive to transform the dead mental patient in the asylum into a living person, responsible for his own health.
>
> **(Basaglia, 2000, p. 74)**

> Certainly one of the most important therapies to fight madness is freedom. When a man is free, possessed himself and his life, it will be easier for him to fight madness.
>
> **(Basaglia, 2000, p. 89)**

Here, Basaglia posed the idea (with limitations and cautions) that recovery of responsibility for one's own health within a whole life is combined with the goal of emancipation and recovery of power. The contradiction 'between what we are and what we would like to be', between a denied individual and his objectification in the positivist and reductionist vision of disease, can be the engine of that struggle for the affirmation of a subjectivity towards the objectivity of the medical condition, ratified by the institution mentioned by Basaglia (2000, p. 22).

Since it is submitted to a process of nullification, within that objectification, the expression of subjectivity is in itself a manifestation of resistance against the institution. Deinstitutionalization has produced the visibility of the suffering subjects, inside and beyond the illness (Rotelli, 1988a). They finally appear as concrete individuals who take part in social relationships, seeking to thwart fates of exclusion. We could say that only starting from this perspective, all therapeutic and care practices can be organized, based on the entirety and integrity of the person and his/her body, in real life.

The notion of recovery is based on the recognition of the importance of elements and factors associated with one's subjectivity in repositioning one's relationship not only with the disease, but with life. Therefore, it is primarily a construct of the individual, a personal fact, and, as such, it is a non-linear and multidimensional process or path (Mezzina, 2012, 2015). In 'personal recovery', as opposed to 'clinical recovery' (Slade, 2009; Unger, 2010), the person *himself/herself* remains a determinant of the process not only through his/her capacity for self-determination, resilience, and coping with the illness, but also through personal change and the simultaneous acceptance of responsibility.

However, recovery, or healing, cannot be seen only as an individual path. This would underlie an ethic of individual redemption from a condition, the illness, still seen as guilt. We can maintain that, apart from the correct emphasis on singularity and subjectivity, recovery is above all an interpersonal and social fact. Precisely because it respects the individual, recovery lies in the whole living experience within a given social and cultural context, what Basaglia defined as 'the social body' to which everyone should be part (Ongaro Basaglia and Basaglia, 1979).

Social factors: external resources and opportunities for individuals

Social factors of recovery are often described by the epidemiological term, 'social determinants' of health (Marmot, 2005; WHO and Calouste Gulbenkian Foundation, 2014). Basaglia wrote: 'Recoverability has a price, often very high, and is therefore an economic and social rather than a technical and scientific fact' (Basaglia, 1969). In this sense, he viewed healing as a social class fact. There are a number of personal, family, and environmental factors that allow for healing and recovery if the prognosis is favourable. 'We cannot understand what is disease as long as the primary needs of men are not met' (Basaglia, 1975). Even outside the realm of mere survival, material resources and tools for inclusion are obviously necessary. However, they are not sufficient in themselves in the path towards autonomy and improvement of the most objective components of the quality of life (Borg et al., 2005). Money, a home, and a job are essential vehicles for recovery, because they represent opportunities for the reconstruction of one's identity and social bargaining capacity. 'He who does not have, is not' recalled Basaglia. Many years later, an association was found between employment and recovery rates in the course of the twentieth century (Warner, 1985, 2005).

However, Basaglia wonders how social factors affect a subjectivity that is recovering. This is to say, how extrinsic factors relate to intrinsic factors, although theories of recovery divide them in a somewhat mechanistic manner sometimes (Jacobson and Greenley, 2001). In defining how social factors prove subjectively useful one must, on the one hand, work around the probabilistic–statistical construct of 'determinants' and, on the other hand, bypass the sociological and controversial construct of need. The recovery process should find answers to needs but, as Basaglia recalls, these needs are always mediated by the social organization. People do not express their needs, but that which they introject as a need (Basaglia, 1980). This, however, contains the contradiction between the individual and the constructed nature of the need, and its political and collective dimension.

Regarding the process of deinstitutionalization, Franco Basaglia wondered how he could differentiate between the tools and resources made available after disassembling the asylums into their individual situations. It was precisely the subjectivity of individuals that gave them a meaning that was from time to time specific. These were identified in life projects (Portacolone et al., 2015), through the opportunities and alternatives that could be implemented: for example, economic aid can be used for different personal purposes (Basaglia, 1983). This raises the importance of the subjective factor or of subjectivity itself. How are aid factors subjectivized or how do they become subjectively relevant factors (Davidson and Strauss, 1992)?

Health and illness: their dialectics in everyday life

In this discussion, the dimension of daily experience is taken as central. This is in contrast to the scant attention it usually receives from services and in the field of research, as compared to the attention paid to symptomatic behaviours. It is a matter of recognizing the scope of life's practical issues, how individuals experience situations, face obstacles, and challenges, and adapt their goals and ideas along the way, in a creative manner. Not unlike in total institutions as described by Goffman (1961), the crucial requirements for recovery of the material conditions of life outside institutions are a job and an income. A home and social relationships involve daily life and its routines. We must also consider the role of chance and events as opportunities for change, for new interests, and new emerging meanings (Borg and Davidson, 2008). It is in this everyday life dimension that we can find the essential contradictions of the recovery process. This is Basaglia's greatest challenge to the theory and practice of medicine. 'Healing' must not exclude or cancel suffering, but recognize it as part of the human experience, within a process of recovery and reprocessing.

Reciprocally, if we look at the illness, healing will be included in it, to dig the space of life out of it. That provides ground for the option not only of healing 'from' the illness, which is inherent in the medical discourse, but also to recover 'in' the illness (Davidson and Roe, 2007). In other words, 'a life despite symptoms' was one of the great teachings of the school of deinstitutionalization. People, even within a disease or a ratified diversity, could live in the community, long for a normal life, and be entitled to receive a response to primary needs and relationships.

A central assumption of the late Basaglia is that a peculiar aspect of human beings is that health and illness are in a constant dialectical relationship with one another. These two constructs certainly relate to each other within a framework defined by the 'norm', which is explicitly expressed in terms of participation in productive life. In this sense, Basaglia took us back to that constitutive component of healing, from a social perspective, which is reclaiming one's life back:

> That which is commonly intended as healing is therefore together the expression of the patient's acceptance of his condition of being defrauded and dispossessed of the possibility of living the disease dialectically, and consequently one's body as experience. The medical ideology and practice contributes to deepen the fracture, support the alienation of the self as a value, and technically confirm them as the main condition beyond which lies health.
>
> **(Basaglia, 1975, p. 377)**

Services and the issue of power: deinstitutionalizing the institutional relationship

The movement that built up in the 1960s, by Basaglia and others (e.g. the organization called 'Psichiatria Democratica') (see Figure 3.2), emerged on the wave of the anti-asylum fight and revolved around the problem of redefining the psychiatrist's social mandate, questioning his power and the direction in which he asserts such power as an 'functionaries of consent' (Basaglia and Ongaro Basaglia, 1975). Institutional critical practice moved from the 'most brutish' aspects of psychiatric oppression in the asylum to the political, social, and economic conditions that shaped it in the 'outside space'.

It is remarkable that the public health role of psychiatry is now also recognized—and advocated—by the psychiatric establishment (e.g. the WPA-Lancet Commission). It is important that the role of psychiatry and the psychiatrist in society, in the domain of law, and in the issue of human rights is clearly stated. Here, the contradiction of the psychiatrist's role as an authority between human rights and prevention of violence 'poses a constant challenge', especially after the CPRD states 'a general task to stand up for the rights, dignity and inclusion of people with mental disorders' (Bhugra et al.,

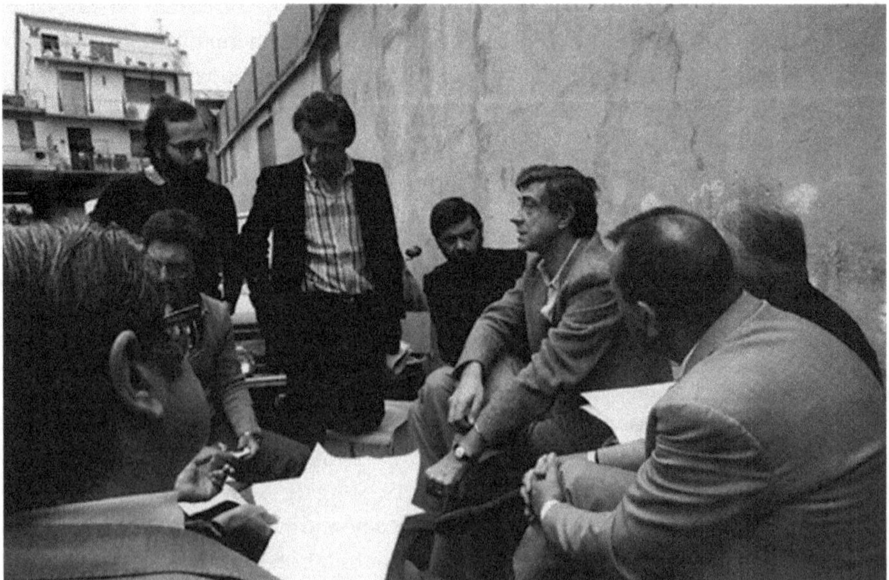

Figure 3.2 Franco Basaglia at a Psichiatria Democratica congress with other psychiatrists, Arezzo, 26 September 1976.
Courtesy of Emilio Tremolada

2017). Hence, there is a political obligation to advocate and lobby for the improvement of societal factors, both as an individual and through larger organizations.

Exposing the care–guardianship binomial, as the mandate as well as the key contradiction of psychiatry, is maybe the most important operation of empowerment during deinstitutionalization. It is no longer buried in the confinement of lunatic asylums under the technician's protection, and its practical overturning is seen in giving bargaining power back to the patients as social parties.

'Deinstitutionalizing' meant fighting against the institutional mechanisms that oppress not only, of course, the patient but also the patient's guardian-therapist. The coercive system was broken up by the overcoming of the hierarchical structure of power and the horizontal separations of the staff roles, the criticism of medical expertise, and the change of the operational organization. It is precisely in the mutual subjectivation of the patient as an independent person who expresses his needs, and the professional as an independent person who can listen to him, relate to him, and try to find a solution, that the two can actually come close to each other, can 'be on the same side', far beyond a mere therapeutic alliance. In the new scenario of community care which has resulted from the closure of the mental hospital and the re-conversion of resources to community-based services, deinstitutionalization can be seen as a change in relations of power. Priority is given to the user's needs and actions, but in order for them to become 'visible', the distance in the institutional relationship must be criticized and radically reduced.

In order to transform the actors of the institutional scene and the link between knowledge and power, Basaglia examined the 'pedagogy of power' (Basaglia and Gallio, 1992). By this he meant the ways in which all the actors involved, including the patient/user, can learn to use power for the transformation of existing conditions. Power is something that can be divided, shared, delegated, or offered as a choice in a strategy of empowerment. Dismantling the psychiatric hospital's apparatus of oppression and its hierarchy, the power transfer was either a bottom–up or a top–down process.

In the shift from institutions to community, the professionals' work aimed at letting users get hold of real assets (financial support, canteens, work, social services, housing, etc.). 'Deinstitutionalizing' then means also removing the effects of the incapacitation of the person due to the years of internment in the asylum. Likewise, 'rehabilitation' (as reclaiming resources and powers) (Rotelli, 1993) means rediscovering how to use the body and mind that had been expropriated and made totally dependent, with the person eventually regaining a social role and the related power, ultimately one's autonomy and independence. 'Exchange' is the key word here.

The steps of returning to social exchange are several, and they relate to the 'social factors' previously mentioned. Financial support and disability pensions are required as income, given illness-induced unproductivity, while social cooperatives include attempts to bring patients back into the labour market. Similarly, patients have the right to housing outside the boundaries of the asylum and to holidays and leisure. Real exchanges, direct social relations, can be thus reopened (Rotelli, 2015). Outside the psychiatric institution, the professional and the patient go through newly born community services as places of reproduction of subjectivities, and thus start to access general welfare.

> Any type of organization that does not take into account the patient in his free personal way of inhabiting the world will fail its purpose, because it will act on that subject as a negative force, even though seemingly aimed at his healing.
>
> **(Basaglia, 1965, pp. 289–90)**

Crucial questions arise here. If it is true that recovery as a personal fact (if not even strictly individual for some) may occur outside the codified systems of care, what is its relationship with micro and macro social contexts? What is the role of the services in this regard, if they are usually organized around the disease? In contrasting the damage produced by the institutions and all the iatrogenic effects related to the a so-called 'therapeutic' sphere of action, what should we ask from the services so that they may facilitate recovery (i.e. the reacquisition and recovery of the self)? Apart from a mere technical role, can services function as mediators and act as agents for that emancipation of the subject?

We may talk about a 'deinstitutionalization of the therapeutic relationship' connected with the recovery of the decision-making power of the person over his/her own life. The shift from the relationship of domination/control to a real therapeutic relationship must be seen as a two-way relationship, towards a discovery of the whole person and their subjectivity. From this point of view, we have not only seen a change in the balance of power, but a possible new relationship has been defined in place of the diagnostic objectification that excludes it. The globality of the person has been rediscovered, beyond exclusively technical interpretations (Mezzina, 2015). Once again, this has corresponded to treating the other equally and with reciprocity, even 'breaking the rules or the roles' (Topor, 2001).

The challenge of recognition and participation

Basaglia insisted on giving the patient the opportunity to speak, stating that 'it is the content of experience that should be transmitted' (Basaglia, 1980, p. 480). The narrative of recovery is an 'I say', where the words are back in the mouth of the subject who lives the experience. Basaglia looked at it again and defined it in terms that differ from psychiatric categorizations:

> It is only in this direct contact, without the mediation of the disease and its interpretation, that the subjectivity of those who suffer from mental disorders may emerge: a subjectivity that may only emerge in a relationship that, eventually out of the objectifying categories of positivist psychiatry, whose most concrete result has been the mental hospital, manages not to lock the abnormal experience in a

> further objectification and preserve it linked and closely connected to the individual and social history.
>
> **(Basaglia, 1980, p. 472)**

We are again confronting the almost obsessive question of whether that contact advocated by Basaglia since his earliest writings is really made possible in deinstitutionalization, or whether it is only an idealized contact, as he feared:

> In order to cope with the disease, we should be enabled to deal with it outside the institutions, not only outside psychiatric institution but outside any other institution that has the function of labelling, codifying and establishing. But does an 'outside' where we can act before institutions destroy us exist? The face of the disease that we know is always 'institutional'.
>
> **(Basaglia, 1968, p. 516)**

As a precondition, we should ask: 'Who listens? What is his/her power position with respect to the individual who speaks and to what extent does this power determine the meaning of the word?' (Ongaro Basaglia and Basaglia, 1979, p. 433). There must be a mutual recognition with somebody who takes the risk and makes his/her power available. According to Basaglia, this implies that the therapist is challenged by the patient, as well as the patient being challenged by the therapist, so that each one is recognizable by the other: 'Therapy makes sense when there is a reciprocity between the patient and the doctor' (Basaglia, 2000, p. 41). This process of redefinition of the demand for care, of decoding, and, therefore, deinstitutionalization of the illness itself (Rotelli, 1990), takes place today in the conditions posed by the new community scenario. Within it, the person can walk his/her path, if the service is capable of necessarily taking its share of positive risk regarding the person as a whole, his/her abilities, his/her health in the dialectic interface between illness and life (see Figure 3.3).

Reappropriation of health cannot really take place on an individual level, but is something that belongs to social and political processes and changes. The entire deinstitutionalization movement highlighted the need to cross the participatory dimension of the transformation process. Similarly, reconstructing, understanding, enabling the connection between the 'self' and collectivity, between own and shared, is also one of the most fascinating aspects of the question of recovery. In this sense, the same participatory dimension, when posed with evidence, indicates that the person is emerging from isolation, from the rupture of meaning and language that results in desocialization.

For many who have experienced suffering, the balance between socialization and independence remains difficult and precarious, with solitude sometimes as a choice. What then is the meaning of 'recovering a social life'? Some have mentioned a 'lived citizenship' as the unveiling of the intimate social nature of even the most personal recovery (De Leonardis, 1990; Mezzina et al., 2006).

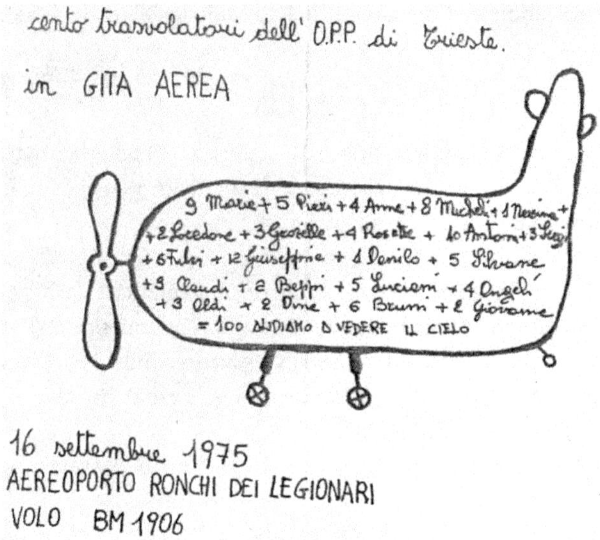

Figure 3.3 Ugo Guarino poster for the patient flight, which took place eventually on 16 September 1975.
Courtesy of Claudio Erné

Social integration, intended as adaptation to reality, seems rather linked to a sort of pedagogy of the social game. We should, in fact, understand what the relationship between recovery and unliveable conditions or oppression is, what the prerequisites of any 'coming out'" of madness are. Healing often takes place within antinomian pairs: either to accept society in terms of values and a prevalent ruler, or to antagonize it. Another issue is what contribution individuals can make to changing the rules and dominant ideas on the contradiction between health and disease, for example by breaking the disability–stigma nexus. This means, for those who suffer, working towards a disintrojection of deviance, towards abandoning the role of the sick person.

A post-reform stage was necessary, a reformulation of the theme of needs and the response to them, as laid out by Basaglia, in terms of citizenship rights. One of the most frequently used conceptual frameworks in policy and guidance documents on the topic of recovery (Le Boutiller et al., 2011) is the promotion of citizenship, to support the reintegration of people into society as citizens (i.e. enjoying rights, inclusion, employment), and not separated from a change of the services ('whole system change'). This is why it is important to grasp the link between psychiatry critical practices and the new leadership, empowerment, the entrance of the users of the services as collective subjects, on the policy scene (WHO, 2013).

Even in official documents (WHO, 2010), empowerment is depicted as a multidimensional social process that determines changes in the lives of individuals and in the circumstances of their health. That is why we prefer today, with Basaglia, to use both recovery *and* 'emancipation' to emphasize those aspects of 'non-freedom' related to the disease condition—personal and social misery, the loss of rights, and the prevention of access to socially usable resources.

Expanding civil rights

At the end of the 1970s, in Trieste, as well as in Perugia and Arezzo, the process of phasing out the old asylums was almost complete. This opened the way to the enforcement of Reform Law 180 of 13 May 1978, to which Basaglia contributed. So, the new model of community care was designed to coincide with the transformation of the psychiatric hospital. Today, 40 years after Law 180, deinstitutionalization throughout Italy has been completed, even if it took about 20 years for the closure of all asylums and another two decades to close all large forensic hospitals.

Basaglia spoke of 'anomia' in the asylum, where there are no constitutional rules, a prelude to the irreversible loss of rights. The legislative abolition of the false mental disorder/dangerousness equation raises the issue of psychiatric assistance regarding social rights, too. This includes the use of welfare services aimed at guaranteeing the fundamental right to mental health, protected by Article 32 of the Constitution of the Italian Republic (1948). Hence, the seminal character of Law 180 implied some corollaries. These included laws for welfare state provision and the social inclusion or integration of people with severe mental illness: the law on social co-operatives (381/1991); the law on the support administrator (6/2004); the law on integration of welfare and health care services (328/2000) (Mezzina, 2018).

Basaglia pointed out the insertion into the legislation of a civil and constitutional element that should have been implicit in it and was not—the *recognition of human rights* (Basaglia, 1979; Piccione, 2013). With the end of the asylum, the right to mental health, precisely because it aims to emancipate the person from need, constitutes the precondition for the exercise of civil liberties (Piccione, 2013).

The paths of inclusion, of the enlargement of the participatory democracy of services and rights, was initiated by Law 180. People with mental health problems have increasingly come into play as protagonists in reclaiming their full rights, intervening in the debate on the disease, on healing, on the paths of recovery, and on the quality of service responses (Piccione, 2013). Practices of deinstitutionalization, as a way to realize human rights, have penetrated a range of institutional areas, from medicine to schools, to prisons, to shelters for the elderly, to institutions for minors and for people with disabilities, and, more generally, to the entire ambit of welfare policies.

The Legislation of 1978 was based on the 'discovery' of rights and the centrality of the person as envisaged within the Italian Constitution. Today, human rights are recognized as key tools in mental healthcare (WHO, 2017) and are conceptualized as universal rights guaranteed also to vulnerable individuals. Subjectivation can be seen as the assumption and recognition of the fundamental human rights of an individual or of a group, which allow them to become historical actors (Touraine, 2015).

Total institutions have been clearly identified by Basaglia and this anti-institutional movement as the source of a culture of oppression and violation of human rights, of stigmatization and social exclusion, and must be overcome. The return of the dignity of the person with a mental disorder is achieved precisely through the idea that he has to self-determine in the context of care. In addition, the public health system must always offer assistance adaptable to individual subjectivity and needs, without replacing it with the undesired prejudice depriving the illness from understanding and choice. The mental disorder cannot undermine the right to self-determination (Piccione, 2013).

From this perspective, the most important step forward during last 10 to 15 years has been the United Nations' CRPD. This is the first high-level, international, legally binding standard which aims to promote, protect, and ensure the full and equal enjoyment of all human rights and fundamental freedoms by all persons with disabilities, including those with mental health conditions ('psychosocial disabilities'), and to promote respect for their inherent dignity. Such persons are definitely considered capable of claiming those rights and making decisions regarding their lives based on their free and informed consent. They are also active members of society, according to principles of non-discrimination and full and effective participation and inclusion in society (Mezzina et al., 2018).

In order to apply the CRPD in a concrete way, democracy and equality must be ensured, challenging social exclusion, and acting on social determinants of health to achieve greater equity and stability of home, work, and income. The defence of the dignity of human beings must not be separated from the pursuit of social justice, from an active struggle against inequalities, privileges, and injustices (Touraine, 2015).

The problem of the 'practically true': Trieste, moving forward

The closure of the asylums, which Law 180made possible, realized the return to people of the paramount right of having a life worth living. After the sudden conclusion of the work in Gorizia (Foot, 2015), the experience of Trieste represented, eventually, the 'practically true' invoked by Basaglia, using Sartre's words. He was 'obsessed' with practice as verification of theory. Trieste became internationally known when, as a WHO pilot area, its process resulted in the first closure of a psychiatric hospital in Europe (see Figure 3.4) (Bennett, 1985; Rotelli, 1988b; Dell'Acqua and Cogliati Dezza, 1986), dismantling the apparatus and the institutional norms that build on the person as a patient, as an object of the psychiatric institution. In a nutshell, the work in Trieste is marked by the first years (1971–1974) of transformation of the asylum and the creation of a state of rights for the inmates: opening of wards and gates, assemblies, review of the status of hospitalization and increase in voluntary admissions, establishment of hospitality, economic subsidies, creation of the first working cooperative for patients, and review of guardianships. This was followed by a phase

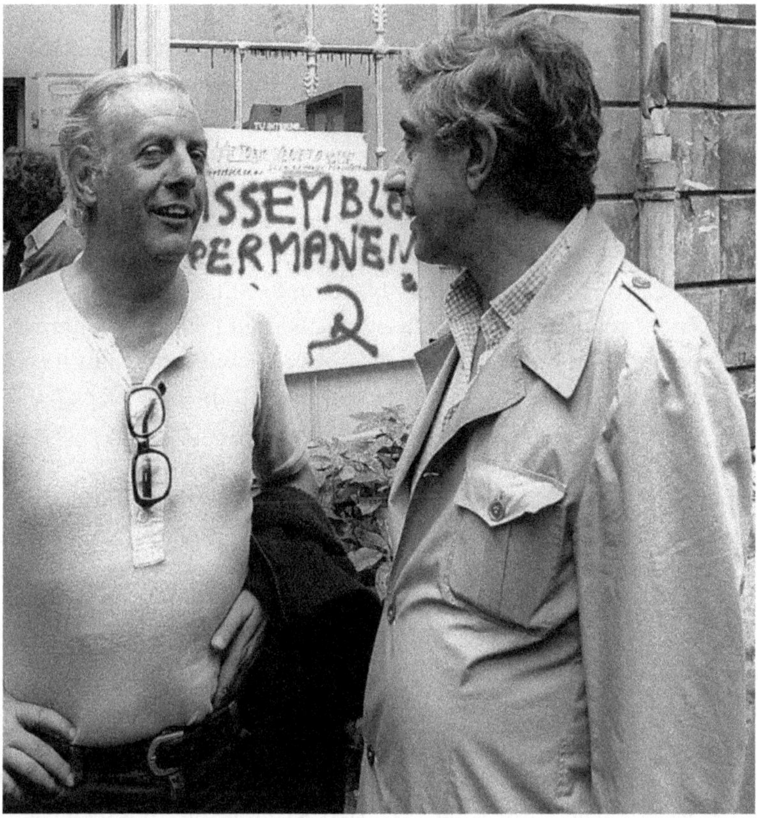

Figure 3.4 The actor, painter, and writer Dario Fo with Franco Basaglia, Trieste. Dario Fo shared Basaglia's aims and intervened in the debate on the overcoming of the psychiatric hospital.
Courtesy of Claudio Erné

of the opening of community mental health centres (1975–1978), together with the search for housing solutions for an increasing number of discharged patients (group apartments). Finally, the asylum was totally substituted by a comprehensive community service network (1978–1980), with all centres organized to offer round-the-clock access and beds (Gallio et al., 1983; Dell'Acqua, 2010).

In fact, Trieste has continued an autonomous elaboration from Basaglia, that develops his premises further, with completion marked by systematization/rationalization. The reduction of political involvement in the 1980s, and the attacks on the law and the legislative attempts to change it, led to a strong defence from within the psychiatric field. This meant strengthening the service model, making the alternatives a reality, and changing the language.

Nowadays, many people, unaware of the history of Trieste, see its outcome: a completely alternative system of services to asylums and a different approach to care and social inclusion. Trieste today is a city that has had no asylums for the past 40 years, with a totally open-door system. It has shown that it is possible to act in a new way to foster recovery and social inclusion in the community, while embracing a human rights approach. The Mental Health Department was recognized as a WHO Collaborating Centre in 1987 and is considered to be a sustainable model for service development because of its demonstration of cost effectiveness (WHO, 2001).

The process of changing the thinking, the practice, and the services, invoked by Basaglia as a real deinstitutionalization and not a mere dehospitalization (Rotelli et al., 1986), led from a clinical model—based on the illness and its treatment—to a wider concept of community mental health focused on the person within the social fabric. The organization is based on fully accessible, 24-hour community mental health (CMH) centres, with a few community beds in each of them, providing 'hospitality' instead of 'hospitalization' and working around the life stories of people in care. Today, the personal healthcare budget system helps to tailor individual recovery and social inclusion pathways, entering daily-life domains, especially for those with complex social care needs (about 150 people a year). One quarter of the department's budget directly supports people in their daily life (Mezzina, 2010, 2014, 2016). Total expenditure is (2018) 37% that of maintaining one mental hospital; 94% of this budget is spent in the community, and only 6% funds a six-bed general hospital-based service that acts as an emergency first-aid station at night and operates with an external crisis team. In the whole region of Friuli Venezia Giulia (1.2 million inhabitants), just six forensic beds are available in three community facilities that are managed with an open-door policy. The wide range of responses includes providing job training and placement for about 200 service users annually, with about one in ten becoming full-time members of social cooperatives (or employed in the labour market) each year. Day centres, social clubs, and community agencies and associations, including sport and cultural ones, are active partners for human development and social inclusion (Mezzina, 2014).

The shift from residential facilities to transitional and supported housing, for about a hundred clients, is aimed at the highest level of independent living (Ridente and Mezzina, 2016; Zero Project, 2015). Beyond psychiatry, the integration of mental health services into a system of healthcare districts for community-based medicine (elderly, young and adolescent, disabled, specialized medicine, etc.) supports the right to adequate care and extends the fight against institutionalization of the elderly and adolescents, while promoting community engagement and development (in the so-called micro-areas project) (Mezzina, 2016). All this constitutes the system of support and opportunities for recovery.

In terms of human rights, it has to be noted that Trieste has one of the lowest rates of involuntary treatment in Italy, and such occurrences are mostly managed in CMH centres operating an open-door policy. Stemming from psychiatry, a regional deliberation in 2017 proscribed mechanical restraints in all healthcare and social care facilities, including nursing homes and general hospitals.

If 'freedom is therapeutic' was the original motto in the Trieste experience, nowadays, it is particularly relevant that principles such as open doors, hospitality, negotiation, and alternatives to coercion are embedded in the service vision and culture. 'Freedom first' (Muusse and Van Rooijen, 2015) emphasizes that personal liberty is not the outcome but a precondition for care which overturns control mechanisms and supersedes them with people empowerment. Thus, services also recognize the value of participation of all stakeholders, through networking, forms of co-production, cooperation, and exchange.

Trieste, after being a vanguard and pioneer of psychiatric reform in Italy and in the world, as recognized by the WHO, as well as the best example of the realization of the law, is now a human rights banner for the United Nations (UN, 2018). A rights-based approach must indeed be valued when considering 'the person as a whole'. Healing 'recognizes' the person and, thus, refers to shared basic values of humanity. Recognition of the 'human commune' beyond the disease was brought into the open by the Husserlian 'epoché' of Franco Basaglia. The person calls into question a whole life (in all domains), whole systems, and a whole community (IMHCN, 2017).

We cannot escape the contradiction between suffering subjectivity and the institution just by denying it or transforming it, or even reinventing it (Rotelli, 1988a). We should create a service in which a complex interaction mixes the 'existence suffering' (and the disease itself) with life, through experiential situations and contexts. According to the conceptualization of Rotelli, 'the institution which we have been debating for the last twenty years is not the mental hospital, but madness . . . To us, on the contrary, the subject has always been "the patient's existence suffering and its relation with the social body"' (Rotelli, 1988a, p. 189). An institutional apparatus, totally referring to 'illness', was set out in this artificial separation. It was necessary to dismantle this apparatus (to deny those institutions) in order to connect again with the patients' existence (i.e. his or her life as a whole), as much as with their 'ill existence' (Rotelli, 1988a). Also, however, new institutions must be constantly dismantled and reconstructed so that innovation, creativity, and change become possible.

Recovery and human rights are connected

In the light of Basaglia, social control of behaviours and related social exclusion, with a great number of human rights violations, still affect both the caring and the healing process worldwide. If exclusion predominates, freedom stands out as a priority requirement, as a precondition of recovery and full citizenship. In itself, mental illness is described as 'non-freedom' and 'non-choice', as a trap for individual subjectivity. Then, the nexus between recovery and emancipation—as achievement of human rights—cannot but consist of a process of opening up a range of possibilities that enable suffering individuals to see their hopes come true. It is a promise, or rather, a right for everybody—including those who keep feeling bad—to a different management of their illness and their life. This human rights–recovery nexus is nowadays confirmed by the Quality Rights Programme of the World Health Organization (WHO, 2017).

The emphasis on factors and determinants that are internal and external to the person, subjective and social, versus naturalistic factors related to the 'disease', is combined with the requirement to obtain collective solutions to a whole set of needs and, simultaneously, to demand rights. This requires a process that sees the person with mental health issues as a protagonist of change in services, culture, and knowledge. This cannot happen in a mechanistic and extrinsic, hetero-determined way, but through the significance of said factors in the recovery process, within the world of an individual. Precisely because they are identified with this world, these factors must be contextualized, and so become founding elements of a reconstruction of subjectivity, as Basaglia declared.

Thanks to the research and experiences around the theme of recovery, we today understand that this illness object is still revealed as a precarious construct that confirms Basaglia's criticism to traditional psychiatry. It constantly changes over time and can be seen as an open process. It is an irregular and jerky process that occurs in parallel with life, with its facts and lived experiences, with changes and significant social transitions. In this longitudinal, irreversible vision of one's biography, we already see a concept of historicity of the existing that refers to recovery as a self-narrative. A narrative that materializes for the first time, that is as a reflective awareness of one's path, collected by witnesses who are the peers, the significant others, the operators.

This brings us back to Basaglia's theoretical elaborations:

> Disease and abnormality, like any other human contradiction, can be used as a means of re-appropriation or alienation of one's self, therefore as an instrument of liberation or dominion ... The significance of each action is determined by the value we recognize to man and the use we want to make of it, hence we infer the use we will make of his health and his disease, of his normality and his abnormality ... If the value is man, health and normality cannot be the norm, because the human condition is that of being healthy and ill together, normal and simultaneously abnormal.
>
> **(Basaglia, 1975, p. 380)**

According to this framework, the notion of recovery—the two aspects of the 'clinical' and the 'personal'—seems amenable to systemic reason, that of being clinician and patient, respectively (Mezzina, 2015). Together, they confirm a dominant culture that sees the world of psychiatry (namely, the institutional world) and the world of life (i.e. the world of people and their communities) as separate and incommunicable, with the former trying to dominate, interpret, and control the latter. A vision of recovery, in the wake of Basaglia, should include both these poles in a dialectical process of transformation of the observer and of the observed. The visions and proposals of both—the therapeutic and life spheres—engage in a confrontation, a full-contact match that will deeply transform both of them. This will happen in the awareness that the definition of the institution as reality/ideology embraces both. Therefore, it is not the cure but the transformation of this relationship that we still deal with today. It is the creation of new balances of power and opportunities of existence for those who suffer and as a precondition of care work.

Provisional conclusions (what we have learned so far)

While the medical model of treatment is an insufficient support for the process of subjectivation, one of the main purposes of Franco Basaglia was to pose the question of suffering subjectivity within the institution with its oppression of the mentally ill, and to have attempted the difficult practice of liberation from this regime. This meant trying to free one's subjectivity from the objectification performed by institutions, even those intended as organizations within micro- and macro-social systems, and moving them towards more humane care. Dismantling and deconstructing the institution is then a precondition for recovery of individuals, by placing them within a real-life, whole-life context. Their (rediscovered) subjectivity acts, in turn, as a weapon against institutions themselves. But what will happen when a total institution disappears? Is this subjectivity liberated?

It was not enough to rediscover an individual with their singularity, as anthropophenomenology claimed, on behalf of professionals. A whole person has the same rights as everyone of us; personal liberty from the institution is just a first step. Thus, consciousness about universal human rights was the new, decisive element that came into play. The new frontier that Basaglia anticipated was not only about fighting against asylums on the one hand ('changing the service') and, on the other hand, advocating rights, but a convergence of both actions. Basaglia would have supported today's double deinstitutionalizing/human rights based strategy, and reconnected it to a recovery vision based not only on individual strengths and efforts, but also on a profound system change that involves culture. Worldwide, deinstitutionalization, as such, is probably the most important strategy that can contribute to a human rights approach.

Basaglia spoke about fundamental human rights, and the so-called Basaglia Law 180 abolished, at the root, the differences, in terms of rights, established for psychiatric conditions. The claim and struggle for (social rights) entitlements (e.g. income, work, a home) has been dictated by the historical contingencies of the struggle for welfare and also by the imperative of guaranteeing the social reproduction of weak subjects, whom we would now call 'vulnerable'. But Basaglia's gaze went further, to the horizon of the human and an ethical affirmation of universal rights, without passing through economic, social, and political intermediaries (Touraine, 2015).

The rights payable

The outcomes are the rights due, as stated in the UN CRPD. They are represented by individuals themselves, for whom these rights become real, and who see their 'recovery' inextricably linked to their citizenship. But in mental health, can an approach based on rights and ethics be effective, generate evidence? Can the 'three Es'—Ethics, Evidence, Experience— (Thornicroft and Tansella, 2009) be interconnected?

The person in the world of life

This approach is centred on the person or, holistically, on the entirety of the sphere of life. It starts from shared values—freedom and humanity above all, and it is an approach to the whole system. How come it is effective? Perhaps because it produces a shared and coherent, readable and cohabitated world, to which each one is called to contribute and to be responsible. A world where there is continuous exchange, and not a donation but a production of meaning, of an intersubjective meaning, which implies an exit from alienation and social re-inclusion. The knowledge of complexity is also the knowledge of normality, and, as such, is suspended between the trivial and extraordinary. Today, complexity is understood as a co-determination, co-evolution of services and people in the field of healthcare: complicity and alliance and dialogue.

The illness outside brackets

A central theme of Basaglia's reflection has been that of putting mental illness in 'brackets'. This is a Husserlian epoché that may perhaps pave the way to that contact with the suffering subject that, in the final stage of this reflection, becomes an event outside institutions (Basaglia, 1967). On the one hand, it is not true that the illness in the community is still in brackets: in the recovery vision, it is instead fully recognized as part of the person, of his horizon, of his situation. There is no longer the parallel world, the parallel code, the segregated and segregating language of psychiatry. People speak themselves, as illness speaks to health, refers to it, and revives it. On the other hand, 'bringing the illness between brackets' is, today, equivalent to talking about the rights of vulnerable people, starting from the social model of disability. The primacy of the treatment that psychiatry always claims for itself is no longer an 'indirect way' to recover, but, rather, the primacy of human rights and quality of life. What can be more clearly discerned, in the post-institutional age (if by institution we refer to the total, to the asylum), is perhaps what, in the social context, leads from the illness to the person.

Empowerment and political action today

Responding to needs was the first political reclaim, supported by a critical approach to psychiatry. Then we can assume that by moving from advocacy of patient rights, on the part of clinicians, to self-advocacy, responsibility has been shared or even shifted.

This was declared by the CRPD, and the new (even vulnerable) social actors are recognized and entitled with rights. It requires their real empowerment—so their subjectivity can become truly political. To defuse a risk confined within the specific field of psychiatry and within the search for sectorial rights, our societies, starting from their dimension of community, must be mobilized by a strategy that includes two-way movement, a dialectical movement between persons with disabilities and the social context (Davidson et al., 2010).

If we now declare the right to be a citizen, it links to the right to have a life, recognizing that the whole person requires opportunities for the prospect of a whole life. Thus we need social and human development that could converge, not conflict, with substantive, individual rights. We need an unarmed psychiatry, for which tools for change are rights, opportunities, and, finally, empowerment.

Basaglia's real outcomes are the subjectivities of those who were considered as objects, within their tangible, unique lives. Moreover, until there is civil awareness and real participation of all citizens in community mental health as a whole transformation for society, the dream of Franco Basaglia will not have been completely realized.

References

Barton, R. (1959). *Institutional Neurosis*. Bristol: Wright.

Basaglia, F. (1964). The destruction of the mental hospital as a place of institutionalization. Thoughts caused by personal experience with the open door system and part time service. First international congress of social Psychiatry, London. Reprinted in: L. Toresini and R. Mezzina (eds), *Beyond the Walls. Deinstitutionalisation in the European Best Practices in Mental Health*. Meran: Alphabeta, 2010.

Basaglia, F. (1965). Potere e istituzionalizzazione. Reprinted in: *Scritti I, 1953–1968, Dalla Psichiatria Fenomenologica all'esperienza di Gorizia*. Torino: Einaudi, 1982, pp. 283–93.

Basaglia, F. (1967a). Prefazione a 'Che cos'é la psichiatria?'. Reprinted in: *Scritti I, 1953–1968, Dalla Psichiatria Fenomenologica all'esperienza di Gorizia*. Torino: Einaudi, 1982, pp. 384–93.

Basaglia, F. (1967b). Esclusione, programmazione e integrazione (Appunti sulla realtà psichiatrica italiana). Reprinted in: *Scritti I, 1953–1968, Dalla Psichiatria Fenomenologica all'esperienza di Gorizia*. Torino: Einaudi, 1982, pp. 410–23.

Basaglia, F. (1968). Il problema della gestione. Reprinted in: *Scritti I, 1953–1968, Dalla Psichiatria Fenomenologica all'esperienza di Gorizia*. Torino: Einaudi, 1982, pp. 512–21.

Basaglia, F. (1969). Introduzione a 'Morire di Classe'. Reprinted in: *Scritti II, 1968–1980, Dall'apertura del manicomio alla nuova legge sull'assistenza psichiatrica*. Torino: Einaudi, 1982, pp. 73–9.

Basaglia, F. (in collaboration with Giannichedda, M.G. and Ongaro Basaglia, F.) (1975). Il concetto di salute e malattia. Reprinted in: *Scritti II, 1968–1980, Dall'apertura del manicomio alla nuova legge sull'assistenza psichiatrica*. Torino: Einaudi, 1982, pp. 362–81.

Basaglia, F. (1979). Prefazione a 'Il Giardino dei Gelsi'. Reprinted in: *Scritti II, 1968–1980, Dall'apertura del manicomio alla nuova legge sull'assistenza psichiatrica*. Torino: Einaudi, 1982, pp. 467–72.

Basaglia, F. (1980). Conversazione: a proposito della nuova legge 180. Reprinted in: *Scritti II, 1968–1980, Dall'apertura del manicomio alla nuova legge sull'assistenza psichiatrica*. Torino: Einaudi, 1982, pp. 473–85.

Basaglia, F. (1983). Lezione-conversazione con gli infermieri. In: G. Gallio, M.G. Giannichedda, O. De Leonardis, and D. Mauri (eds), *La libertà é terapeutica. L'esperienza psichiatrica di Trieste*. Milano: Feltrinelli, pp. 41–7.
Basaglia, F. (2000). *Conferenze Brasiliane*. F. Ongaro Basaglia and M.G. Giannichedda (eds). Milano: Raffaello Cortina.
Basaglia, F. and Ongaro Basaglia, F. (1971). La malattia e il suo doppio. Reprinted in: *Scritti II, 1968–1980, Dall'apertura del manicomio alla nuova legge sull'assistenza psichiatrica*. Torino: Einaudi, 1982, pp. 155–84.
Basaglia, F. and Ongaro Basaglia, F. (1975). Crimini di pace, Einaudi, Torino. In: *Scritti II, 1968–1980, Dall'apertura del manicomio alla nuova legge sull'assistenza psichiatrica*. Torino: Einaudi, 1982, pp. 237–338.
Basaglia, F. and Gallio, G. (1992). La vocazione terapeutica. Per un'analisi critica della 'via Italiana alla riforma psichiatrica' (1950–1978). In: A. Debernardi, R. Mezzina, and B. Norcio (eds), *Salute Mentale. Pragmatica e Complessità*. DSM USL n.1 Triestina, Centro Studi e Ricerche Regionale per la Salute Mentale, Regione Autonoma Friuli-Venezia Giulia, pp. 549–96.
Bennett, D.H. (1985). The changing pattern of mental health care in Trieste. *International Journal of Mental Health* 14:7–92.
Bhugra, D., et al. (2017). The WPA–Lancet Psychiatry Commission on the Future of Psychiatry. *Lancet Psychiatry* 4:775–818.
Borg, M. and Davidson, L. (2008). The nature of recovery as lived in everyday experience. *Journal of Mental Health* 17(2):129–40.
Borg, M., Sells, D., Topor, A., Mezzina, R., Marin, I., and Davidson, L. (2005). What makes a house a home: the role of material resources in recovery from severe mental illness. *American Journal of Psychiatric Rehabilitation* 8(3):243–56.
Bracken, P., et al. (2012). Psychiatry beyond the current paradigm. *British Journal of Psychiatry* 201:430–4.
Ciompi, L. (1984). Is there a schizophrenia? The long term course of psychotic phenomena. *British Journal of Psychiatry* 145:636–40.
Davidson, L. and Roe, D. (2007). Recovery from versus recovery in serious mental illness: one strategy for lessening confusion plaguing recovery. *Journal of Mental Health* 16(4):459–70.
Davidson, L. and Strauss, J.S. (1992). Sense of self in recovery from severe mental illness. *British Journal of Medical Psychology* 65(2):131–45.
Davidson, L., Mezzina, R., Rowe, M., and Thompson, K. (2010). A life in the community: Italian mental health reform and recovery. *Journal of Mental Health* 19(5):436–43.
Davidson, L., Rakfeldt, J., and Strauss, J. (2010a). *The Roots of the Recovery Movement in Psychiatry—Lessons Learned*. Chichester: Wiley.
De Leonardia, O. (1990). *Il terzo escluso. Le istituzioni come vincoli e*. Milano: Feltrinelli.
Dell'Acqua, G. (2010). Trieste: history of a transformation. In: L. Toresini and R. Mezzina (eds), *Beyond the Walls. Deinstitutionalisation in the European Best Practices in Mental Health*. Meran: Alphabeta, pp. 424–47.
Dell'Acqua, G. and Cogliati Dezza, M.G. (1986). The end of the mental hospital: a review of the psychiatric experience in Trieste. *Acta Psychiatrica Scandinavica* 316:45–69.
Foot, J. (2015). *The Man Who Closed the Asylums*. London: Verso Books.
Gallio, G., Giannichedda, M.G., De Leonardis, O., and Mauri, D. (1983). *La libertà é terapeutica. L'esperienza psichiatrica di Trieste*. Milano: Feltrinelli.
Goffman, E. (1961). *Asylums. Essay in the Social Situation of Mental Patients and Other Inmates*. New York: Anchor Books, Doubleday.
Harding C.M., Zubin, J., and Strauss, J.S. (1987). Chronicity in schizophrenia: fact, partial fact, or artifact? *Hospital & Community Psychiatry* 38(5):477–86.

International Mental Health Collaborating Network. (2017). *Whole Life, Whole Community, Whole Systems Approach*. Available at: www.IMHCN.org

Jacobson, N. and Greenley, D. (2001). What is recovery? A conceptual model and explication. *Psychiatric Services* 52:482–5.

Le Boutillier, C., Leamy, M., Bird, V.J., Davidson, L., Williams, J., and Slade, M. (2011). What does recovery mean in practice? A qualitative analysis of international recovery-oriented practice guidance. *Psychiatric Services* 62(12):1470–6.

Maccacaro, G.A. (1978). Appunti per una ricerca su: epidemiologia della istituzione psichiatrica come malattia sociale. *Fogli d'Informazione* 50:306–10.

Marmot, M. (2005). Social determinants of health inequalities. *Lancet* 365:1099–104.

Mezzina, R. (2005). Paradigm shift in psychiatry: processes and outcomes. In: S. Ramon and J.E. Williams (eds), *Mental Health at the Crossroads. The Promise of the Psychsocial Approach*. Hants, England: Ashgate.

Mezzina, R. (2010). Outcomes of deinstitutionalisation in Trieste. In: L. Toresini and R. Mezzina (eds), *Beyond the Walls. Deinstitutionalisation in the European Best Practices in Mental Health*. Meran: Alphabeta.

Mezzina, R. (2012). Che cos'è guarigione? L'oggetto oscuro della nostra (e vostra) ricerca. In: I. Marin and S. Bon (eds), *Guarire si può. Persone e disturbo mentale, 180—Archivio Critico della Salute Mentale*. Merano: Alphabeta Verlag, pp. 7–23.

Mezzina, R. (2014). Community mental healthcare in Trieste and beyond. An 'open door-no restraint' system of care for recovery and citizenship. *Journal of Nervous and Mental Disease* 202:440–5.

Mezzina, R. (2015). Tra soggettività e istituzioni: da Franco Basaglia alla recovery. In: A. Maone and B. D'Avanzo (eds), *Recovery. Nuovi paradigmi per la salute mentale*. Milano: Cortina, pp. 195–215.

Mezzina, R. (2016). Creating mental health services without exclusion or restraint but with open doors—Trieste, Italy. La santé mentale en France et dans le monde. *L'Information Psychiatrique* 92(9):747–54.

Mezzina, R. (2018). Forty years of the Law 180: the aspirations of a great reform, its success and continuing need. *Epidemiology and Psychiatric Sciences* 27:336–45. doi:10.1017/S2045796018000070

Mezzina, R., Borg, M., Marin, I., Sells, D., Topor, A., and Davidson, L. (2006). From participation to citizenship: how to regain a role, a status, and a life in the process of recovery. *American Journal of Psychiatric Rehabilitation* 9(1):39–61.

Mezzina, R., Rosen, A., Amering, M., and Javed, A. (2018). The practice of freedom: human rights and the global mental health agenda. In: K.D. Fountoulakis and A. Javed (eds), *Advances in Psychiatry*. New York: Springer, pp. 483–515.

Muusse, C. and Van Rooijen, S. (2015). *Freedom First. A Study of the Experience with Community-Based Mental Health Care in Trieste, Italy, and Its Significance for The Netherlands*. Utrecht: Trimbos Instituut.

Ongaro Basaglia, F. and Basaglia, F. (1979). Follia/delirio. Reprinted in: *Salute/malattia. Le parole della medicina, 180—Archivio Critico della Salute Mentale*. Merano: Alphabeta Verlag, pp. 119–47.

Piccione, D. (2013). *Il pensiero lungo. Franco Basaglia e la Costituzione*. Merano: Alphabeta Verlag.

Portacolone, E., Segal, S.P., Mezzina, R., Scheper-Hughes, N., and Okin, R.L. (2015). A tale of two cities: the exploration of the Trieste public psychiatry model in San Francisco. *Culture, Medicine and Psychiatry* 39:680–97.

Priebe, S., Burns, T., and Craig, T.K.J. (2013). The future of academic psychiatry may be social. *British Journal of Psychiatry* 202:319–20.

Ridente, G. and Mezzina, R. (2016). From residential facilities to supported housing: the personal health budget model as a form of coproduction. *International Journal of Mental Health* 45:1–12.

Rotelli, F. (1988a). The invented institution. *Per la Salute Mentale/For Mental Health* 1(88):189–96.

Rotelli, F. (1988b). Changing psychiatric services In Italy. In: S. Ramon and M.G. Giannichedda (eds), *Psychiatry in Transition. The British and Italian Experiences.* London: Pluto Press.

Rotelli, F. (1990). Modelli scientifici e complessità. Reprinted in: *Per la normalità. Taccuino di uno psichiatra negli anni della grande riforma.* Trieste: Asterios, 1999, pp. 70–3.

Rotelli, F. (1993). Ri-abilitare la ri-abilitazione. Reprinted In: *Per la normalità. Taccuino di uno psichiatra negli anni della grande riforma.* Trieste: Asterios, 1999, pp. 104–13.

Rotelli, F. (2015). *L' istituzione inventata. Almanacco Trieste 1971–2010. 180—Archivio Critico della Salute Mentale.* Meran: Alpha & Beta.

Rotelli, F., De Leonardis, O., and Mauri, D. (1986). Deinstitutionalization: a different path. The Italian mental health reform. *Health Promotion* 2:151–65.

Scheper–Hughes, N. and Lovell, A.M. (eds) (1987). *Psychiatry Inside Out: Selected Writings of Franco Basaglia.* New York: Columbia University Press.

Slade, M. (2009). *Personal Recovery and Mental Illness. A Guide for Mental Health Professionals.* London: Cambridge University Press.

Thornicroft, G. and Tansella, M. (2009). *Better Mental Health Care.* Cambridge: Cambridge University Press.

Topor, A. (2001). *Managing the Contradictions. Recovery from Severe Mental Disorders.* Stockholm: Stockholm University, Department of Social Work.

Touraine, A. (2015). *Nous, sujets humains.* Paris: Editions du Seuil.

Unger, R. (2010). *Moving Beyond Clinical Recovery and Personal Recovery: Reclaiming the Possibility of Full Recovery.* Available at: http://recoveryfromschizophrenia.org/2010

United Nations. (2006). *Convention on the Rights of Persons with Disabilities.* United Nations General Assembly Resolution, 13 December 2006, A/RES/61/106. Available at: www.ohchr.org

United Nations. (2017). *Report of the Special Rapporteur on the Right of Everyone to the Enjoyment of the Highest Attainable Standard of Physical and Mental Health.* Human Rights Council, 35th session, 6–23 June 2017.

United Nations. (2018). *Consultation on Human Rights and Mental Health: 'Identifying Strategies to Promote Human Rights in Mental Health'.* 14–15 May 2018, Room XVI, Palais des Nations, Geneva, Switzerland. Available at: www.ohchr.org

Warner, R. (1985/2005). *Recovery from Schizophrenia. Psychiatry and Political Economy*, 3rd edn. London/New York: Brunner–Routledge.

Wing, J.K. (1962). Institutionalism in mental hospitals. *British Journal of Social and Clinical Psychology* 1(1):38–51.

World Health Organization and Calouste Gulbenkian Foundation. (2014). *Social Determinants of Mental Health.* Geneva: WHO.

World Health Organization. (2001). *Stop Exclusion—Dare to Care. World Health Day 2001.* Geneva: WHO (Department of Mental Health and Substance Abuse). WHO/NMH/MSD/WHD/00.2

World Health Organization. (2010). *User Empowerment in Mental Health—A Statement by the WHO Regional Office for Europe.* With the support of the European Commission Health and Consumers Directorate-General.

World Health Organization. (2013). *Mental Health Action Plan 2013–2020*. Geneva: WHO.
World Health Organization. (2017). Quality Rights Programme. Available at: www.who.int/mental_health/policy/quality rights/en
Zero Project. (2015). For a World Without Barriers. Available at: https://zeroproject.org/practice/mental-health-department-whocc-italytrieste/

4
Basaglia's legacy and Italian mental healthcare today

Angelo Fioritti

Introduction

Whilst psychiatry is perennially and necessarily in crisis (Binswanger, 1957), the development in Italian psychiatry between 1962 and 1978 is without any doubt one of the crises that led to the most radical change in the discipline's history. Law 180 of 1978 marked something that had never happened before, and is probably unrepeatable. The historical studies of recent years (Foot, 2014; Babini, 2014) draw attention to the uniqueness in the medical history of the Italian anti-institutional movement. This, despite its complexity and the variety of opposing positions, led to a total rejection of places, methods, and conceptions consolidated over two centuries, which constituted the pillars of asylum practice. It was an ethical, political, and professional uprising that found careful and prepared public opinion, courageous and enlightened political leaders, and a professional body aimed largely at change, albeit with different accents and nuances.

Franco Basaglia, a Venetian psychiatrist of vast medical, philosophical, and humanistic accomplishment, dominates this process. Basaglia was the main reference of the Italian anti-institutional movement throughout the 1960s and 1970s. He is an example of how to intertwine intellectual production and political action, and to involve professionals and intellectuals from very different backgrounds. A great figure in world psychiatry, he occupies a prominent place both in the history of psychiatry and in the political and social culture of the twentieth century (Burns, 2013).

In this chapter, I will try to analyse the way in which the process that brought about the 1978 reform developed, and then summarize the vicissitudes of mental health services in Italy from 1978 to today. Finally, I will review the current situation, identifying how Basaglia's legacy influences the present day.

Other chapters in this book provide aspects of Basaglia's biography (see Chapter 1), an outline of his thought and its international influence (see Chapters 5 and 6), and a description of his action and his legacy in Trieste (see Chapter 3).

Before 1978—how we came to Law 180

Many scholars agree that Italian psychiatric reform is the most radical and complete process of deinstitutionalization (DI) to have taken place in the Western world, among the many that began in the 1960s and 1970s. Many attribute this greater radicalism to the deterioration of post-war Italian psychiatric hospitals, deeply marked by the preceding 20 years of fascism which had led to a break in scientific relations with other European countries. This repressive orientation was not free from the political use of internment and a drift toward pseudo-scientific racist theories, especially in its colonial psychiatric practice (Benevelli, 2010).

In the climate of conquered post-war freedom and in the gradual awareness of the horrors just passed, the anti-institutional critique crossed vast sectors of Italian society, questioning family, Church, schools, institutions for minors, and mental hospitals. The latter embodied the epitome of repression and dehumanization, to be fought with greater vehemence. The fight against mental hospitals became the goal of an entire generation, that of 1968, and for which *L'Istituzione Negata* (Basaglia, 1968) became the cult book, an indispensable reference point.

The process that led to Law 180 went through various stages (Pulino, 2016). It started with the indignation of public opinion over the inhuman conditions of asylums (Cerletti, 1949; Del Boca, 1966), giving way to resonance with the Gorizia experience conducted by Basaglia (1962–1968), a therapeutic community within a mental hospital inspired by the work of Maxwell Jones in Scotland. Then there were the programmes aimed at humanizing and downsizing psychiatric hospitals in Arezzo, Parma, and Perugia and the start of alternative community services in Reggio Emilia. The final steps took place all in 1978. In January, Basaglia announced that the Trieste psychiatric hospital of which he was director was going to close, the first in the world, within the year. In May, Law 180 was approved and admission to all psychiatric hospitals was forbidden in Italy. In December, Law 833, establishing the National Health System (NHS), was also approved and psychiatry was fully integrated within it. The celebrated slogan appearing on the walls of Trieste Hospital—'Freedom is therapy'—had found its way into reality.

The anti-institutional movement was not just an Italian phenomenon: its connections with European and American experiences were very evident. But in Italy it connected to the battles for civil rights, for divorce, for abortion, and for the construction of the NHS. Also, especially in Italy, the professional body of psychiatrists did not have a harsh attitude of contrast and resistance. Indeed, they participated in and promoted change, in some cases accepting it passively—something rarely seen in other countries.

It would be an error to focus only on Law 180 and its implications for mental health. The second half of the 1970s brought radical changes in many sectors of Italian civil society, mostly inspired by an anti-institutional vision. The report of the Falcucci Commission[1] on the integration of disabled pupils in schools, published in 1975, was

[1] Available at: https://www.edscuola.it/archivio/didattica/falcucci.html

equally, if not more, revolutionary than Law 180. It led to Presidential Decree 970 of 1975 and eventually to Law 517/1977, which determined the closure of all the special classes and 'socio-psycho-pedagogical institutes' (truly shameful asylums). All disabled children had the right to attend ordinary schools, which in their turn tackled the task of preparing specific programmes for these children. This reform is still the basis on which the Italian school system rests.

Law 658 of 1975 ('Discipline of narcotic drugs and psychotropic substances. Prevention, treatment and rehabilitation of the related states of drug addiction') introduced the distinction between consumer and dealer, and provided for clinical and rehabilitation services for drug addiction. It acknowledged the complete failure of previous attempts to tackle the rampant epidemic of heroin addiction with mandatory hospitalization in mental hospitals. The 40-year success of addiction services in Italy results from the same spirit from the same time. The capillary network of addiction services (SerT) integrated into the NHS is a rarity in Europe, the network of therapeutic communities run by non-governmental organizations (NGOs) is the most widespread and extensive in the world, and the integration between socio-medical approaches of NHS services and psycho-educational vision within the private sector is unknown in most countries.

After Law 180, a completely new phase of Italian psychiatry opened up, with the progressive dismantling of psychiatric hospitals (the final one only closing in 1997) and the construction of the community mental health services network, according to a departmental model organized with different levels of provision. The conceptual scheme that led to both the deconstruction of the asylum and construction of community psychiatry was the DI paradigm (Basaglia, 2005), the implications of which for the present and the future of Italian psychiatry will be considered later.

It is beyond the purpose of this chapter to provide a detailed historical analysis of that period. What is certain is that the 1978 Italian reform represents an irreversible jump, a discontinuity in the linear process of the history of psychiatry, marking a watershed, between before and after. Its consequences were of utmost importance for the subsequent development of Italian psychiatry.

The making of community mental health in Italy, 1978–2018

Forty years after the reform of 1978, Italy still has a radical community psychiatry system, one of the few countries in the world where community psychiatry has been *the* national policy for such an extended period. DI and development of the community mental healthcare network occurred nationally within a complex balance between federal and regional powers for planning, managing, and evaluation. Since 1999, planning and managing of health services have been within the competence of regional administrations, making it technically inappropriate to talk either of a NHS or of 'Italian psychiatry'. In effect, this has produced 20 different regional systems, making the peninsula a unique site for scholars in mental health policy and services evaluation to explore commonalities and differences.

The NHS is tax-funded, covers all citizens, and absorbs 6.7% of total gross domestic product (GDP). A further 2.2% of GDP is spent on private health services by citizens on a voluntary additional basis (ISTAT, 2017). According to the Italian Ministry of Health, the mental health sector is provided with about 5% of national health expenditure. However, the Italian Society of Psychiatric Epidemiology (SIEP) found that real costs absorbed by mental health services account for 3.5% of all NHS costs, with large variability and plausible disparities between the regions (Starace et al., 2018).

The NHS is currently organized through 121 Aziende Sanitarie Locali (local health trusts (LHTs)) and 71 Aziende Ospedaliere (hospital trusts (AOs)), the latter selling hospital services to the former, which are both providers and purchasers. Each LHT cares for a geographically defined population of, on average, 500,000 inhabitants. They have full economic accountability and reasonable autonomy in planning, managing, and evaluating services. Each LHT includes one Department of Mental Health (DMH) that provides comprehensive psychiatric care for the population. It manages the local network of services on a unitary basis, and these must provide at least the following minimum set of services required by national policy documents:

1. community mental health centres,
2. day-hospital/day-care rehabilitation centres,
3. general hospital psychiatric units,
4. non-hospital residential, medium-, and long- term facilities.

A recent comparison among G7 countries of mental healthcare facilities and staff availability (Barbui et al., 2018) found that Italy has nearly eight psychiatrists, 20 nurses, two social workers, and less than three psychologists per 100,000 population. These are low figures in comparison with other G7 countries where, for example, there are 22 psychiatrists in France, 102 nurses in Japan, 18 social workers in the USA, and more than 45 psychologists per 100,000 population in France and Canada. The same study showed that the number of beds in psychiatric hospitals ranges from eight (UK) to 208 (Japan) per 100,000 population, and that Italy is the only country to have no beds in mental hospitals. At the same time, Italy has fewer beds in psychiatric wards in general hospitals, but more beds in community residential facilities and supported housing programmes. Analysing historical data over the last 40 years, this work shows also that the DI process did not affect either the rate of compulsory admissions (which declined in absolute figures from about 20,000 in 1978 to 9,000 in 2015), nor the age-adjusted suicide rate (which declined from 7.1 to 6.3 per 100,000 in the same period).

Without any doubt, Italy is running the most community-orientated system in developed economies, and Basaglia's influence has been crucial both in the passing of Law 180 and in the developments of the system in the following 40 years. His vision and his reputation have inspired and supported the process of closing the mental hospitals that lasted until 1997. This deconstruction varied in different parts of Italy but, in every context, it was possible to avoid discharging patients without alternative accommodation, with few family re-entries and negligible abandonment in streets. In most of the asylum-closing programmes, community residential alternatives were provided. These facilities and programmes initially hosted the most disabled population from psychiatric hospitals, later reorganizing themselves towards new needs emerging from the changes in user profiles. Achievements and limitations of this sector of mental healthcare have been widely reported and debated in the international literature (de Girolamo et al., 2002, 2005).

The process of construction of community services overlapped in the beginning with that of DI, and continued until 2008. Many regions successfully managed to transfer human and financial resources from the hospital to the community (Fioritti et al., 1997), while in some, they were lost in the change, which explains today's resource disparities. A north–south divide is visible in all sectors of regional health services, despite equity in allocation of resources by the national government. These differences have also been widely studied by scholars in social sciences, who have mostly attributed them to different civic traditions in a country that only became a unified nation in 1861 (Putnam, 1993).

In addition to Basaglian philosophy, the development of community services has also been supported by the spread, amongst professionals and administrators, of a public health and psychiatric epidemiology approach. Michele Tansella has been a key figure in this, not only with professionals (Tansella et al., 1987; Tansella and Burti, 1999) but also in advising the Ministry of Health and helping draft the National Mental Health Plan which, at the end of the 1990s, sought to reduce local inequalities (Decreto Presidente della Repubblica, 1999).

Despite many different local nuances, the professional culture of Italian mental healthcare services tried to integrate (often in a very lively, debated, and conflictual way) Basaglian practices, conceptual tools from psychodynamics, elements of social psychiatry and epidemiology, and medico-biological notions, especially with reference to the use of prescription drugs. All in all, practice came first and went in search of its theories.

One crucial aspect for the life and culture of mental health departments was their full integration into the NHS, and the subsequent sharing of both their advantages and crises. Until 1992, LHTs were public administrations governed directly by local municipalities, without any real financial accountability. Since 1992, they have become 'public companies' with a system of governance and financial responsibility similar to the private sector. The tools for planning, budgeting, and evaluation of professionals and performances are now applied to all components of the NHS, including mental health services. This meeting between management and social psychiatry was not an easy one, and often experienced as frustrating by professionals. Some psychiatrists have engaged with this new phase of institutional life by taking on key managerial positions of importance, as Franco Rotelli did when becoming Chief Executive Officer (CEO) of two different LHTs, giving rise to original and creative experiences both for general and psychiatric healthcare (Gallio and Cogliati Dezza, 2018). The author of this chapter, at different stages of his career, has served as Medical Director of two LHTs, with only partial success in reconciling cultures and professional practices from the fields of mental health, public health, and management.

Since 2008, the Italian NHS and their DMHs have shared the vicissitudes arising from the convergence of dramatic socio-demographic changes and the financial crisis. This past decade represents a significant phase in the life of the DMHs and will be discussed later.

Many authors have highlighted the great variability between regions and questioned the overall value of the Italian experience, often seen as 'patchy and confused' (Freeman et al., 1985). What Italian psychiatric services have in common is that they are universal, tax-funded, fully integrated within the NHS, and espouse a public-health approach. They have liberal regulations about involuntary admissions, offer a guaranteed minimum set of services, reflect scepticism about 'programmes', and are also broadly psychosocial in orientation, with minimal degrees of subspecialization. This is also where the differences start.

The need for specialization is tackled differently by each regional system. There are few specialized services for dual diagnosis (either substance abuse or learning disability), eating disorders, or personality disorders. Specialized clinics for specific disorders such as anxiety or obsessive-compulsive disorder are virtually unknown and confined to a handful of university departments, mostly geared to research in collaboration with foreign centres. Remarkable differences can be found in standards (e.g. number of beds, allocation of resources to each unit within the department) and integration of private services within DMHs, as well as in integration with child psychiatry, drug abuse, learning disabilities services, and provision of specialized care for eating disorders.

The picture emerging helps frame the puzzling differences in service provision along three major dimensions (Fioritti and Amaddeo, 2014; Lora et al., 2014):

1. high-versus low-resource regional systems (basically a north–central/south gap);
2. radical community versus balanced-hospital/community systems, with Trieste and Lombardy at the two ends of the spectrum; and
3. 'generic' versus 'partially specialized' systems, with Campania and Emilia-Romagna at the two ends of the spectrum.

Forensic psychiatric hospitals were not included in the reform process in 1978. It was only in 2008 that a bill, calling for the transfer of all health services from the prison administration to the NHS, provided for the progressive closure of forensic psychiatric hospitals. Psychiatric care of mentally ill offenders is currently provided within the network of the NHS departments, with some 500 beds allocated, in small-size residential facilities, to provide care for the most difficult patients. Admissions to forensic hospitals have been forbidden since April 2015, and the last patient left such units in April 2017—the last tile of the mosaic of DI imagined by Basaglia has been put in place (Barbui and Saraceno, 2015).

Where do we go now?

Forty years later, the balance sheet for Italian psychiatry would seem at first glance quite positive (Fioritti, 2018). Looking at objective elements, Italy has carried out the largest and most radical dehospitalization process in the history of psychiatry, implementing at the same time a widespread system of community services throughout the country, albeit with very varied degrees of solidity and quality. The long-standing division between ordinary services and forensic services has been overcome, returning the mental healthcare of the mentally ill to the NHS. All this without significant evidence of abandonment, criminalization of the mentally ill, homelessness, social alarm, or suicide increase—at least so far. Overall, Italy is the country with the lowest degree of formal coercion of the mentally ill for those who record this practice. Yet the air breathed inside and around Italian psychiatry is by no means characterized by optimism and pride in these accomplishments. Uncertainties, fears, and frustrations prevail—very different from the bold enthusiasm of 40 years ago.

The profound transformations that have affected Italian society over the decades, and which are reflected in the NHS, play an important role. For over 10 years, mental health services have been asked to do much more, with much less, and in a much less protective society (Starace, 2016). For eight consecutive years, NHS funding has remained unchanged, which, in the face of rising costs, equals an effective reduction of about 15%. A survey by the Italian Society of Psychiatry found that, in the past decade, staff allocated to community services had been reduced by about 50%, with the provision of professionals per 1,500 inhabitants reducing from 0.8 to 0.4. In many regions, mental health funds have fallen far below minimal thresholds, in some cases reaching comparable rates to developing countries (Starace et al., 2018).

At the same time, the spectre of needs has expanded and diversified, under the combined effect of greater psychosocial vulnerability (e.g. first- and second-generation migrants, growing population of the poorest in the cities, the effect of early use of drugs) and the growing availability of costly technical interventions that are underpinned with scientific evidence (e.g. psychotherapies in personality disorders, behavioural therapy in autism). These are problems that afflict all contemporary societies, but in Italy, more than elsewhere, they seem to overstretch the plan that 40 years ago was set up with the NHS and with DI in psychiatry.

Taking into account the socio-demographic and economic dynamics that affect Italian society (e.g. population ageing, growing inequality, reduction of social capital), the entire NHS should strive to increase community care for citizens with chronic diseases and disabilities, who today crowd the general hospitals, inappropriately, with considerable waste of resources. The DMHs are an example of how increased community care is possible, useful, and beneficial, for the population and for society. Furthermore, the intertwining of the most complex and problematic cases of physical, mental, and social problems should lead to a reallocation of resources from traditional medical care to multi-professional case management. This would rely on organizations and methodologies that the DMHs have developed through the last four decades. All this should result in a strengthening of the role and prestige of DMHs in local realities.

All in all, this is not happening. The crisis in welfare financing is pushing citizens with social, economic, disability, and youth problems towards the services of the DMHs. They have needs which are not met elsewhere and that mainly represent the material, educational, and relational impoverishment of contemporary Italian society.

As in many other parts of the world, the social and political climate has rapidly changed and the legendary solidity of Italian communities (Putnam, 1993) is giving way to isolated, frightened, distrustful, impoverished individuals or households, who demand security and liberation from the complexities of everyday life. The space and time to work on the construction and maintenance of social networks is reduced day by day. The difficulties that the holistically and psychosocially set-up DMHs encounter in their work are perceived as inefficiencies and boring complaints. This is visible in the interinstitutional dialectics with Justice, municipalities, social services, local administrations, and local communities.

Reductionist and simplistic biomedical and neurobiological recipes have begun to exert a certain attraction for public opinion. More generally, stakeholders and experts who sell high-tech proposals and programmes in healthcare (usually aimed at small populations with ultra-specialized needs) are more likely to obtain funding than those who maintain a public health perspective addressed to the general population. The age-old quarrel over autism is the clearest example of such conflicts. Reintroducing special classes in schools is no longer a taboo, and the idea that we need to reopen long-term care places for mental illnesses is being proposed again by political forces currently in government.

Basaglia and the DI paradigm have meant, and continue to mean, much more to Italy than the closure of psychiatric hospitals. DI is a social and political construct designed to reformulate relations between individuals and society, balancing power relationships in favour of vulnerable individuals. It implies an attitude of constant awareness of the iatrogenic, destructive, and dehumanizing effects of institutional interventions, and a continuous effort to minimize them. For this reason, any DI-based programme is necessarily a political programme. It also includes a technical component that outlines how to achieve this balance, working on the environment (e.g. rules, access to care, opportunities, support, safeguards, promotion of open social networks) and on the individual (e.g. awareness of rights, promotion of health, control of care processes that concern him/her). The DI paradigm has also had a profound influence on national and regional policies for drug dependency, disability care, approach to juvenile deviancy, and other populations.

DI developed in Italy of the 1970s, in an era that Becker and Fangerau (2018) have defined as a 'unique—enabling—time in history … a window of operative opportunity'.

DI and Basaglia's legacy have persisted to the present, but are now challenged by dramatic, hectic, and unforeseeable changes in our society and our culture. Basaglia was the most attentive and acute interpreter of his times and managed successfully to integrate, into his action, suggestions, ideas, and professional and political positions. The zeitgeist of our time calls for a broad reanalysis of where we are now, in order to understand what DI can be in the future and how this legacy can be brought forward.

All this poses important questions about the future of Italian mental health services. The challenges of today and tomorrow must be tackled with the tools of today and tomorrow. It does not make much sense to lament the styles and modalities of a glorious past, but it is wiser to roll up one's sleeves and carry the ethical foundations of the profession into the forms of our time. Freedom, care, encounter, quality, protection, citizenship, and human and civil rights require highly professional staff and adequate provision of resources. Professional challenges must be tackled with confidence and firmness. Looking ahead, we should be aware of a past that should encourage us to go further, and not burden the future.

References

Babini, V.P. (2014). Looking back: Italian psychiatry from its origins to Law 180 of 1978. *Journal of Nervous & Mental Disease* 202:428–31.

Barbui, C., Papola, D., and Saraceno, B. (2018). Forty years without mental hospitals in Italy. *International Journal of Mental Health Systems* 12:43.

Barbui, C. and Saraceno B. (2015). Closing forensic psychiatric hospitals in Italy: a new revolution begins? *British Journal of Psychiatry* 206:445–6.

Basaglia, F. (2005). *L'utopia della realtà.* Torino: Einaudi.

Basaglia, F. (ed.) (1968). *L'istituzione negata.* Milano: Baldini Castoldi Dalai.

Becker, T. and Fangerau, H. (2018). Fortieth birthday of the Italian mental health Law 180. Perception, reputation abroad, and a personal suggestion. *Epidemiology and the Psychiatric Sciences* 27:314–18.

Benevelli, L. (2010). *La psichiatria coloniale italiana negli anni dell'Impero (1936–1941).* Lecce: Argo.

Binswanger, L. (1957). *Der Mensch in der Psychiatrie.* Pfullingen: Günter Neske.

Burns, T. (2013). *Our Necessary Shadow.* London: Allen Lane.

Cerletti, U. (1949). La fossa dei serpenti. *Il Ponte*:1371–7.

Decreto Presidente della Repubblica (1999). Progetto obiettivo *Tutela della Salute Mentale 1988–2000.* 10 November 1999.

de Girolamo, G., Picardi, A., Micciolo, R., Falloon, I., Fioritti, A., and Morosini, P. (for the Italian PROGRES Study Group) (2002). Residential care in Italy: a national survey of non-hospital facilities. *British Journal of Psychiatry* 181:220–5.

de Girolamo, G., et al. (for the PROGRES Study Group) (2005). The severely mentally ill in residential facilities: a national survey in Italy. *Psychological Medicine* 35(3):421–31.

Del Boca, A. (1966). *Manicomi come lager.* Torino: Edizioni dell'Albero.

Fioritti, A. (2018). Is freedom (still) therapy? The 40th anniversary of the Italian mental health care reform. *Epidemiology and the Psychiatric Sciences* 27:319–23.

Fioritti, A. and Amaddeo, F. (2014). Community mental health in Italy today. *Journal of Nervous & Mental Disease* 202:425–7.

Fioritti, A., Lo Russo, L., and Melega, V. (1997). Reform said or done? The case of Emilia-Romagna within the Italian psychiatric context. *American Journal of Psychiatry* 154:94–8.

Foot, J. (2014). *The Man Who Closed the Asylums.* London: Verso Books.

Freeman, H.L., Fryers, T., and Henderson, J.H. (1985). *Mental Health Services in Europe. Ten Years On.* World Health Organization: Geneva.

Gallio, G. and Cogliati Dezza, M.G. (2018). *La città che cura. Microaree e periferie della salute.* Merano: Alphabeta Verlag.

Istat (2017). *Statistiche Report: Anni 2012–2016.* Available at: https://www.istat.it/it/files/2017/07/CS-Sistema-dei-conti-della-sanit%C3%A0-anni-2012-2016.pdf

Lora, A., Starace, F., Di Munzio, W., and Fioritti, A. (2014). Italian community psychiatry in practice: description and comparison of three regional systems. *Journal of Nervous & Mental Disease* 202:446–50.

Pulino, D. (2016). *Prima della legge 180. Psichiatri, amministratori e politica (1968-1978).* Merano: Alphabeta Verlag.

Putnam, R.D. (1993). *Making Democracy Work. Civic Traditions in Modern Italy.* Princeton, New Jersey: Princeton University Press.

Starace, F. (2016). The mental health paradox, between increased demand and cutback of resources. *Journal of Psychopathology* 22:219–20.

Starace, F., Baccari, F., and Mungai, F. (2018). Salute mentale in Italia. La mappa delle diseguglianze. *Quaderni di Epidemiologia Psichiatrica* 2. Available at: http://siep.it/wp-content/uploads/2017/05/La-Salute-Mentale-in-Italia-SIEP-2017.pdf

Tansella, M. and Burti, L. (1999). The Italian psychiatric reform. In: H. Freeman (ed.), *Century of Psychiatry, Vol. 2.* London: Mosby-Wolfe Medical Communications, pp. 257–60.

Tansella, M., De Salvia, D., and Williams, P. (1987). The Italian psychiatric reform: some quantitative evidence. *Social Psychiatry* 22:220–4.

5
Basaglia's international influence

Benedetto Saraceno and Sashi P. Sashidharan

Introduction

In this chapter, we consider the impact of Franco Basaglia's work on professional thinking and mental health service development internationally. Basaglia's writing, clinical practices, and institutional strategies inspired and determined the most radical reformation of psychiatric care ever seen in the Western world (Mosher, 1982). However, the impact of his work in transforming mental healthcare outside of Italy appears to be limited. We explore the reasons for this and argue that Basaglia's work deserves greater international recognition.

Basaglia's work outside Italy

Outside of Italy, the two countries where Basaglia's work has had a critical influence in challenging institutional models of care are Spain and Brazil. In Spain, towards the end of Franco's rule, Basaglia's work became part of the cultural and social movements that challenged institutional hierarchies and the prevailing political order, including the traditional organization of mental health services. Basaglia visited Spain five times between 1973 and 1980, and had a significant impact on the emergence of a new psychiatry there. In many Spanish provinces, young mental health professionals were inspired by Basaglia and started a process of reforming the local mental health services (most notably in Asturias and Andalusia). However, it was only in the province of Oviedo that there was a concerted move to close down the mental hospital and develop community-based services (Jordá et al., 1993). The other Spanish experiences had a more limited impact on transforming the mental health system or sustaining the radical processes of deinstitutionalization (Rendueles, 1997; Garcia, 1995; Desviat, 1994).

Basaglia's work had a greater impact in Brazil, resulting in extensive and sustained reform of mental healthcare (Castadelli and Ventriglio, 2016; Ministerio da Saude Brasil, 2005). Brazil, like Spain, was emerging from the dark times of military dictatorship when Basaglia visited the country in 1979. Through a series of lectures (Basaglia, 1979), he inspired the early stages of Brazilian Psychiatric Reform. This became one of the most successful and innovative experiences in a large country (Various Authors, 2011) cited as a reference model by the WHO (2001).

There was a radical transformation of psychiatric care in many Brazilian cities and states, from a predominantly institutional model to community-based services. This change was achieved through the mobilization of public opinion in favour of progressive deactivation of asylums. Over a 20-year period, the number of psychiatric beds in Brazil was reduced, and large hospitals (with more than 400 beds) were downsized. This marked the process of humanization of mental healthcare which was followed by deinstitutionalization. There were only 148 community mental health centres in Brazil in 1998, but by 2010, the number had increased over ten-fold, to 1,620. By 2006, community mental health expenditure was higher than hospital expenditure: the per capita hospital cost had decreased by 45% while the extra-hospital cost had increased by 354% (Weber Gonçalves et al., 2012).

Impact of Basaglia's work

The reforms in Spain and Brazil were modelled on the transformation of mental health services in Italy during the 1970s. The changes in dynamics and momentum of the deinstitutionalization movement in Italy, eventually leading to the closure of all mental hospitals, came about as a direct result of the seminal work of Franco Basaglia and colleagues, first in Gorizia, later in Parma, and finally in Trieste. The groundbreaking Law 180, with directives for closure of all psychiatric hospitals (not just long-stay wards), was passed in 1978. All mental health services were relocated in the community, configured around small community mental health centres. However, deinstitutionalization meant more than the process of phasing out mental hospitals. In the words of Franco Rotelli, Basaglia's successor as the Director in Trieste, this involved the modification of psychiatry's cultural, theoretical, and scientific paradigms: breaking the clinical paradigm was the true aim of the deinstitutionalization project.

Community mental health services offered a more consensual and humanistic form of mental healthcare that took into account both people's preferences and needs. According to Rotelli, the psychiatric hospital had been criticized for a long time in cultural terms, but the 'small difference' in Italy was that this denunciation was taken seriously, 'in concrete, real terms'. The consequences were far-reaching. Rotelli reminds us that 'today, this choice still needs to be made and constitutes the primary characteristic of deinstitutionalisation' (Rotelli, 1994, p. 89). The outcome of the 'small difference' that Basaglia and colleagues made by their work in mental hospitals in Gorizia, Parma, and, later, in Trieste, eventually resulted in the complete transformation of mental healthcare in Italy, from an outdated institutional model to a comprehensive community-based system. After his premature death in 1980, Basaglia's vision and thinking continued to influence mental healthcare in many centres in Italy. The most notable example of this is the internationally renowned experience of Trieste, described as the best mental health system in the world (Allen, 2015).

Basaglia became the director of mental health services in Trieste in 1971, following his seminal work in Gorizia and Parma. He initiated a comprehensive deinstitutionalization programme soon after he took charge of the vast asylum, San Giovanni.

A series of fundamental reforms followed, including rapid reduction in the number of inpatients. By 1978, the number of patents in the hospital had been reduced by over 90%, eventually resulting in the successful closure of San Giovanni. A comprehensive community mental health programme was introduced which extended the scope and potential of mental healthcare in the city. This service has continued to thrive and evolve further over the years (Muusse and van Rooijen, 2015).

Basaglia's successors as mental health directors at Trieste—Franco Rotelli, Peppe Dell'Acqua, and Roberto Mezzina—have been remarkable ambassadors of the 'Trieste model'. Over the last four decades, the Trieste model of mental health reform and care has influenced mental health professionals all over the world. Franco Rotelli, the immediate successor to Basaglia, played a significant role as mentor in Brazilian experiences of mental health reform, such as in the city of Santos. This was the first psychiatric hospital to close in Brazil. The Argentinian experience of Rio Negro in Patagonia and the mental health reforms in Balkan countries were similarly influenced by the Trieste model. The continuing evolution of the Trieste experience has had a significant impact in other countries as well, including England. For example, in Birmingham, England, the replacement of an outdated and increasingly toxic mental healthcare system, reliant on hospital-based services, with specialist community mental health teams in the 1990s was inspired by the work of Basaglia and the Trieste experience. This model of care, successfully implemented in Birmingham, was subsequently adopted as the template for mental health services across England. The collaboration with Trieste was an important part of the work in Birmingham. This included reciprocal study visits. Psychiatrists and other mental health staff from Trieste spent various periods of time working alongside colleagues in the new community teams in Birmingham, sharing experience and expertise.

Over the years, an international network of innovative experiences has been established based on the Trieste model, and Trieste is now one of WHO's international collaborative centres. Through these arrangements, the Trieste experience is shared and further developed, with many innovative mental health programmes across the world, in over 40 countries to date. Currently, the staff from Trieste are actively engaged in collaborative projects in South America, Wales, India, and China.

Lack of international recognition

Despite Basaglia's groundbreaking achievements, in both the theory and practice of deinstitutionalization, his work is poorly known outside Italy. His contribution to mental health is largely ignored in the international psychiatric literature, especially in English-speaking countries. One reason for this is that much of Basaglia's writing is not generally available in English. Many of his seminal texts, including *L'Istituzione Negata* (Basaglia, 1968), are still not translated into English. The lack of translation of *L'Istituzione Negata* is especially important. This is the central text of Basaglia's thinking and of the deinstitutionalization movement in Italy, and has been influential in initiating mental health reform in other countries, such as France and Germany.

Apart from the book by Scheper-Hughes and Lovell (1987), little of Basaglia's work is accessible to English-speaking psychiatrists. Even an analysis of Basaglia's work by an English historian, originally written in English, was published only in Italian and not in English (Foot, 2014). The first comprehensive account of Basaglia's life and work in English was not published until 2015 (Foot, 2015). Apart from these, there are a few essays (usually by Italian authors) in English which present his thinking and vision in a cursory and non-systematic manner. The two exceptions are the 'Extracts from the theory of Franco Basaglia' by Maria Grazia Giannichedda (1988) and a chapter by Anne Lovell in a book concerned with broader themes in relation to mental health-care and social policy (Lovell, 1985). By comparison, several translations of Basaglia's writing are available in Spanish and Portuguese; the French translations are fewer, but the debate around his thinking and work is still quite vivid in France. Generally, Basaglia's work is acknowledged more in sociological and anti-institutional literature than in psychiatry itself.

There is a further 'silencing' of Basaglia's work within English psychiatry. In Britain, for example, his contributions are systematically ignored and his work often treated with condescension; a classic example of this is the superficial and contemptuous series of papers by Jones and Poletti (1984, 1985a, 1985b, 1986). These papers encapsulate the disbelief, animosity, and colonial attitude prevalent in much of British psychiatry in the 1980s towards Basaglia's vision and his anti-institutional thesis. His work was portrayed as a mixture of failures and tricks inspired by a radical, political ideology that had little to do with mental health or psychiatric care. As noted by Cohen and Saraceno, 'some observers have assumed, mistakenly, that Basaglia and his colleagues either eschewed the notion of therapy altogether or were badly trained' (Cohen and Saraceno, 2002). Partly, this lack of interest in Basaglia's work and the distortion of his thinking in the international literature are the product of a fundamental distrust of German phenomenology that is evident in mainstream British psychiatry in particular. A phenomenological approach, more than a biomedical psychiatric approach to the patient, characterized much of Basaglia's early work.

Although Jones and Poletti's impressionistic reports were severely criticized at the time by Italian psychiatrists, as nothing more than 'a superficial and unbalanced report of a journey to Italy, perfused with an old-fashioned and unrealistic colonial attitude' (Tansella, 1986), these polemical papers no doubt contributed to the negative reactions to Basaglia's work and Italian reforms in England. Within mainstream professional debates that followed, Basaglia was simply dismissed as an anti-psychiatrist and his reforms characterized as leading to 'chaos' (Foot, 2014).

Misunderstandings (distortions) of Basaglia

Apart from the absence of much of Basaglia's writings in English, the negative portrayal of his work, and, more generally, that of the Italian experience of deinstitutionalization, we identify three areas of common misunderstanding or distortions which have contributed to the silencing of Basaglia's work. These can be summarized as follows: Basaglia belonged to the movement of anti-psychiatry, his approach was driven by ideology, and his work was essentially inspired by a philanthropic impetus. All three assertions are inaccurate.

First misunderstanding: Basaglia belonged to the anti-psychiatry movement

Basaglia was not an anti-psychiatrist, as he was often portrayed. Although he had great respect and admiration for leading figures in anti-psychiatry in the 1960s, such as R.D. Laing and David Cooper, there was a fundamental difference between Basaglia's work and the intellectual adventures of Laing and Cooper. Basaglia recognized that the anti- psychiatry 'enterprise', however radical it seemed, was essentially condemned to remain a highly sophisticated production of cultural dissent. It was an individualistic enterprise, a personal 'trip', fundamentally disconnected from a more collective praxis of liberation. Basaglia's work, on the contrary, was premised on collective action, a collective praxis of transformation of mental health systems with radical implications for public health (Saraceno, 1988).

While Laing and other anti-psychiatrists gave moral and psychological legitimacy to psychotic experience, Basaglia's primary concern was the patient and his/her status as a citizen denied their full rights by the ideology of psychiatry and its dominant power. While anti-psychiatrists were concerned with the dominance of reason over unreason, Basaglia's focus was the dominance of psychiatric power and the unequal dynamic between the institution of psychiatry and the psychiatric patient. For Laing, it was important to establish the legitimacy of 'madness'. He argued that psychiatry could never accept or normalize the subjective experience of 'the other'. This resulted in psychiatry's violence towards 'the other', those deemed 'mad'. The only way to challenge this was to comprehend madness differently; it had to be welcomed, witnessed, and made legitimate. Laing recognized the 'mad' as someone able to produce 'another' kind of reason. However, this was deemed as a 'wrong reason' by the dominant reason (what Michel Foucault called 'de-raison') (Foucault, 1972). Legitimizing madness involved allowing/helping the person experiencing psychosis to go through his or her experience, including making available a place where he or she may regress with no constraints from the norms of psychiatry. In some ways, we can hear echoes of this approach in elements of what we now recognize as the recovery movement in mental health.

In contrast, for Basaglia, legitimacy was essentially to do with the body: the body of the patient that is institutionalized in the asylums. The person, therefore, should be liberated from such confinement and helped to acquire a social identity that restored his/her rights to affectivity, dignity, a social life, and economic independence. Basaglia was concerned with the freedom to rebuild social connectedness rather than the freedom to experience madness. The person with mental disability, incarcerated in the asylum, needed full access to the real world where people exchanged emotions, entered relationships, and could acquire knowledge, goods, and money. This enabled the person to 'negotiate' their social inclusion and to ensure and enjoy their rights. (Interestingly, in ancient Latin, negotiating is the opposite of being paralysed in a forced idleness: *otium* as the opposite of *neg-otium*.) Arjun Appadurai (2002) and Amartya Sen (1992) have argued in a similar vein that institutions, in general, prevent or diminish people's 'capacity to aspire', 'capacity to functioning'. In this context, we note the fundamental differences between Laing and Basaglia are, to some extent, reflected in the subtle tensions currently emerging between the recovery-focused approach in mental health and the call for regulations to restore the full rights of people with psychosocial disability, as recommended by the United Nations Convention on the Rights of Persons with Disability (United Nations, 2006).

Laing and the intellectual adventures of anti-psychiatry were driven by the utopia of a 'self' whose sociality, it was argued, was essentially confined by the psychology and dynamics of family interactions. For Laing, 'society has as its maximum extension a constellation of families … has no concrete temporal connotation, no economic specificity but it is shaped as an eternal dimension' (Vegetti-Finzi, 1986). This meant a journey towards fuller individuation, self-actualization, and self-knowledge. Basaglia's work had little to do with this utopian vision of anti-psychiatry but, instead, was concerned with the concrete process of liberation of the body: from the body humiliated and neglected by the institution to the social body, and from a private and dehumanized to a collective and human experience. For anti-psychiatrists, the legitimacy of madness trumped dominant reason. For Basaglia, psychosis was not a source of creativity and the 'art of madness' was an invention of psychiatrists: 'The work of the patient loses any meaning once it has been completed because its true and intrinsic value is just represented by the overcoming of the inability to communicate by the patient himself… the work of the patient becomes a Kitsch, a thing, a fashionable thing'[1] (Basaglia, 1964).

Basaglia's primary concern was not the existence of mental illness, or otherwise, but rather the moral and scientific legitimacy of psychiatry, and acceptance of the burden and responsibility of being a psychiatrist. Basaglia's colleague and successor as Director at Trieste, Franco Rotelli, addressed the paradox of denying the legitimacy of psychiatry and assuming responsibility as a psychiatrist. He wrote:

> in spite of knowing nothing about madness, I do not resign from myself, I do not resign from my role as a psychiatrist: I simply denounce the lack of scientific legitimacy (of psychiatry) and its political legitimacy. Indeed, I have a power and I recognise this. I decide to use this power first of all to demonstrate the inconsistency

[1] English translation of the following original: 'L'opera del malato perde ogni significato nel momento in cui è compiuta, proprio perché il suo vero, intrinseco valore sta nel superamento dell'impasse della capacità a comunicare di chi l'ha dipinta … L'opera del malato è ormai diventata un *Kitsch, una* cosa, una cosa mondanizzata'.

> of my knowledge which was granted to me by an arbitrary society. I use this power to provide time and means to those who are institutionalised to get out from their condition of oppressed, neglected, underserved, to promote their emancipation, to defend them from a society which wants them excluded and institutionalised, to assert the right and the right, to accompany them within the body of a society which has lost them.
>
> **(Rotelli, 2005)**

Second misunderstanding: Basaglia's approach was driven by ideology

Reducing Basaglia's contribution to pure ideology denies that there was any scientific basis to his work. It is probably hard, from a biomedical perspective, to recognize the scientific method which Basaglia relied on to develop his analysis and models of his anti-institutional praxis. His analytical insights and models of intervention are never true forever, but are fragile and dynamic exactly because they are not driven by ideology but arrived at through trial and error. The practice of anti-institutional psychiatry (not anti-psychiatry) is a revolution that is characterized by a deferment of its own fulfilment to avoid the loss of its intrinsic power of liberation. For Basaglia, any theoretical formulation, if not linked to a tireless transformation of reality, was meaningless and amounted to nothing more than simple crystalized institutional engineering.

Basaglia considered his project as 'civitas', the building of a community of citizens in constant and dynamic transformation. If this mission was not kept alive constantly, he argued, the efficiency and the bureaucracy of the organization would work against the needs of the patients and, eventually, reproduce the logic of institutions. In 1971, Basaglia wrote:

> the asylum with its purpose of exclusion and segregation ... the therapeutic community with its liberalization of institutional relationships ... the Community Mental Health Centres ... are institutional answers, maybe innovative but always technically matching with explicit economic demands and they turn out to be effective only once economy needs them.[2]
>
> **(Basaglia, 1971)**

In other words, psychiatry is primarily concerned with serving society at large, rather than patients. It achieves this by containing, managing, and controlling vulnerable

[2] English translation of the following original: 'Il manicomio, con la sua finalità esclusoria e segregatrice ... la Comunità Terapeutica, con relativa liberalizzazione dei rapporti istituzionali ... i Community Mental Health Centers ... si tratta [sempre] di risposte istituzionali di tipo innovatore che corrispondono tecnicamente a delle esplicite domande economiche e che risultano efficaci solo nel momento in cui l'economia le esige.'

populations. It would be a parody to call this a scientific enterprise. Basaglia refused to codify any model. His ultimate aim was to ensure the continuity of transformation processes: 'When new techniques start to be codified into an organic discipline . . . the margin of freedom needed to grant the process of transformation is no longer there'[3] (Basaglia, 1967).

The transient nature of Basaglia's model of change and transformation is in contrast to the logic of dominant order and rationality (what Michel Foucault called 'bourgeois reason', due to its utopian optimism) that is persistent and pervasive. Basaglia follows the logic of the scientific method, grounded on the provisional status of any model rather than the permanent crystallization that characterizes all ideologies. In this sense, psychiatry is more often driven by ideology than science and, therefore, cannot be considered as an entirely scientific enterprise.

By comparison, the research hypothesis and the logic of *L'Istituzione Negata* are coherent, well-grounded, and, most importantly, subject to verification. He wrote that 'psychiatry in love with itself and, as a consequence, with the disease as an abstract entity generated by itself, has continued formulating ideological interpretations without any concern about reality check or refutation'[4] (Basaglia, 1967). In contrast, Basaglia confronted the challenges he faced and sought solutions to them as a scientist, not as an ideologue or politician. He devised 'a research protocol' to transform Gorizia, then Parma, and, eventually, Trieste in 'natural laboratories'—the experiment of an idea or hypothesis, and not driven by ideology.

Third misunderstanding: Basaglia was driven mainly by philanthropic concerns

The third distortion of Basaglia's work is that he was essentially concerned with doing good for the people who were institutionalized. Of course, Basaglia's work had enormous benefits for people 'annihilated by the asylum'. Often, this is seen as the main reason for what he did; that his work and thinking amounted, primarily, to a fight against the scandal of the asylum. However, this was only one aspect of his vision. According to Basaglia, it was not just the psychiatric institution that was in need of change but also the institution of psychiatry. Both required radical transformation.

He approached this through strategies to challenge the monologue of reason about madness. He argued that overcoming the asylum represented the best way to negate the legitimacy of such a monologue. This went beyond any philanthropic objective of simply improving the living conditions of people who were institutionalized in the asylum.

[3] English translation of the following original: 'Nel momento in cui le nuove tecniche incominciano, invece, a strutturarsi in una scienza organica . . . il margine di libertà necessario al processo di trasformazione viene a mancare.'

[4] English translation of the following original: 'la psichiatria . . . innamoratasi di sé stessa e quindi della malattia come di una entità astratta da essa stessa partorita, ha continuato ad elaborare le sue interpretazioni ideologiche senza preoccuparsi di trovare una verifica o una smentita nella realtà.'

Engineering the mechanics and dynamics of institutions to ensure more humane care was not enough. His critique went beyond the asylum.

Forty years ago, Basaglia was affirming that continuing to accept psychiatry and its definition of mental illness actually means accepting the inhuman world where we live. This conviction represented a true 'manifesto' amounting to a political rather than a philanthropic commitment. He developed this theme further in a book, *Crimini di Pace* (*Crimes of Peace*), a collective work including Noam Chomsky, Michel Foucault, Ronald Laing, Robert Castel, and others (Basaglia et al., 1975). Their focus was the role of intellectuals in facilitating, maintaining, and defending oppression in all its forms. The oppressive practices in the asylum—mandated, approved, and facilitated by psychiatry—amounted to a crime. Such a crime needed to be confronted and eradicated, which meant changing psychiatry. Basaglia set out a vision, a praxis, and a radical new ethic for psychiatry which is still valid half a century later and remains an invitation and challenge to contemporary psychiatry to move beyond its current politically correct formulations and actively engage to ensure and restore the rights of its patients.

Our understanding of the complex interactions of genetic, neurobiological, psychological, and social factors which underpin mental health problems has significantly increased since Basaglia's time. However, central issues of the patient's subjectivity and the nature of the relationship between patient and psychiatry remain major impediments to deinstitutionalization. It is still the case that, in psychiatry, the fundamental relationship between the clinician and patient is characterized by the lack of recognition of the patient's subjectivity. This relationship is also framed by the substantial difference in power between the psychiatrist and the patient. The work of psychiatry continues to be dominated by an urgency for classifying rather than understanding the patient experiences. Although, compared to 50 years ago, psychiatry today provides a generally more sympathetically articulated and humane approach, the distance between the patient and the psychiatrist is still marked by the same asymmetry of power. However, the biomedical model, the lingua franca of modern mental healthcare, assumes the experience of illness as its own property: 'medical ideology . . . assumes the illness experience neutralizing and negating it, reducing the patient's experience to the object of its own competence . . . and it forces the patient to live his illness not as his own personal experience but as an accident which science can make objective'[5] (Basaglia et al., 1975).

Implications of the misunderstandings about Basaglia's work

The three distortions of Basaglia's thinking and work that we have identified reflect ignorance of his work and ongoing refusal to engage with it. This is likely to persist

[5] English translation of the following original: la ideologia medica assume per sè l'esperienza della malattia, neutralizzandola e negandola fino a ridurla a puro oggetto di sua competenza . . . inducendo il malato a vivere la malattia come puro accidente oggettivabile dalla scienza e non come esperienza personale.

and prevent a full appreciation of the significance of his legacy, especially amongst English-speaking psychiatrists. Through prevailing condescension by the psychiatric establishment, Basaglia's work and achievements are marginalized. In an article published by the French journal of philosophy *Les Temps Modernes*, one of the authors of this paper (Saraceno, 2012) defined the distortions of Basaglia's work as typical of the British psychiatric establishment. This was meant as a provocation to initiate engagement with Basaglia's work and a wider debate, but this has not happened. Basaglia's work continues to be ignored in the mainstream international psychiatric discourse. There remains a fundamental resistance to the challenging nature of Basaglia's work, borne out of the professional reluctance to move beyond theory and commit oneself to a meaningful transformation of reality.

Like Antonio Gramsci, Basaglia believed that theory is a reflection on reality and understanding of the mechanisms of transforming that reality. Basaglia's long intellectual journey and his anti-institutional vision can be understood as amounting to '*Gramscian* existentialism', a concern for individual human subjectivity to be closely linked to a requirement for collective transformation of the social environment. The crisis of psychiatry is grounded on the loss of subjectivity and, as any other science, reflects what Husserl defined as the crisis of European sciences which, losing the meaning of a real relationship with the human being, have deserted the primary meaning of their own existence. Overcoming the crisis of psychiatry and the violence inherent in the relationship between the patient and psychiatrist is only possible 'by the acceptance of a dialectic way of thinking that contains its own critique and its own overcoming'[6] (Basaglia, 1967). Basaglia combines the need to recover the lost subjectivity of the patient with a requirement to transform the reality that surrounds that subjectivity. In this way, he links the phenomenology of Jaspers, Schneider, Binswanger, and Minkovski,[7] the existentialism of Sartre with political commitment to the transformation of reality that he took from Gramsci. That is, theory is impossible if not linked to a radical change of the reality.

Basaglia's cultural, professional, political, and personal journey is marked by acknowledgement of the indivisibility of theory/transformation. Every possible theoretical model should be, by definition, a practice waiting for a theory, and every theory should be a reflection on reality. According to Basaglia, psychiatry must recognize the 'other', but it should also ensure that this recognition leads to a practice of transformation. Basaglia fully acknowledged that institutional annihilation, the misery caused by 'the care' provided to patients, was the key determinant of a patient's

[6] English translation of the following original: 'risulta soltanto nell'accettazione di un pensiero dialettico che comporti in sé stesso la propria critica e il proprio superamento'.

[7] Karl Jaspers published, in 1913, the fundamental *Allgemeine Psycopathologie* which moves the gaze of psychiatry from the brain and its illness to the internal world of the patient and to his or her personal experience. The anthropological phenomenology of Ludwig Binswanger does not consider psychotic experience as incomprehensible or meaningless but, on the contrary, as a way of 'being in the world', even if quite foreign to the common way of living and feeling. Basaglia, even if recognizing himself as part of the school of phenomenology of Jaspers, Binswanger, Minkowski, and, in Italy, Cargnello and eventually Borgna, goes well beyond the process of existential analysis (*Daseinalyse*).

career. The patient's career took them down a steep descent towards the impoverishment of institutional chronicity. However, 'knowing' this was not enough. The 'gestalt' of the theory/practice which characterizes the patient journey is forgotten or underestimated.

Too often, people use Basaglia's 'words' out of context, isolated from the fundamental and intimate dyad of theory/practice and robbed of their original meaning. This results in his words becoming generic, vague, and vacuous. As an example, let us consider a word which is central in Basaglia's thinking, 'deinstitutionalization'. This word has complex meanings but is often used in current psychiatric discourse as being synonymous with 'dehospitalization'. Thus, a complex and comprehensive concept about change and transformation is rendered an administrative term, akin to using the word 'revolution' to indicate nothing more than the simple action of turning over an omelette.

The tendency to decontextualize and simplify Basaglia's words risks a progressive dilution of his core concepts and actions. Very soon, one forgets the complex reflection and analysis of the ideology of psychiatry and its oppressive practices that Basaglia offered. What is left is a presumption of Basaglia's vision and practice as nothing more than philanthropic indignation about the inhuman condition of people in large asylums and reasonable adjustments to reorganize mental healthcare (e.g. a little bit more community mental health, additional outpatient clinics, fewer beds). The theoretical rationale, his complex vision, and the transformative challenge inherent in his practical work are set aside and replaced by a purely administrative task—a philosophical legacy transformed into mere bureaucracy.

Global mental health and Basaglia

Every year, the World Health Organization (WHO) publishes its most authoritative document, *The World Health Report*. In 2001, the WHO devoted its report to mental health (WHO, 2001). In this important public health document, the WHO recognized the significance of the mental health services in Trieste. This experience has been considered as the best achievement of Basaglia's vision and work and has been sustained for nearly half a century.

In 2002, Cohen and Saraceno wrote: 'Today, Trieste remains one of the best examples of the Italian mental health reforms' that were first initiated by Basaglia and his colleagues in Gorizia. The Ospedale Psichiatrico Provinciale has been closed for 20 years. Community mental health centres offer services to the city and province of Trieste, 24 hours a day, every day of the year. The provisions include general hospital beds for the care of individuals suffering from acute psychiatric crisis. There is a network of social cooperatives providing employment and residential facilities, which allows many people with severe mental illness to live and work in the community. Family support services make it possible for users of psychiatric services to live with their families. Most importantly, deinstitutionalization in Trieste meant more than merely transferring treatment techniques to non-hospital settings. The transformative work in Trieste (as in Gorizia and Parma previously) signified a rejection of the former practices of Italian psychiatry which were rooted in the narrow biological treatment of psychopathology. The WHO's identification of the Trieste experience as a model for public health was a significant endorsement of Basaglia's work.[8] This recognized the global relevance of Basaglia's philosophy and the practice of deinstitutionalization as a model for mental health reform across the world.

In the last decade and a half, following publication of the WHO's *World Health Report*, there has been a renewed focus on downsizing psychiatric hospitals in many countries, including in low- and middle-income settings. At the same time, concerns about the human rights of people treated in psychiatric facilities have been highlighted, resulting in various initiatives to address these problems. We have already argued that the simple reduction of the hegemonic role of the psychiatric hospital does not mean that Basaglia's vision has been realized, as downsizing the hospital and scaling up services simply reflects a process of 'modernization' of psychiatric care. Reduction in the size of institutions and improvement of the living conditions of people in psychiatric facilities are often little more than rationalization and better management of resources (smaller institutions spread across a territory). This hardly signals a change of paradigm.

Basaglia's vison calls for a serious critique of the psychiatric paradigm and a challenge to the hegemonic role of psychiatric institutions. Sadly, the adjustment to mental health services across the world in the last 40 years (downsizing the hospital, scaling up services) has not been accompanied by any serious challenge to traditional psychiatry or its biomedical approaches to mental health. There are exceptions, as shown by the evolution of innovative practices, based on local knowledge and tailored to local conditions, in some settings. In these places, a hospital-based system of care has been transformed into a community-based system with an emphasis on the rights of people with mental health problems, social aspects of care, support for families and carers, housing, and income. These innovative experiences have not all been inspired by Basaglia or his successors. However, they have been driven by the moral imperative and humanistic principles that were at the heart of Basaglia's work. Until then, such issues, the moral indignation about the inhuman treatment of mentally ill people, were often hidden by the mental hospital.

Basaglia and his colleagues were convinced of the many therapeutic opportunities and resources available within the community. It is unfortunate that, despite the overwhelming evidence of the success and durability of revolution in mental healthcare initiated by Basaglia and colleagues over half a century ago, national psychiatric establishments and other professional interest groups, such as the World Psychiatric Association, continue to champion outmoded models of psychiatry. Psychiatry remains heavily compromised by conflicts of interests, including the pharmaceutical industry.

[8] For the service model and service organization in Trieste, see Mezzina (2018).

Basaglia's commitment to restore the rights of people in mental hospitals was linked to a notion of freedom that went beyond legal status. His idea of freedom was, in many ways, strikingly similar to that offered by Amartya Sen (1999), that freedom is the foundation, rather than the result, of human and economic development. In much the same way, Basaglia realized that freedom was a prerequisite for effective care, rather than a condition one strives for through treatment. Giving freedom to the patient meant relinquishing a degree of power, which will compel the practitioner to examine his or her role in the institution. We believe this vision of Basaglia remains unique and relevant today.

Conclusion

The revolution in mental healthcare (Foot, 2015) started in Gorizia in the early 1960s by Basaglia and his colleagues, and subsequently sustained through well-developed community programmes, amounts to the most significant mental health reform in the twentieth century. Arguably, the importance and impact of this are on a par with the more celebrated and widely known revolutions in psychiatric care, such as Phillippe Pinel striking the chains off the mentally ill more than two centuries ago or 'moral treatment' that led to reform and development of the asylum system in Western Europe and North America in the eighteenth and nineteenth centuries. These 'revolutions' changed the concept of 'mad' to 'patients' needing treatment. The contemporary equivalent of this is the transformation of psychiatric patients to citizens, with the emphasis on restoring their rights and ensuring social inclusion. This owes much to Basaglia's work. His legacy, however, remains poorly understood, particularly within Anglo-American psychiatry. We have explored some of the reasons for this here, including misinformation and distortions regarding his work. It is time to challenge and change this.

We believe that Basaglia's work is still relevant, although many of the degradations and depredations that characterized the 'manicomi' of his day are no longer a feature of modern mental healthcare. However, mental health services across the world are still dominated by institutional models of psychiatry with disproportionate emphasis on control and custody of the mentally ill rather than care or cure. The polarization of the rights of patients and their mental health needs is still evident in much of contemporary psychiatry. We believe that the remarkable movement that Basaglia inspired, and the revolution in mental healthcare that came about as a result, remain the best template for resolving these contradictions at the heart of psychiatry.

References

Allen, F. (2015). World's Best and Worst Places to be Mentally Ill. *Psychiatric Times* 30 December 2015. Available at: http://www.psychiatrictimes.com/couch-crisis/worlds-best-and-worst-places-be-mentally-ill/page/0/1

Appadurai, A. (2002). Deep democracy: urban governmentality and the horizon of politics. *Public Culture* 14(1):21–47.

Basaglia, F. (1964). Kitsch ed espressione figurativa psicopatologica. In: *Il Verri. Psicopatologia dell'espressione.* Milano: Feltrinelli Editore, pp. 27–34.

Basaglia, F. (1967). Crisi istituzionale o crisi psichiatrica? Reprinted in: *Scritti I, 1953–1968.* Torino: Einaudi, 1982, pp. 442–54.

Basaglia, F. (1968). *L'Istituzione Negata.* Torino: Einaudi.

Basaglia, F. (1971). Riabilitazione e controllo sociale. Reprinted in: *Scritti II, 1968–1980.* Torino: Einaudi, 1982, pp. 199–208.

Basaglia, F. (1979). *A psiquiatria alternativa: contra o pessimismo da razão, o otimismo da prática: conferências no Brasil.* San Paulo, Brasil: Brasil Debates.

Basaglia, F. and Basaglia Ongaro, F. (1975). Il tecnico del sapere pratico. In: *Crimini di pace.* Torino: Einaudi, pp. 3–111.

Basaglia, F., Ongaro, F., and Giannichedda, M.G. (1975). Il concetto di salute e malattia. Reprinted in: *Scritti II, 1968–1980.* Torino: Einaudi, 1982, pp. 362–81.

Castadelli-Maria, J.M. and Ventriglio, A. (2016). The impact of Basaglia on Brazilian Psychiatry. *International Journal of Social Psychiatry* 62(5):411–14.

Cohen, A. and Saraceno, B. (2002). The risk of freedom. In: A. Cohen, A. Kleinman, and B. Saraceno (eds), *World Mental Health Casebook.* New York: Kluwer Academic/Plenum, pp. 191–220.

Desviat, M. (1994). *La reforma psiquiátrica.* Madrid: Dor.

Foot, J. (2014). Franco Basaglia and the radical psychiatry movement in Italy, 1961–78. *Critical and Radical Social Work* 2(2):235–49.

Foot, J. (2014). *La Repubblica dei matti. Franco Basaglia e la psichiatria radicale in Italia, 1961–1978.* Milano: Feltrinelli Editore.

Foot, J. (2015). *The Man who Closed the Asylums: Franco Basaglia and the Revolution in Mental Health Care.* London: Verso.

Foucault, M. (1972). *Histoire de la Folie à l'âge classique.* Paris: Gallimard.

García, R. (1995). *Historia de una ruptura. El ayer y el hoy de la psiquiatría española.* Barcelona: Virus Editorial.

Giannichedda, M.G. (1988). Crisis and identity: extracts from the theory of Franco Basaglia. In: *Psychiatry in Transition: British and Italian Experiences.* London: Pluto, pp. 252–60.

Jones, K. and Poletti, A. (1984). The mirage of a reform. *New Society* 1137:10–1.

Jones, K. and Poletti, A. (1985a). The Italian transformation of the asylum: a commentary and review. *International Journal of Mental Health* 14:195–212.

Jones, K. and Poletti, A. (1985b). Understanding the Italian experience. *British Journal of Psychiatry* 146(4):341–7.

Jones, K. and Poletti, A. (1986). The Italian experience reconsidered. *British Journal of Psychiatry* 148:144–50.

Jordá, E., et al. (1993). Evaluación del resultado de la desinstitucionalización de pacientes mentales crónicos: un estudio de cohorte. *Revista de la AEN* 45:113–23.

Lovell, A. (1985). From confinement to community: the radical transformation of an Italian mental hospital. In: P. Brown (ed.), *Mental Health Care and Social Policy.* Boston: Routledge & Kegan Paul, pp. 375–86.

Mezzina, R. (2018). Forty years of Law 180: the aspirations of a great law, its success and continuing need. *Epidemiology and Psychiatric Sciences* 27(4):336–45. Available at: https://doi.org/10.1017/S2045796018000070

Ministerio da Saúde Brasil (2005). *Reforma psiquiátrica e política de saúde mental no Brasil.* Brasilia: Ministerio da Saúde.

Mosher, L.R. (1982). Italy's revolutionary mental health law: an assessment. *American Journal of Psychiatry* 139:199–203.

Muusse, C. and van Rooijen, S. (2015). *Freedom First—A Study of the Experiences of Community-Mental Healthcare in Trieste, Italy and Its Significance for the Netherlands*. Utrecht: Trimbos Institute.

Rendueles, G. (1997). De la coordinadora psiquiátrica a la Asociación Española de Neuropsiquiatría. De conspiradores a burócratas. In: V. Aparicio (ed.), *Orígenes y fundamentos de la Psiquiatría en España*. Madrid: ELA, pp. 287–308.

Rotelli, F. (1994) Alternative territorisli e miseria della psichiatria. In: F. Rotelli, *Per la Normalità*. Trieste: Asterios Editore, p. 89.

Rotelli, F. (2005). Foucault, Trieste e Totò. In: R. Rotelli (ed.), *Per la Normalità*. Mantova: Microtest Collana Dentro Fuori, p. 56.

Saraceno, B. (2012). La 'distorsion anglaise': remarques sur la réception de la pensée de Franco Basaglia. *Les Temps Modernes* 668:55–63.

Saraceno, B. (1988). Introduzione. In: R.D. Laing (ed.), *L'io e gli altri. Psicopatologia dei processi interattivi*. Firenze: Sansoni Editore, pp. 7–26.

Scheper-Hughes, N. and Lovell, A.M. (1987). *Psychiatry Inside-Out. Selected Writings of Franco Basaglia*. New York: Columbia University Press.

Sen, A. (1999). *Development as Freedom*. New York: Alfred Knopf.

Sen, A.K. (1992). *Inequality Reexamined*. Oxford: Oxford University Press.

Tansella, M. (1986). Community psychiatry without mental hospitals—the Italian experience: a review. *Journal of the Royal Society of Medicine* 79:664–9.

United Nations (2006). *Convention on the Rights of Persons with Disabilities*. New York: United Nations. Available at: http://www.un.org/disabilities/convention/conventionfull.shtm

Various authors (2011). Reforma Psiquiãtrica no Brasil: ideas, atores e instituições políticas. *Ciência & Saúde Coletiva* 16:12.

Vegetti Finzi, S. (1986). *Storia della psicoanalisi*. Milano: Mondadori.

Weber Gonçalves, R., Sulpino Vieira, F., and Godinho Delgado, P.G. (2012). Mental health policy in Brazil: federal expenditure evolution between 2001 and 2009. *Revista da Saúde Pública* 46(1):51–8.

World Health Organization (2001). *The World Health Report 2001—Mental Health: New Understanding, New Hope*. Geneva: WHO.

6 The impact in Latin America of Basaglia and Italian psychiatric reform

José Miguel Caldas de Almeida

Introduction

The first steps towards reforming mental healthcare in Latin America date back to the 1960s. They consisted mainly of experimental projects in the community, based in most cases on inter-sectoral cooperation, and depending to a large extent on the presence of a leader and on circumstantial political and administrative support (González Uzcátegui, 1992). Despite the lack of resources available and limited political support, some of these projects had an impact on society and helped the dissemination of the new concepts of community mental health that had, by that time, emerged in the USA and Europe.

There is evidence that Franco Basaglia was aware, by the end of the 1960s, of these early mental healthcare reform initiatives in Latin America and was interested in establishing contact with the people behind them. In 1969, after the Gorizia period and before initiating his work in Parma, he 'decided to take a break and spent six months in New York with his family studying a huge psychiatric hospital, before embarking on a study-tour of Latin America' (Foot, 2015). According to Foot, the objective of this tour of Latin America was 'to carry out research into anti-institutional movement there'. Was he just interested in knowing more about what people fighting for mental healthcare reform were doing in that part of the world? Did he have reason to believe that he would find, in Latin America, a fertile ground for the dissemination of the reforms he had started to develop in Gorizia? Or was he expecting to find, in Latin America, answers to the conceptual and strategic questions he had just been confronted with in the last phase of the Gorizia reform? Unfortunately, it is impossible to answer these questions because the book that should describe his visit to Latin America was never published.

What is certain is that his interest in Latin America continued in the following years and he would eventually make several visits to Brazil in 1978–79. During these visits, he gave an impressive number of conferences in Rio de Janeiro, São Paulo, and Belo Horizonte, and had the opportunity to discuss (with hundreds of people interested in mental healthcare reform) the main conceptual and operational implications of this process, to present in a systematic way the reforms carried out in Italy, and to share with the audiences his views on the relationships between the psychiatric reform and other political and social movements.

The Brazilian Conferences (Basaglia, 2000) were a real tour de force. In 10 days, Basaglia gave 14 conferences in three cities, which covered all topics that are relevant to psychiatric reform. Every conference was followed by a long period of discussion with the audience, in which Basaglia, stimulated by the (often very challenging) questions raised by the participants, developed, with evident enthusiasm, his views on multiple issues directly or indirectly associated with psychiatric reform. The reading of the text of the conferences and the discussions with the audiences that followed each of them is one of the best ways to discover the richness of Basaglia's thought and to understand the roots, the context, and the vicissitudes of Italian psychiatric reform. (Unfortunately, as far as I know, these texts have only been published in Portuguese, French, and Italian). These texts also allow us to understand why Basaglia decided to develop such an undertaking and to make such a personal investment in the conferences.

The questions of the participants reveal that Brazil, in 1979, was a country with all the problems, needs, and contradictions that make a profound psychiatric reform almost obligatory. The psychiatric system was mostly based on a huge number of psychiatric hospitals, where thousands of patients lived in terrible conditions and were submitted to all kinds of human rights violations. The military regime was ending. Despite the repression, the capacity of the government to control the aspirations of the different layers of society was rapidly diminishing. A strong dynamic of change was asserting itself in the country, animated by an active worker movement and the pressures of a growing urban youth fighting for social and political change.

In every conference, participants asked Basaglia what should be done to overcome the problems of mental healthcare in Brazil. Responding to this question, Basaglia repeatedly said that he had not come to Brazil 'to bring a European recipe for Brazilian problems' and that he believed that it was the Brazilians who should 'find solutions to their problems'. However, he always left a message of hope and a promise of cooperation. He also repeatedly stressed that the series of conferences aimed at something much broader than just discussing the reform of psychiatric services in Brazil: something that also included the creation of a cement that could unite people who wanted to work differently in different parts of the world. In his opinion, this cement was necessary to create the international unity that was indispensable to emancipate people with mental disorders, and, at the same time, to use these actions to diminish 'the misery of the world'.

As he summarized in one of the conferences:

> When we say no to the asylum, we say no to the misery of the world and we join all of the people in the world fighting for a situation of emancipation. Right now, we are not just a psychodrama society, nor a social psychiatry society. We are united people struggling for a real freedom in the world.
>
> **(Basaglia, 2000)**

Through this statement, we can understand that what motivated Basaglia, in his commitment to psychiatric reform, was not only the moral obligation he felt, as a psychiatrist, to contribute to the improvement of the quality of psychiatric care and to the overcoming of the exclusion and violations experienced by people with mental disorders throughout history; nor was it not only the excitement of action, nor the satisfactions associated with the overcoming of obstacles and the access to fame. What counted to him, above all, was the opportunity this struggle offered him to feel united with others in the fight against 'the misery of the world' and in favour of the emancipation of human beings.

With this statement, Basaglia also said to the participants in the Brazilian Conferences that he firmly believed in the power of international cooperation in all processes of social change; and he left a clear proposal for cooperation in the future. The cancer that killed him, in 1980, prevented Basaglia from participating in the proposed cooperation, but the Trieste team, led by Franco Rotelli, followed up his efforts, developing, throughout the 1980s, a process of cooperation that would eventually play a very important role in the growth of the Brazilian movement for mental healthcare reform—a movement that led to the implementation of one of the most interesting and profound national transformations of a psychiatric system in the world.

This cooperation was not limited to Brazil: it subsequently extended to Argentina and other Latin American countries. Simultaneously, former collaborators of Basaglia and mental health professionals from other regions of Italy also started providing technical support for mental health reforms in Latin America. Benedetto Saraceno, a psychiatrist who had initiated his training in Trieste, and was working for the Institute Mario Negri in Milan, was one of those Italian mental health professionals who became involved in the support provided for such reforms in Latin America. In the 1980s, he started a regular collaboration in Nicaragua and El Salvador that eventually led to the establishment of a partnership with the Mental Health Unit of the Pan American Health Organization (PAHO), coordinated by Itzhak Levav (Saraceno et al., 1990).

This collaboration was the first step in a process that made possible the organization, for the first time in history, of an international initiative aiming at the reform of mental healthcare in one region of the world, with the participation of governments and different stakeholders in the region, as well as international consultants from places with experience in mental healthcare reform, under the coordination of a WHO regional office. This process, formally initiated at a conference held in Caracas in 1990, resulted from the conjunction of several factors: a set of important successful reforms initiated in the 1980s (in countries such as Argentina, Brazil, Chile, Nicaragua, and El Salvador, among others), the technical cooperation offered by professionals and services from European countries with mental healthcare reform experience, and the coordination of PAHO.

The early death of Basaglia deprived him of seeing put into practice, in Latin America, his idea of a large international collaboration between people from different countries committed to a common goal: the replacement of psychiatric hospitals by community-based services capable of respecting the human rights and of promoting the emancipation of people with mental disorders. However, his vision, his ideas, and the innumerable lessons learned from Italian psychiatric reform played a fundamental role in this process. In the course of its development, other influences and contributions would enrich the support offered to Latin American countries interested in reforming their mental health services. However, the influence of Basaglia's conceptualization of mental health reform has remained, until today, an essential component of this process.

In some countries—Brazil is the best example—these concepts were imparted directly by Basaglia and, subsequently, by the Trieste team. Almost 30 years after his visits to Brazil, Basaglia continues to be recognized in this country as the father of psychiatric reform. His name has remained forever associated with the 'luta antimanicomial' (the fight against asylums), and mental healthcare reform in Brazil is undoubtedly the Latin American reform that most faithfully replicates the Trieste model.

In other countries, Basaglia's influence was not directly transmitted by him personally or by his collaborators from Trieste, but through people from other parts of Italy or from other Southern European countries that had also developed mental health reforms and had established, in the 1980s, close connections with several regions of Italy. In fact, for some time, there was even a Permanent Conference for Psychiatric Reform of Southern European Regions, including Trieste, Livorno, Arezzo, Andalusia, Asturias, and Lisbon—regions that would subsequently participate in the Latin American process.

PAHO's Mental Health Unit, as the leader of this entire process, ensured the liaison with governments and with the WHO Department of Mental Health and Substance Abuse, in Geneva, provided technical and administrative support (through its headquarters in Washington DC and the offices that existed in every country in the region) and facilitated support from other PAHO units relevant to mental health reform (e.g. Health Services, Health Promotion, Emergencies, Human Rights, Chronic Diseases).

The Caracas Declaration

In November 1990, a Regional Conference for the Restructuring of Psychiatric Care in Latin America was held in Caracas, Venezuela, with the involvement of governments, mental health related institutions, and international entities and experts. At the end of the Conference, the participants approved a declaration calling for a shift from hospital-based care to community-based care, for the integration of mental health into primary care, and the protection of the human rights of people with mental disorders.

The Caracas Declaration became a landmark in the mental healthcare reform process in the region. According to the Declaration, psychiatric care should be provided by community-based services, with the capacity to guarantee accessible, decentralized, comprehensive, participatory, and continuous care. Additionally, psychiatric hospitals should be progressively closed down. In this process, the integration of mental health into primary healthcare should play a key role, both at treatment and prevention levels. Another fundamental aspect of the Declaration was the importance it attached to the protection of the human and civil rights of people with mental health problems (Levav et al., 1994; Caldas de Almeida and Horvitz-Lennon, 2010).

The influence of Italian psychiatric reform is clearly visible in the high priority attributed to the replacement of the psychiatric hospital with community-based services, and in the central importance of ending the violations of patients' human rights. However, these objectives appear, here, closely associated with something that was not present in the Italian reforms of the 1960s and 1970s: the idea of giving primary care services a key role in the new mental healthcare systems. The central role of primary care in the Caracas Declaration was associated with the huge impact the Declaration of Alma Ata had in Latin America after 1978,[1] and with the increasing notion, supported by studies carried out both in high- and low-income countries, that not only were mental disorders highly prevalent in primary care services, but also that many of these cases could be effectively treated at this level of care.

The Caracas Declaration was the culmination of a process set in motion by several developments: the recognition of the failures of traditional psychiatric hospitals to meet the complex needs of people with mental disorders and of their frequent association to patients' human rights violations; the demonstration that it is possible to replace psychiatric hospitals with community-based specialized services and give people with severe mental disorders access to better care and to full citizenship; and the replacement of several authoritarian regimes by democratic governments whose firm commitment to respecting human rights focused attention on the plight of psychiatric patients (Levav and González Uzcátegui, 2007).

In order to put into practice the principles of the Caracas Declaration, PAHO promoted the Initiative for the Restructuring of Psychiatric Care in Latin America, with the active collaboration of the mental health units of the countries of the region and important contributions from several European institutions that offered technical and financial support (Levav et al., 1994). Through this Initiative, local and international resources were mobilized, research activities were developed, training workshops on community mental health for leaders and professionals were promoted, and technical assistance was provided to many countries for the development of mental health policies, plans, and services.

Formal agreements were established between PAHO and regions from Italy and Spain (including Friuli Venezia, Emilia Romagna, Andalusia, and Asturias), which made possible the organization of visits of professionals from Latin America to

[1] The Declaration that resulted from the International Conference on Primary Health Care, held in Alma Ata in 1978, was the first international declaration stating the importance of primary healthcare and outlining the world governments' roles and responsibilities to the health of the world's citizens. It emerged as a key milestone in the field of global public health and had a profound influence on health policies adopted all over the world, particularly in low- and middle-income countries.

innovative services in Europe, as well as the establishment of schemes of technical assistance to mental healthcare reforms developed in Latin American countries. These latter schemes, through which international experts were charged with ensuring regular support to a mental health reform carried out in a specific place, proved to be particularly effective and, in many cases, they have endured for many years.

As a result, throughout the 1990s, some countries (including Chile, Cuba, El Salvador, Guatemala, and Panama) made important advances, particularly in the integration of mental health into primary care, while others (such as Argentina, Brazil, and Belize) were particularly successful in the development of integrated mental health services in the community. The reforms carried out in the province of Río Negro, in Argentina (Collins, 2008; Cohen and Natella, 2009), and in the city of Santos, in Brazil (Tenório, 2002), deserve a special mention for having created a system of services in the community with a strong component of psychosocial rehabilitation and the active participation of users. Some countries of the region passed mental health legislation and improved the protection of the human rights of people with mental disorders. Among the entities that have collaborated with PAHO in these efforts, a special reference should be made to the Italian mental health services of Trieste and Emilia Romagna, the Mario Negri Institute in Milan, the specialized services of the Spanish autonomous communities of Andalusia, Asturias, and Galicia, as well as of the city of Madrid.

2001 and a new momentum for mental healthcare reform

The year of 2001, with WHO's historic decision to devote several of its major global initiatives to mental health (World Health Day, World Health Report, and key meetings of the World Health Assembly), marked the beginning of a new phase in mental healthcare reform worldwide. The moto of the 2001 World Health Day—'Stop exclusion. Dare to Care'—eloquently expresses the two main and inseparable dimensions of WHO's vision for mental health at the beginning of the new millennium: to eradicate human rights' violations, discrimination, and social exclusion of people with mental disorders; and to improve access to quality mental healthcare. In its turn, the title of the 2001 World Health Report—*Mental Health: New Understanding, New Hope*—indicated that, according to WHO, the best hope for making the new vision of mental health a reality was the creation and dissemination of new knowledge (WHO, 2001a).

The new priorities of WHO, announced in 2001, represented strong support for the principles enshrined in the Caracas Declaration. At the same time, they were an encouragement in the development of further efforts towards its full implementation. In this context, the PAHO Directing Council, which included representatives of all the governments in the Americas, analysed, in September 2001, the situation of mental healthcare in the region, based on the results of the first regional survey conducted as part of the ATLAS project (WHO, 2001b). According to these data, considerable progress had been made in policy, plans, and legislative development: 70% of the countries in the region had, in 2001, a national mental health policy, and 80% had national action plans, more than 70% of which were established after 1990; and the proportion of countries in the region that had specific mental health legislation had increased from 22% in 1990 to 30% in 2001. Psychiatric hospitals, however, continued to be the basic structure of the mental health system in most countries. More than 70% of the countries had less than 20% of psychiatric beds in general hospitals. Although 70% of the countries had community services, in most cases these covered only a small part of the population in need.

All the information available at the time showed that, in the course of the 1990s, the leading principles of the Caracas Declaration had been adopted by many countries of the region, several valuable experiments had taken place, advances had been made, and lessons had been learned about both successes and obstacles. The experience gained, however, showed that it was necessary to pay more attention to several issues. One of these issues was the role of psychiatric units in general hospitals in the context of mental healthcare reforms—a role that had been undervalued in many countries. Another issue was the importance of integrating, within deinstitutionalization programmes, new services and psychosocial programmes that might diminish the risk of creating a new generation of persons affected by psychiatric disorders of long-term course and disability. The participation of service users and their families in the planning and management of mental health services and programmes also emerged as a subject requiring much more support. Finally, it became agreed that it would be necessary (1) to improve collaboration with the social sector; (2) to strengthen the development of particular services and programmes to meet the specific needs of women, children, the elderly, refugees, disaster victims, and indigenous peoples; (3) to develop the capacity to monitor and evaluate services; and (4) to develop epidemiological studies and services research (Caldas de Almeida, 2005).

Recent developments

Since 2001, numerous new activities have been developed to strengthen international cooperation on mental healthcare reform in Latin America. At the macro level, several big conferences have been organized to enlarge partnerships, mobilize resources, and build consensus at the political and technical levels. These have led to the Brasilia Principles on the Development of Mental Health Care in the Americas, approved in 2005 (PAHO/WHO, 2006); the Strategy and Plan of Action on Mental Health, approved by the 49th Directive Council of PAHO in 2009 (PAHO/WHO, 2009); and the Plan of Action on Mental Health 2015–2020, approved in 2014 (PAHO/WHO, 2014).

The strengthening of the national capacity of countries to develop mental health policies, plans, and services continues to be, to this day, the main goal of the collaborative process initiated in Latin America 40 years ago. Strategies and methods, however, have changed, in accordance with the evolution registered in needs, priorities, available information, resources, and tools. The provision of on-site technical advice has had an important impact on the development of policies and services. While in the first phase, this advice was provided mostly by consultants from Europe, after 2001, it started being increasingly delivered by consultants from Latin American countries where successful reforms had taken place. Another important change occurred with the new creation of PAHO sub-regional mental health coordinators for Central America, South America, and the English Caribbean—a measure that significantly improved the coordination of cooperation activities. Finally, thanks to the creation of new mechanisms to finance inter-country collaborative projects, it has become much easier to promote the sharing of experiences and competencies among countries.

In the area of training, new programmes have been created to develop the capacities of the leaders of reforms and services, and to train professionals with the mh-GAP tools. In relation to research, programmes to build capacity for mental health services research in Latin America have been promoted with the support of the US National Institute of Mental Health (NIMH) and several universities, and multi-centre studies have been carried out in the context of an international NIMH initiative.

Over recent years, many other collaborative projects have been carried out in specific areas indirectly related to mental healthcare reform: for instance, epidemiological studies have been developed; information systems improved; guidelines for the treatment of severe mental disorders, depression, and other mental disorders disseminated; promotion and prevention programmes scaled up; and initiatives for the participation of users and the protection of their human rights implemented.

Achievements and barriers

Following the Caracas Declaration, a significant number of Latin American countries approved mental health policies, plans, and legislation inspired by the principles set forth in the Declaration. By 2001, the countries of the region that had, during the previous 10 years, formulated and approved a national mental health policy, developed a national mental health plan, and passed mental health legislation were, respectively, 40%, 47.7%, and 20% of all countries (WHO, 2001b). Further progress took place in the following decade: between the years 2001 and 2011, the proportion of countries that had approved a national mental health policy increased to 66.7%, the proportion of countries that had developed a national plan for implementation increased to 72.2%, and the percentage of countries that had promulgated mental health legislation increased to 35.3% (Minoletti et al., 2012). These advances in policy and legislation development represented a great achievement but, overall, what was the impact of these efforts on the reform of mental healthcare?

The first conclusion we can draw from the available data is that the level of implementation of the new policies, plans, and legislation varied significantly in the region; and consequently, there were marked differences in the degree of restructuring of mental health services in Latin American countries. Some countries developed national mental health processes that resulted in profound changes to the psychiatric hospital-based model that existed at the beginning of the 1990s. On the opposite extreme, a small number of countries made little progress in the reform of their mental health services. The large majority of the countries, which were somewhere between these two extremes, made important advances in the implementation of reforms, but this implementation was only partially successful, either because key components of the reform were not taken into consideration or because the reforms were only implemented in a part of the country.

The Latin American countries that truly reformed their mental health services at the national level, in accordance with the Caracas principles, were Brazil, Chile, and Panama. Belize should also be included in this group because, although it is an English-speaking country, it is located in Central America and implemented national reform that was greatly influenced by the Caracas Declaration. The magnitude of the changes registered in the countries that implemented national reforms, compared with the average changes made by the other countries in Latin America, show, in a very impressive way, the impact the national reforms had on the restructuring of services.

While psychiatric hospital beds were completely abolished in Belize, and the number of these beds in Brazil, Chile, and Panama was reduced (for the three countries combined) by 62.2% in the first decade of the new millenium, the average reduction in the number of mental hospital beds in the other countries of the region in the same period was only 23.9% (Minoletti et al., 2012). In turn, the four countries replaced the psychiatric hospitals with beds in general hospitals, community mental teams and centres, and group homes. The number of psychiatric beds in general hospitals, outpatient facilities, and day facilities (day centres and day hospitals) is now two to seven times higher in Brazil, Chile, and Panama than in other Latin American countries. To achieve this change, these three countries have increased, significantly, the percentage of public mental health expenditure allocated to general hospitals, outpatient facilities, and community services—by 67.7% in Brazil, 88.0% in Chile, and 56.0% in Panama (Minoletti et al., 2012). In these countries, users and family organizations were also encouraged to participate in the elaboration of policies, plans, and legislation.

Reform in Brazil

We will describe and analyse psychiatric reform in Brazil in some detail because it was undoubtedly the Latin American reform that was most deeply influenced by Basaglia's thought. From the outset, fighting the exclusion of people with mental disorders and closing down psychiatric asylums were the main goals to be attained. In order to replace the psychiatric hospitals with a network of community-based services, the chosen strategy was to develop a network of centres for psychosocial care (CAPS), which basically replicated the Trieste model of mental health centres (Ministry of Health of Brazil and Pan American Health Organization/WHO, 2007).

Beginning in the 1980s, the reform was part of the redemocratization process that also started at that time in the country. To address the generalized violation of the human rights of patients in psychiatric hospitals, the reform initially focused on the improvement of the living conditions in these institutions and on deinstitutionalization. Based on a strong mobilization of both professionals and large sectors of Brazilian society, the reform was focused not only on ensuring the access of persons with mental problems to national care networks, but also on the development of a new cultural sensibility about the mentally ill, and the production of new scientific and cultural knowledge that might contribute to care innovation.

The implementation of the reform has been closely associated with the social and cultural changes that have occurred in Brazil since the 1980s. It has also been associated with the creation of the Brazilian Unified Health System (SUS) and the development of the complex process that led to the decentralization of health administration in the country. Another important characteristic of the Brazilian reform has been the participation of all sectors of society in this process: national mental health conferences with thousands of participants, including professionals, users, and families, had a key role in the development of mental health policy; social and cultural activists were often important allies; and users' participation was significantly encouraged.

As an evaluation conducted by Fiocruz and the Gulbenkian Foundation has shown (2015), since 2001 Brazil has made solid advances in the deinstitutionalization process, with a drastic reduction in the number of beds in psychiatric hospitals: from 53,962 in 2001 to 25,988 in 2014. This process, however, was the result of changes that had begun in the previous decade, when audits carried out by the authorities led to the closing of innumerable psychiatric hospitals that did not comply with the minimum requirements established, or which had been the objects of complaints of human rights' violations. This movement resulted in the approval of the law of psychiatric reform in 2001, which together with the political support gained at the Third National Mental Health Conference, which was held the same year, made it possible to embark on bed reduction and on other actions specifically aimed at long-stay patients, such as the setting up of residential services.

It should be noted that deinstitutionalization was a planned and progressive process: between 2002 and 2011, macro hospitals with more than 400 beds, that had accounted for 30% of the entire bed total, suffered a gradual reduction to 10.5% of the total; in contrast, the smaller hospitals of up to 160 beds, that had accounted for only 22% of the bed total in 2002, gradually increased their share, so that by 2011 they had reached 52% of the bed total.

Simultaneously, community-based services were created to replace the hospital-based services. The CAPS constituted the core of these services. They were designed to respond to the main care needs of patients who suffer from grave and persistent mental disorders. From 2002 onwards, CAPS-I, set up to serve children and adolescents, were launched and incorporated into the SUS health network, and CAPS-AD were set up to provide care for patients with problems related to alcohol and substance abuse. In 2006, there were 673 CAPS for adults and 66 special CAPS for children and adolescents. In 2014, there were 2,209 CAPS.

Therapeutic residential services, which can house up to eight patients, also became an important resource for the deinstitutionalization of long-stay patients. In 2004, there were 265 residential services with 1,363 residents. In 2014, there were 697 services with 4,180 patients.

An interesting and innovative strategy for deinstitutionalization was the 'Returning Home' programme, created through a national law approved by Congress in 2003. Within this programme, financial support could be provided to deinstitutionalized patients who had been interned uninterruptedly for a minimum of one year. In addition to this support, these patients were also entitled to benefit from a case management programme provided by the CAPS of their residential area. In 2003, 206 patients had been included in the programme. By 2014, the number had increased to 4,349 patients.

In the course of this process, the budget for psychiatric hospital care was reduced from 95% of the total to less than 30%, thus enabling the financing of the substitute network to be 15 times bigger than before (Fiocruz and Gulbenkian Foundation, 2015).

Can we say that the Brazilian reform process has been a complete success? According to the conclusions of the Fiocruz and Gulbenkian Foundation evaluation (2015), the reduction of the number of beds and the transition from a markedly hospital-centric scenario to a balanced model, combining inpatient resources and community services, were carried out in a proper and effective manner. It was also found that there was significant incorporation of financial and human resources. Nevertheless, it was recognized that important gaps still exist in aspects of financing and human resources. There was a large consensus on the considerable advances made in the area of legislation and norms. In addition, the CAPS and other responses, such as the 'Returning Home' project, were generally considered to have been innovative responses to the challenges found in the development of community services. Finally, the existence of a strong network of primary care health services was considered a solid basis for expanding care capacity and overcoming the huge care gaps that still exist.

Several important barriers to the advancement and consolidation of the reform were also identified through the different sources of information and analysis. Financing, although directed correctly to the community services, was considered still insufficient. Human resources development was considered one of the most important problems. Training of health professionals was considered insufficient and inadequate. Participants also cited significant precarious states in services in the community, especially in regard to physical conditions of services, supplies, and working conditions. Fragilities were also pointed out in relation to the quality of information produced by the services, the integration of mental health into primary care, and the sustainability of users' associations. Finally, the risks of neo-institutionalization were acknowledged, especially in services related to alcohol and substance abuse, the elderly, and vulnerable children and adolescents.

Reform in Chile

Chile's national mental health reform was also closely associated with the re-democratization of the country. It was based on the same principles adopted in Brazil, but the Italian reform didn't have a direct influence on it. In its roots we can find influences from the rich public health traditions of the country, the primary care movement, the Caracas Declaration, and the reform in Andalucía, Spain. Strategically, it presents several important particular traits: the process of deinstitutionalization has been less radical than in Brazil, while the creation of inpatient units in general hospitals and the integration of mental health into primary care have had a more important role.

Chile has had three national mental health plans until now (Ministerio de Salud de Chile and Pan American Health Organization/WHO, 2006; Farmer, 2008; Araya et al., 2009; Minoletti et al., 2012). The first, in 1993, introduced innovative practices in the community and the integration of mental health into primary care. The second, in 1999, established a more elaborate model, according to which mental healthcare (including mental health promotion, and the prevention and treatment of mental disorders) is provided within each geographical sector by a network of integrated services and facilities. At the centre of the network there is a primary care centre and a community mental health centre, which communicate with each other through defined strategies, and which coordinate the other facilities in the network. The model developed in Chile is based on the following principles:

- sectorization;
- coordination and continuity of care;
- primary care is the main provider of mental health services;
- the community mental health centre provides essential care to people with severe mental disorders and maintains a collaborative relationship with primary care;
- inter-sectoral collaboration;
- participation of users in the planning and evaluation of the care network.

The third plan, launched in 2017, has, as its main objectives, to support the optimal development of the mental health services network, making it more accessible, equitable, and responsive to the mental health needs of the population, using both a human rights and a recovery-based approach.

The implementation of the plans, coordinated by high-quality teams in the Ministry of Health, successfully led by Alfredo Penjeam, Alberto Minoletti, and Rafael Sepulveda, led to profound changes in the mental health system. Between 1999 and 2006, the fraction of the health budget allocated to mental health almostdoubled, from 1.2% to 2.1%. In the same period, the percentage of the mental health budget allocated to psychiatric hospitals decreased from 57% to 33% (Ministerio de Salud Chile, 2006). By 2004, Chile's public mental health network already included an impressive array of services: 472 primary care centres with mental health professionals, 38 community mental health centres, 58 outpatient clinics, 40 day hospitals, 18 psychiatric units in general hospitals, 25 day centres in the community, and 96 group homes for people with severe mental illness (Ministerio de Salud Chile, 2006). Further advances have been made since then, which have ensured continued improvement of people's access to good-quality mental healthcare and made possible a progressive refinement of the model previously established. In some areas, however, important goals have not yet been attained. The approval of a new mental health law is one of those goals, despite the many efforts made in that direction for many years now.

Reform in Belize

The Belize reform, also initiated in the 1990s, was extremely successful. It enabled a poor country, in less than 20 years, to close down a terrible psychiatric asylum, which was the only psychiatric service the country had at the beginning of the process, and replace it with an integrated mental health network based on the community and the general hospital. The network included an inpatient unit in the general hospital, day hospitals, residential facilities, an integrated assertive community service for severe mental patients, and community teams formed by nurses specifically trained to provide essential mental healthcare throughout the country, under the supervision of a psychiatrist. These achievements resulted from a virtuous conjunction of factors: political support, the excellent and creative leadership ensured by Dr Claudina Cayetano (for some years the only psychiatrist in the country), the involvement of users and families, the capacity to develop a good mental health plan, and very good use of international cooperation provided by WHO, PAHO, and several donors (Ministry of Health of Belize and Pan American Health Organization/WHO, 2009).

Reform in Panama

Panama was the last of the four countries to initiate its reform: the plan was launched in 2003. It has, therefore, benefitted from the other countries' reform experiences. It has also benefitted from the sub-regional cooperation initiated by PAHO in Central America at that time. The reform has been particularly successful in two areas: the integration of mental health into primary care, and the reallocation of resources from psychiatric hospitals to community care (Ministry of Health of Panama and Pan American Health Organization/WHO, 2006; Minoletti at al., 2012).

Reform in other countries

Integration of mental health into primary care, with a strong focus on health promotion and prevention, has been a major component of mental health reform processes in many countries of the region (Argentina, Costa Rica, El Salvador, Guatemala, Nicaragua, Panama, among others). Cuba deserves a special mention in this regard, as it was the first to integrate mental healthcare into primary care as the foundation of its new mental health system, and to implement this strategy at the national level. The existence of a primary care network covering the entire population greatly facilitated integration. However, a more critical factor in this successful integration was the existence of a detailed mental health plan that made it possible to develop new mental health facilities in the community, create specific mental health programmes, and train mental health professionals (Aparicio Basauri, 2008; Ministerio de Salud Publica de Cuba and Pan American Health Organization/WHO, 2011). This highly decentralized community-care system coexists with more than 20 psychiatric hospitals with 56.7 beds per 100,000 population (Minoletti et al., 2012).

In several countries in the region, mental healthcare delivery was reformed not at the national level, but at the state or provincial level. For instance, in Argentina, the reform undertaken by the Rio Negro province replaced the psychiatric hospital with psychiatric beds in general hospitals and a network of community-based services, including mental health centres and psychosocial rehabilitation programmes distributed throughout the territory (Collins, 2008). New community-based services were also established in the provinces of Buenos Aires and Neuquén (Minoletti et al., 2102).

Future reforms

The launching of new national reforms during the last few years indicates that the process of change in Latin American psychiatric services is ongoing. One of the most interesting and promising reforms is the one recently initiated in Peru, where the implementation of a national mental health plan has already led to the creation of several community mental health centres. The reform has clear and strong leadership (something that was not possible in Peru in the past), enjoys technical support from other more advanced countries of the region (particularly Chile), and is financially supported by a Spanish NGO.

New developments of this sort are greatly needed in Latin America. Despite all the advances made in the last three decades, briefly summarized in this chapter, much more has to be done in the future. Available evidence shows that, for the majority of the population, the goals established in the Caracas Declaration are still far from having been met (WHO, 2014).

In order to fully attain these goals, it is essential to take into consideration the lessons learned in the course of previous reforms in Latin America. Most reforms confirmed that low political priority, inadequacy of funding, and resistance from traditional sectors of professionals are major barriers to their implementation. Again and again, mental healthcare reforms in Latin America showed us that these reforms are complex processes, requiring not only resources and political support, but also strong leadership with robust technical capacity. Without these ingredients, it is difficult to ensure the changes that are needed and to overcome the resistances commonly found in this process. Finally, the Initiative for the Restructuring of Psychiatric Care in Latin America proved that international cooperation is a major facilitating factor in the implementation of mental healthcare reforms in low- and middle-income countries (Caldas de Almeida, 2013).

Last remarks

Latin America is one of the regions of the world where Franco Basaglia's vision of psychiatric reform found a more fertile ground and exerted a more fruitful and lasting influence. The ideas he presented in the Brazilian conferences rapidly spread across Latin America through his writings, technical cooperation activities carried out by his collaborators, and the reforms that started to be implemented in many countries of the region in the 1980s.

In the beginning, these ideas were very controversial, and even today they still face strong resistance. However, some of them—particularly, the recognition that mental patients are people with the same rights and duties as every other citizen, that psychiatric asylums must be replaced with a network of community-based services, and that public mental health services are a key component of mental health systems—were incorporated into the basic principles of the Caracas Declaration, which has remained, until today, the main reference of the mental healthcare reforms in Latin America.

Over time, some limitations of Basaglia's conceptualization of psychiatric reform have become evident. One is the lack of inclusion of common mental disorders and primary healthcare in the mental healthcare reform. Another one is the limited importance attributed to the evaluation of services. Both were inevitable: the main focuses of Basaglia's attention were the problems of people with severe mental disorders and the creation of alternatives to asylums, all the rest were of secondary importance. On the other hand, Alma Ata took place two years before Basaglia's death, and the development of psychiatric epidemiology occurred mostly after the 1970s. Considering that Basaglia continually reformulated his views on psychiatric reform in accordance with the lessons he drew from experience, it is legitimate to think that most probably he would have revised his initial vision with respect to these and other limitations, had he lived longer.

We have also to recognize that some of Basaglia's ideological formulations, clearly associated with the European intellectual context of the 1960s and 1970s, now seem overly dated. It is possible that this may have contributed to some ideological excesses of some of his followers in Latin America, in the initial phase of reforms. However, with time, most reforms in Latin America have progressively incorporated other contributions, such as the ones coming from psychiatric epidemiology, services research, and primary healthcare, and have adopted a solid public mental health perspective. Nowadays, problems of lack of openness to dialogue, when they exist, are due more to the resistance to change and intolerance of traditional sectors of psychiatry than from excesses from sectors related to mental healthcare reform.

At the same time, the core of Basaglia's conceptualization has been largely validated by scientific and clinical evidence. His ideas about the associations between mental disorders and socioeconomic factors have been confirmed by studies on social determinants. The advantages of community-based services have been supported by scientific evidence and clinical reasons. The rights of mental patients, and the linking of deinstitutionalization with other movements in favour of the emancipation of vulnerable people, have been incorporated in the key international human rights conventions and treaties. The crucial importance of taking into consideration the subjectivity of people with mental disorders was fully incorporated in the recovery approach.

Overall, the practical implementation of the new mental health policy and plans, together with the influences received from other sources, led to continuing enrichment of the conceptual basis of the Latin American mental healthcare reform approach, already evident in the Caracas Declaration. This approach, indelibly marked by Basaglia's contributions, made possible the unique process of change that has been ongoing in the region of Latin America in the last decades. It has also been an important conceptual inspiration to the mental health policy initiatives promoted by WHO in 2001, under the leadership of Benedetto Saraceno, and, in my opinion, it continues to be one of the most stimulating and comprehensive approaches in global mental health at the present time.

References

Aparicio Basauri, V. (2008). Cuba: mental health care and community participation. In: J.M. Caldas de Almeida and A. Cohen (eds), *Innovative Mental Health Programs in Latin America and the Caribbean*. Washington, DC: Pan American Health Organization, pp. 62–78.

Araya, R., Alvarado, R., and Minoletti, A. (2009). Chile: an ongoing mental health revolution. *The Lancet* 374:597–8.

Basaglia, F. (2000). *Conferenze Brasiliane*. Milan: Raffaello Cortina.

Caldas de Almeida, J.M. (2005). Estrategias de cooperación técnica de la Organización Panamericana de la Salud en la nueva fase de la reforma de los servicios de salud mental en América Latina y el Caribe. *Revista Panamericana de Salud Publica* 18:314–26. [In Spanish]

Caldas de Almeida, J.M. (2013). Mental health services development in Latin America and the Caribbean: achievements, barriers and facilitating factors. *International Health* 5:15–18.

Caldas de Almeida, J.M. and Horvitz-Lennon, M. (2010). An overview of mental health care reforms in Latin America and the Caribbean. *Psychiatric Services* 61:218–21.

Cohen, H. and Natella, G. (2009). Argentina: el programa de salud mental en la provincia de Río Negro. In: J. Rodríguez (ed.), *Salud Mental en la Comunidad*. Washington, DC: Pan American Health Organization. [In Spanish], pp. 357–68

Collins, P. (2008). Argentina: waving the mental health revolution banner: psychiatric reform and community mental health in the province of Rio Negro. In: J.M. Caldas de Almeida and A. Cohen (eds), *Innovative Mental Health Programs in Latin America and the Caribbean*. Washington, DC: Pan American Health Organization, pp. 1–32.

Farmer, C. (2008). Chile: reforms in national mental health policy. In: J.M. Caldas de Almeida and A. Cohen (eds), *Innovative Mental Health Programs in Latin America and the Caribbean*. Washington, DC: Pan American Health Organization, pp. 44–61.

Fiocruz and the Calouste Gulbenkian Foundation (2015). *International seminar on mental health. Innovations in deinstitutionalization and community care in Brazil.* Rio de Janeiro: Fiocruz and Calouste Gulbenkian Foundation.

Foot, J. (2015). *The Man Who Closed the Asylums. Franco Basaglia and the Revolution in Mental Health Care.* London: Verso Books.

González Uzcátegui, R. (1992). Salud mental en la comunidad en América Latina. Ejemplo de programas. In: I. Levav (ed.), *Temas de Salud Mental en la Comunidad*. Washington, DC: Pan American Health Organization, pp. 291–312. [In Spanish]

Levav, I. and González Uzcátegui, R. (2007). The roots of the Caracas Declaration. In: J. Rodriguez (ed.), *Mental Health Care Reform: 15 Years After Caracas.* Washington, DC: Pan American Health Organization. [In Spanish], pp. 44–9.

Levav, I., Restrepo, H., and Guerra de Macedo, C. (1994). The restructuring of psychiatric care in Latin America. A new policy for mental health services. *Journal of Public Health Policy* 15(1):71–85.

Ministerio de Salud de Chile and Pan American Health Organization/WHO (2006). *Informe WHO-AIMS sobre sistema de salud mental en Chile.* Santiago: Ministerio de Salud de Chile. [In Spanish]

Ministerio de Salud Publica de Cuba and Pan American Health Organization/WHO (2011). *Informe WHO-AIMS sobre sistema de salud mental en la República de Cuba.* Washington, DC: Pan American Health Organization. [In Spanish]

Ministry of Health of Belize and Pan American Health Organization/WHO (2009). *WHO-AIMS Report on mental health system in Belize.* Washington, DC: Pan American Health Organization.

Ministry of Health of Brazil and Pan American Health Organization/WHO (2007). *WHO-AIMS Report on mental health system in Brazil.* Brasilia: Pan American Health Organization and Ministry of Health of Brazil.

Ministry of Health of Panama and Pan American Health Organization/WHO (2006). *WHO-AIMS Report on mental health system in Panama.* Panama City: Ministry of Health of Panama and Pan American Health Organization.

Minoletti, A., Galea, S., and Susser, E. (2012). Community mental health services in Latin America for people with severe mental disorders. *Public Health Reviews* 34(2):pii. Available at: http://www.publichealthreviews.eu/show/a/116

Pan American Health Organization/World Health Organization (2001). *43rd Directing Council Final Report.* Washington, DC: Pan American Health Organization.

Pan American Health Organization/World Health Organization (2006). *The Brasilia Principles: Guiding Principles on the Development of Mental Health Care in the Americas.* Washington, DC: Pan American Health Organization.

Pan American Health Organization/World Health Organization (2009*). Resolution CD49.R17 of the PAHO 49th Directive Council.* Washington, DC: Pan American Health Organization.

Pan American Health Organization/World Health Organization (2014). *Resolution CD53/8 of the PAHO 53rd Directive Council.* Washington, DC: Pan American Health Organization.

Saraceno, B., Aguilar Briceno, R., Asioli, F., Liberati, A., and Tognoni, G. (1990). Cooperation in mental health: an Italian project in Nicaragua. *Social Science Medicine* 31:1067–71.

Tenório, F. (2002). A reforma psiquiátrica brasileira, da década de 1980 aos dias atuais: história e conceito. *História, Ciências, Saúde—Manguinhos, Rio de Janeiro* 9(1):25–59. [In Portuguese]. Available at: http://www.scielo.br/scielo.php?script=sci_arttext&pid=S0104-59702002000100003&lng=en&nrm=isso.

World Health Organization (2001a). *World Health Report 2001: Mental Health—New Understanding, New Hope*. Geneva: World Health Organization.

World Health Organization (2001b). *Mental Health Atlas 2001*. Geneva: WHO Department of Mental Health and Substance Abuse.

World Health Organization (2014). *Mental Health Atlas 2014*. Geneva: Department of Mental Health and Substance Abuse.

7

The optimism of practice

The impact of Basaglia's thoughts on Brazil

Ernesto Venturini, Maria Stella Brandão Goulart, and Paulo Amarante

Introduction

The title of this chapter refers to a book published in Brazil that records Franco Basaglia's public meetings during his visits to the country in 1979—*Alternative Psychiatry: Against the Pessimism of Reason, the Optimism of Practice* (Basaglia, 1979). The book was published posthumously, without an Italian review: Basaglia died nine months after his last visit to Belo Horizonte. It appeared as a sort of spiritual testament. It was followed, five years later, by an Italian edition, *Le Conferenze Brasiliane* (Basaglia, 1984), but only for the third Italian edition (2000) did Basaglia's wife, Franca Ongaro, validate the full content. This edition was followed by numerous translations, with different titles: *The Choice of the Psychiatrist. Balance of a Life's Work*, in German; *Alternative Psychiatry*, in Greek; *Psychiatry and Democracy*, in French; *The Condemnation of Being Crazy and Poor. Alternatives to the Madhouse*, in Spanish; and *Basaglia Conferences—Freedom Is Therapeutic*, in Japanese (Giannichedda, 2018, p. X).

The Brazilian edition of the book was not well received in Italy, in part because of the poor translation, but especially owing to the title of the book, which would be changed. In Italy, of course, Basaglia was not regarded as an 'alternative' to psychiatry. In addition, the correct translation should be a reference to Antonio Gramsci's 'optimism of the will and not of practice'.[1] Would this ambiguity in the book's title foreshadow a dialectical synthesis of what Basaglia represents for the Brazilians? In this shift of meanings, it is possible, perhaps, to build the necessary distance for understanding the impact of the interventions Basaglia made in Brazil.

As an introduction to this chapter, we must reflect on the 'alternative' aspect, as an epistemological break, according to the thoughts of French philosopher Gaston Bachelard, and on the emphasis on action, as an essential dimension of the 'Basaglian'

[1] Gramsci states: 'We need to create people who are sober, patient, who do not despair before the worst horrors and who are not exalted by all nonsense. Pessimism of the intelligence, optimism of the will' (Q 28.11, 2.331–2 [CC, 2.265]). The quotations are taken from: Liguori, G. and Voza, P. (orgs) (2017). *Dicionário Gramsciano*. São Paulo: Boitempo Editorial.

praxis.[2] Alternative discourses crossed the Atlantic and still pulsate with great intensity in Brazil.

What is the critical power of Basaglia that leads us to reflect on its dissemination and importance nowadays? What does it mean to speak of an 'impact', and is such meaning a positive or negative one? And when we refer to Brazil, do we refer to the scientific, cultural, social, or political world? How can we evaluate the results of actions implemented on behalf of Basaglia, but made by various other persons and in other circumstances? Through the challenges of these questions, we have reviewed publications, writings, and records of professional practice, and we will try to discuss the impact—the influence and the strength of a thought and a practice—generically referred to as a collective subject: Franco Basaglia.

It is known that the written work of this memorable psychiatrist is an expression of extended thought and dialogues, especially the anti-institutional perspective documented in the book *L'Istituzione Negata* (1968). This compilation gives voice to those who supported the experience of Gorizia.[3] This is a milestone. Numerous collaborators took part in his writings, amongst whom his partner, Franca Basaglia Ongaro, stands out. This self-taught sociologist, translator of children's literature, chronicler, feminist, co-author of the great majority of texts published under the Basaglia name, played a vital role. After Franco's death, as a Senator for two terms, she built the normative ways of Italian deinstitutionalization. She was one of many non-psychiatrists, 'Basaglians', who undoubtedly carried out the utopia of liberation (Goulart, 2012). Is this 'alternative'?

This collective dimension prevails in Brazil, where Basaglia expressed himself and acted in a very specific way. In the first Italian edition of *Brazilian Conferences*, published in 1984, the authors of the introduction justified its relevance by highlighting that Basaglia refused to play the part of a lecturer who comes from abroad to tell stories and give technical advice. 'On the contrary, he opens up a dialogue, seeking, as he always did, to raise awareness through the explanation of contradictions. Franco Basaglia is, after all, once again, the "detonator of a situation" ' (De Salvia and Rolfe, 1984, p. 6). In fact, the term 'conference' fails to convey the intense scene of discussion and empathy that marked the initial 'impact' of Basaglia's encounter with Brazilian mental health workers, activists, public managers, students, and others. It was a relationship established with a particularly participatory audience. At the end of intense debates, Basaglia pronounced a few words, expressing his desire not to appear the solitary hero: 'I am like a medieval minstrel, who crosses the villages and moves on. When I leave, the stage cannot remain empty' (De Salvia and Rolfe, 1984, p. 6). The

[2] Gramsci considers the philosophy of praxis (philosophy of the act) as the original and independent marrow of historical materialism. Praxis is understood as history, a process that occurs with the interference of the human race in the environmental conditions to achieve their purposes and needs.

[3] Nino Vascon, Lucio Schittar, Antonio Slavich, Agostino Pirella, Letizia Jervis Comba, Domenico Casagrande, Giovanni Jervis, Franca Ongaro Basaglia, and Gian Antonio Gilli are co-authors of this book.

activist character of a political subject takes shape, in search of a 'universal dialectic of liberation' (De Salvia and Rolfe, 1984, p. 5).

The polemical and critical dialogue is the trademark of the book that would become known in Italy as *Conferenze Brasiliane*, not *Alternative Psychiatry*. This has been recently reprinted and expanded (2018), although omitting the previous edition's chapter on Brazilian reality (Nicácio et al., 2000). The introduction by Maria Grazia Giannichedda in fact reveals a dynamic of visits and interventions that occurred concurrently with the debates in two consecutive years, and especially 1979, when he stayed in Brazil for almost a month, in close contact with local social movements. In the Brazilian edition, the book ends with a petition (Basaglia, 1979, p. 148) addressed to the governor of the State of Minas Gerais, proposed by Basaglia: a political act. Basaglia's speech is colloquial, affective, intense, loaded with ethical intentions, and very far from the canons of academia and the editorial parameters of psychiatry of his time. It is this ability to communicate, to listen, and to make him understood that was the hallmark of his fully mature phenomenological and existential perspective; the ability to express complexity and to articulate theory and practice.

Reflecting on these meetings, we have to ask whether the term 'alternative' would be more appropriate? Is Franco Basaglia an anti-psychiatrist? Utopian? An ideologist? Philosopher? Reformist psychiatrist? A skilled articulator? Revolutionary? A radical? Democrat? The specialized literature continuously suggests adjectives that could capture his greatness and undeniable relevance (for example, Basaglia, 1982; Amarante, 1996; Schittar, 1999; Colucci and Di Vittorio, 2001; Goulart, 2007; Foot, 2014).

The great journey: from the pessimism of reason to the optimism of practice

To answer the aforementioned questions, we should go back to the years when Basaglia visited Brazil. His trip occurred at a very important and specific moment in the history of this country. In 1978, there were struggles for redemocratization after 14 years of autocratic rule, and consequently, several new actors emerged. These were social movements that advocated not only the struggle against the 'wild capitalism' implemented in Brazil but also causes related to the totalitarian institutions, to gender and ethnic oppression, and to violence, amongst other things.

Before his professional visit to Brazil, local knowledge about Franco Basaglia and his work was not extensive, but the experience of Gorizia was already being discussed by Giovanni Berlinguer, in his book *Psichiatria e Potere* (1969), and also in snippets of information about the Movement of Democratic Psychiatry. It was, however, a period of rigorous political control under a full dictatorial regime. The left-wing tabloid

Opinião of 30 January 1976 published an article entitled 'Basaglia, the Italian Laing', which noted that

> Considered by many to be even more revolutionary than the Englishmen Cooper and Laing, and yet embarrassed, as he himself acknowledges, accepting *de facto* this situation, Basaglia has not achieved wide dissemination except in circles of specialists. His criticism of the establishment not only in terms of psychiatry, but also social and political, has made him an object of exclusion and little publicity.
>
> **(Araújo, 1976)**

One of the issues addressed by Basaglia in Brazil was the oppression in psychiatric institutions. These came to have great social visibility in 1978, with the emergence of the Mental Health Workers' Movement (MTSM), which exposed and spread knowledge of the extremely violent situations in public psychiatric hospitals. In April that year, a significant group of professionals, working in these places, addressed complaint documents to those responsible for the institutions. The protests resulted in an eight-month staff strike. The complaint, concerning the violence and degradation of the psychiatric institutions, reached the national newspapers and exploded into public opinion. In response, the Ministry of Health fired the 263 people who had signed it. From then on, the MTSM became a very important collective player in the psychiatric reform process.

Franco Basaglia arrived in Rio de Janeiro for the First International Symposium on Psychoanalysis Groups and Institutions, organized by the Brazilian Institute of Group and Institutional Psychology and Psychoanalysis (IBRAPSI), and taking place from 19 to 22 October 1978. Among the international guests at the Symposium were Thomas S. Szasz, Erving Goffman, Robert Castel, Felix Guattari, Gilles Deleuze, and Shere Hite. However, only Basaglia chose to meet the MTSM, which was preparing its first actions.

For the MTSM members, this was, of course, an historic opportunity to meet Franco Basaglia at such a special time—a few months after Law 180 (which would become known as *Lei Basaglia*, in reference to his contribution) had been passed. It was a very critical moment, facing the impasses and expectations that the new law brought for the Italian psychiatric reform process (Venturini, 1979). However, the practical results, as presented to the Brazilian public, were not triumphalistic. Basaglia refused to stand as a model; instead, he urged critical involvement in the construction of truly democratic institutions. In this respect, he found an enthusiastic and empathic response from Brazilians.

One of the aspects that most affected the MTSM participants was the discussion fostered by Basaglia on the risk of social control operated by psychiatry. This was a subject already discussed in Gorizia, where it could be noticed that the inmates of psychiatric institutions were, for the most part, poor and unemployed, from the economically disadvantaged social classes. As a result of this awareness of the psychiatric institution's role in social exclusion, there was also the consciousness of the technicians' role as delegates of a repressive instrument. The influence of Antonio Gramsci and Jean-Paul Sartre was present in the Basaglian démarche, addressing the issues of 'officials of consensus' and 'technicians of practical knowledge'[4] in the construction of hegemony.

The epistemological debate

One aspect raised by the dialogue with Basaglia at the beginning of the Brazilian psychiatric reform process was the epistemological debate: specifically, when he criticizes the presumption of science to be neutral (Basaglia, 1967, 1968, 1985). This last aspect is emphasized and expanded to the concept of disease. This is understood from the 'mental alienation' of Pinel through to the contemporary concepts of 'mental disorder' or 'disturbance' and, obviously, by the notion of 'disease'. Basaglia proposes that psychiatry should stop putting the protagonist of this experience in parentheses in order to deal with the disease. Rather, he argues to put the disease in parentheses to deal with the subjects who suffer and live the experience. This epistemological attitude, founded on the 'epoché' (suspension of judgement) conceived by Edmund Husserl, promotes a fundamental displacement in the relations between professionals and the so-called patients (i.e. people who receive a psychiatric diagnosis). This operation, also called 'reduction' or 'suspension', allows for the desires, aspirations, projects, and expectations of subjects (Venturini, 2016). What psychopathology saw as symptoms is now re-defined as diversities, singularities.

In the political practice of Brazilian psychiatric reform, the possibility of understanding and operating this reversal of meaning causes an innovative result: psychiatric reform is no longer reduced only to the transformation of the care model. It is inside a 'complex social process', the main goal of which is to build 'another social place' for madness. The emphasis is placed on a new social inclusion of the patient. The principle of subject empowerment takes on a new dimension; the person who presents psychic suffering is no longer the object of psychiatry, as a patient, but is a social actor, as a protagonist of his own history. This is evident in the construction of a strong and powerful social movement of 'users' (patients) and their families. The greater social participation resulting from this process is significantly strengthened in Brazil, as its national health system (the SUS—the Unified Health System) has the principles of democratization and participation as amongst its most important pillars.

The Brazilian 'alternative' movement was renamed, in 1987, the 'Social Movement for a Society Without Asylums'. On the tenth anniversary of Law 180, a 'National Day of Anti-Asylum Fight' was established to stimulate reflection on psychiatry and its

[4] Through these concepts—'workers of consensus' (in Gramscian vocabulary) and 'workers in practical knowledge' (in Sartre's terms), Basaglia reflects on workers or social operators, groups, communities, and social organizers who threaten to 'create a more subtle and penetrating social-control network' (Basaglia, 1982, p. 119).

institutions within society. Originally to be celebrated on 13 May (the date the law was passed in Italy), the date was changed to 18 May to avoid coinciding with another celebration—the signing of the 'Lei Aurea', the law that abolished slavery in Brazil. Since 1987, 18 May has become a very important date in the political agenda when social, cultural, legislative, political, and academic activities happen throughout Brazil (see Figure 7.1).

Law 180 explicitly inspired Brazilian mental health legislation. This was particularly true in relation to the bill presented to the Chamber of Deputies in 1989 by Paulo Delgado, deputy of the Workers' Party (PT). The long and controversial debate in the

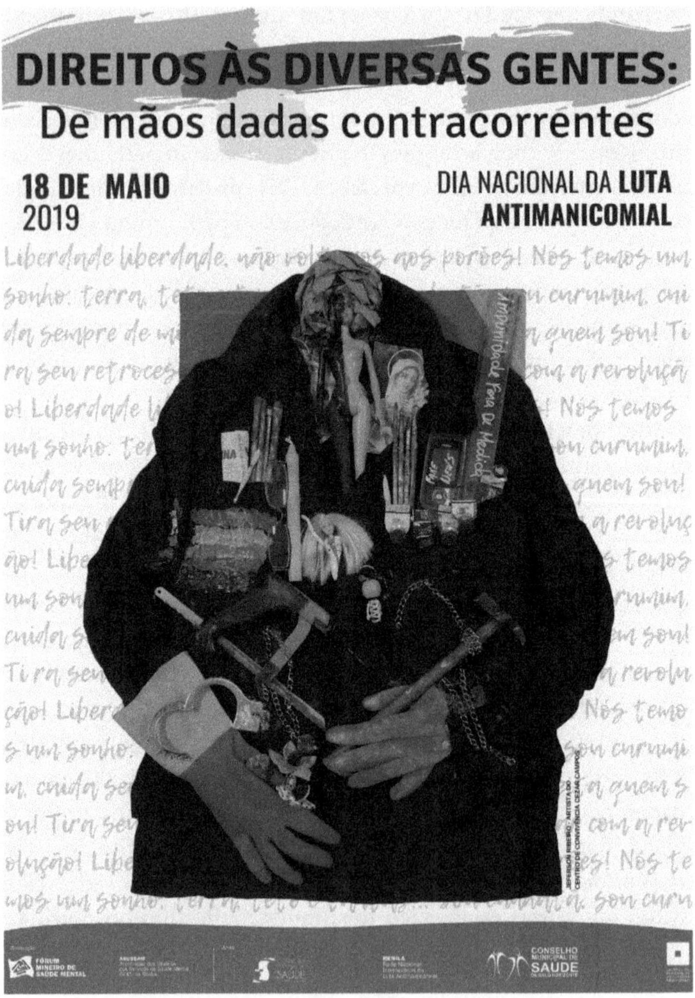
DIREITOS ÀS DIVERSAS GENTES:
De mãos dadas contracorrentes
18 DE MAIO
2019
DIA NACIONAL DA LUTA
ANTIMANICOMIAL

Figure 7.1 Poster to commemorate the 'Day of Struggle against the Psychiatric Hospital'.
Courtesy of RENILA (Rede Internúcleos de Luta Antimanicomial)

Senate led, in 2001, to a law that shows some differences compared to the Italian one. For example, a deadline for the closure of psychiatric hospitals is not defined and the possibility of compulsory internment for mental illness is still decided by Justice. However, the Basaglian intention to create a community health network and to completely close all psychiatric hospitals remains.

The Family Association for Mental Health of the first psychosocial care centre (CAPS) was called the 'Franco Basaglia Association'. Other CAPS (psychosocial attention centres) inspired by the mental health centres in Trieste, and an important foundation in Rio de Janeiro, also bear his name. These brief considerations demonstrate how Basaglia's name has become a sort of 'brand' since his coming to Brazil.

Come and see

In 1978 and 1979, Basaglia toured several cities, including Rio de Janeiro, São Paulo, Salvador, and Belo Horizonte. In this last city, Basaglia was encouraged to visit public psychiatric hospitals in order to check the Brazilian healthcare situation. The most influential visit was to the Public Psychiatric Hospital in the city of Barbacena (Figure 7.2). Accompanied by students, professionals, managers, and journalists, Basaglia was surprised by the institution's level of violence. He reiterated his impressions to the press when he defined the hospital as a 'concentration camp'. This denunciation received a great deal of coverage in the national press (as will be discussed further). At the time, Basaglia was a consultant and researcher for the book published in 1983, *Psychiatry Control and Repression* (Moreira, 1983). This was a severe criticism of the public and private hospitals of the city of Belo Horizonte, which sociologically documented the violence and commerce of madness.

Basaglia's second visit to Belo Horizonte was quite important. He was invited to participate in the Third Psychiatry Congress of Minas Gerais, an event organized by a group of social psychiatrists who had already started to transform care in the region of Minas Gerais (Goulart, 2015). This reform included a therapeutic community and a training course based on social psychiatry concepts. Basaglia invited Robert Castel to present with him. The event hosted a series of protests against the asylums and the release of the film *In the Name of Reason* by film-maker Helvécio Ratton, which featured translated excerpts from Basaglia's book *L'Istituzione Negata*. This widely prized documentary, still watched nowadays, was launched, against the will of local government, in the presence of Basaglia and hundreds of people (Goulart, 2010). After the screening, which turned into an act of protest, a touched Basaglia refused to comment on the film: he preferred that Brazilians should speak.

As a consequence of these meetings, Minas Gerais developed a hospital reform project that impacted the 1980s and resulted in the closure of the psychiatric hospital in Barbacena and the establishment of a public network of mental health teams. In Rio de Janeiro and São Paulo, opportunities for care reorganization were presented, and the practice of deinstitutionalization in several psychiatric hospitals began.

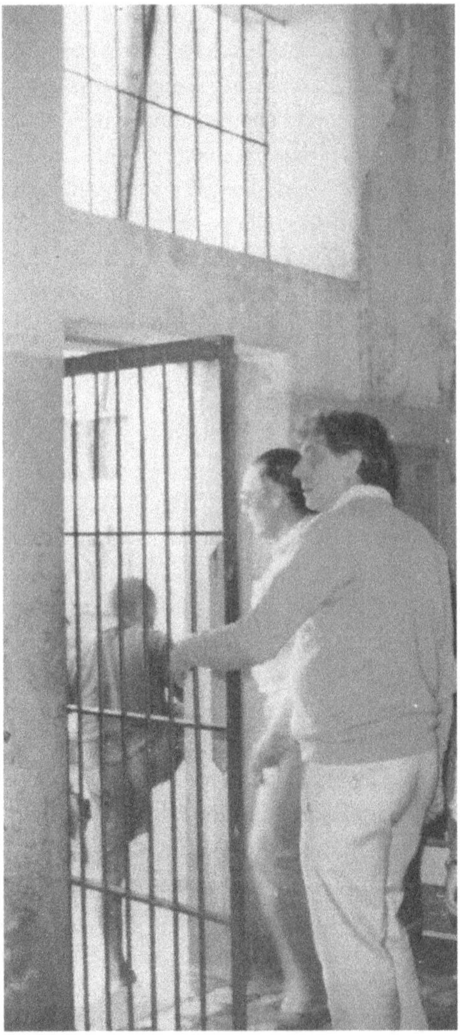

Figure 7.2 Basaglia visiting the Psychiatric Hospital of Barbacena.
Courtesy of Jairo Toledo Furtado

Another hallmark of Franco Basaglia's presence and active participation in Brazil was the invitation he made: 'Venite a vedere' ('Come and see'). He insisted on the relevance of living the experience, consolidated in Trieste. Since the mid 1980s, many people have accepted this invitation and have embraced volunteer activities, and carried out research and training (Goulart et al., 2015, 2017, 2018). This flow resulted in exchanges that supported the closing of the first private hospital in Brazil (Santos, São Paulo), the structuring of psychosocial care networks, and efforts to confront the health market. Later, it took the form of the Valuation and Restructuring Programme of the Psychiatric Assistance in Hospitals (PNASH) of the SUS (2004), which halved private psychiatric beds in Brazil. We can certainly say that Basaglia's good seed resulted in profound psychiatric reform within the Brazilian health system.

Would all this have been possible without this 'democratic' psychiatrist? The Basaglia known in Brazil, and often reinvented as a libertarian, is the key to the shift from the idea of an anti-institutional movement to the practice of the anti-asylum fight. This philosophy guided Brazilian psychiatric reform and shaped its confrontation with the military dictatorship. It reflected the redemocratization that marked the 1980s.

A myth?

It is worth investigating the ways in which Franco Basaglia was perceived and reinvented. Considering him merely as a brilliant and radical person, who created and proposed personal thoughts about psychiatry, can lead to a distorted view of his capacity and work. The myth of solitary leadership erases, among other things, the history of networks of collaboration he mobilized, which had always been part of his professional life.

By thinking about Basaglia from a collective and interactive point of view, we gain a more coherent understanding of his impact. Brazilian records of the 1978 and 1979 meetings (Basaglia, 1979), unlike the subsequent Italian editions, show clearly this collective dimension. They also record the many social and political actors who vividly argued with Franco Basaglia. Many people report his hallmark modus operandi—unrelenting communication, respect for difference, and outrage in the face of violence (in its multiple forms). All this within a dialectic and intense confrontation, including all participants of the meeting. It is this behaviour that positively affected the imagination of Brazilians. On the other hand, such a collective dimension may risk that we consider Basaglia's individual thoughts as less important. We could therefore ask whether there is, in Brazil, broad and direct knowledge of his thoughts as an author. The answer is yes. There is direct knowledge of Basaglia's writings, based on the publication of both his texts and those of Franca Basaglia. Despite the fact that, as we have seen, the first translation dates back to 1979, awareness grew only when the first Brazilian translations were published (Basaglia, 1985, 2005) and the narratives of the anti-institutional experiences that were inspired by him were widely disseminated (Kinoshita, 1987; Rotelli, 1990, 1992; Barros, 1994; Amarante, 1992, 1994, 1995, 1996).

At times, Basaglia's language seems historically dated. For example, the Marxist illusion of the revolutionary power of the proletariat or of the representative of popular power *tout court*,referred to by Basaglia, may be criticized. But any historical updating cannot contradict the substance of the thought, which focuses on the ever-present struggle between oppressors and the oppressed while facing the subject of mental health (Venturini, 2009). The specificity, as well as the innovative and critical intensity, of this thought is linked to what the educator Paulo Freire (a master of Brazilian thought) addressed in *Pedagogy of the Oppressed* (Freire, 1971). Therefore, for Brazilians, there is one more reason to recognize themselves in Basaglia: his thinking is similar and in accordance with the highest points of their own democratic and innovative culture.

However, Basaglia's impact on Brazilian scientific and cultural thinking goes beyond the mere knowledge of the writings attributed to him. When we refer, for example, to mental health professionals working in the public sector, we identify Basaglia's ideas; and when we refer to the patients in public services, we discover how much he is known and loved—with no rhetoric whatsoever. Generally, patients do not know the names of either foreign or Brazilian psychiatrists (except, perhaps, the celebrated Nise de Silveira[5]), but every activist patient knows who Basaglia is, and has something to say about him. This is certainly a positive assessment of his impact, since such knowledge comes through channels other than academic ones.

The Brazilian legislation inspired by Basaglia's principles developed new terms for mental health patients. These include 'bearer of psychic disorder', 'citizen with mental suffering', and 'users'. These terms reveal that the language has evolved to escape biomedical reductionism, enabling expressions to emerge from the social movements of mental health (in the same way that the term 'social operator' was coined in Italy).

The complex cultural and social processes of Basaglia's impact translated into music, theatre, literature, and many other forms of artistic and political expression (Torre, 2018). It is most clearly symbolized by the 'National Day of Anti-Asylum Fight', with placards and T-shirts bearing the name of Basaglia; and in 2015, for example, the parade in Belo Horizonte, organized by the Fórum Mineiro de Saúde Mental and RENILA (Anti-Asylum Fight Centres Network), explicitly paid homage to Franco Basaglia, with colourful costumes, singing, and dancing to a samba song with the theme 'So it is never forgotten, never to happen again: for a Society Without Asylums'. The parade continued in the city, singing the following (see Figure 7.3):

> If Basaglia came here to free me
> Why go back, if we need to progress?
> I called for Xangó and for Tupã
> It was Basaglia who came and showed me
> The tomorrow...

In a celebration in 2015 of the thirty-fifth anniversary of Basaglia's visit to Brazil, organized by RENILA, an 'activist user' (Emilha Maria de Oliveira Marques) shared

[5] Physician and psychiatrist (Maceió, 1905–1999), and Carl Gustav Jung's disciple, Nise de Silveira revolutionized ways of treating the mentally ill, using artistic techniques—painting and drawing—as therapy. She pioneered research on the emotional relationships between patients and animals, and advocated the end of traditional treatments such as electroshock, drug use, and clinical confinement. She founded the Museum of the Unconscious to house the works of her 'clients' (patients) who attended painting and modelling workshops.

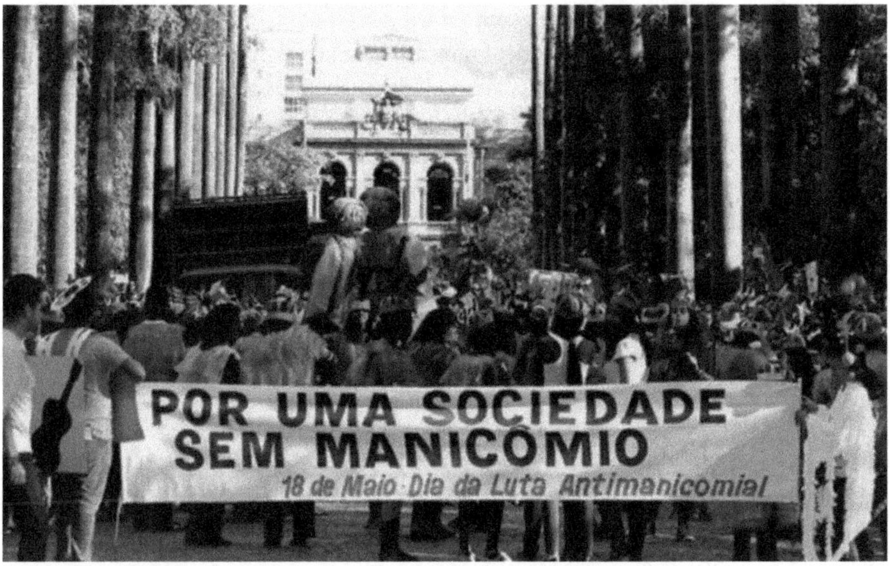
POR UMA SOCIEDADE
SEM MANICÔMIO
18 de Maio Dia da Luta Antimanicomial

Figure 7.3 The parade through the streets of Belo Horizonte in 2015.
Courtesy of Ernesto Venturini

with the participants a kind of 'Basaglian vocabulary', with definitions that show different ways of spreading the work of this democratic psychiatrist:

> *Basaglia*: The guy who frees the loonies
> *Basagliá*: To become like Basaglia
> *Basaglismo*: Basaglian lifestyle
> *Basagliamento*: To subject oneself to the Basaglian lifestyle
> *Basaglianismo*: Study of the Basaglian effect
> *BasagliAção*: Basaglian actions
> *Basagliadô*: Specialist to spread Basaglia's philosophy
> *Basagliagem*: To go from Antibasaglia to Basaglia's agreement
> **(Marques, 2015)**

In these demonstrations, we find a strong adherence to Basaglia's anti-institutional and libertarian discourse, that points to the radicalism of a widely documented historical process.

In Brazil, Basaglia is basically an icon in the fight for democratic freedoms and against the oppressive restrictions of all institutions and disciplines subservient to a repressive power. Like all myths, he expresses potentiality and ambiguity, but his strength is based on the intensity and simplicity of a message which is easily understood by a Brazilian culture marked by slavery, colonial oppression, and ferocious dictatorships (Souza, 2017). It is a message whose meaning is direct and effective. Many of Basaglia's expressions deeply affect the imagination of those who want a fair society and desire radical changes. Prominent among these are 'fight against the institutions of violence', 'freedom is therapeutic', 'mental illness must be put in parentheses', 'optimism of the will', and 'we show that the impossible is possible'. It is a very coherent and simple discourse, which shows however a great ability to communicate.

Nevertheless, the myth is also nurtured by the life and history of the character, Basaglia. He strongly establishes credibility in his work, a man fully committed to public service, a 'civil servant', as Benedetto Saraceno states (2015). He also signifies honesty and courage. Like so many Brazilians persecuted during the military dictatorship, he was arrested during fascism. He was a man who consistently combined thinking and practice, whose ideas and judgements were straightforward, and who presented critical thoughts (Venturini, 2013).

Alternative psychiatry?

However, Basaglia's influence in Brazil, as suggested by the number of citations of his writings in psychiatric publications (with their excessive focus on biochemical reactions and neural receptors), would seem to be virtually nil. If the impact criterion was the intensity of opposition, we should speak of a strong hostile impact, expressed by the Brazilian Association of Psychiatrists, which has a deeply negative opinion about the closure of all psychiatric hospitals. Criticism is based on ideological biases that do not value the great progress made in implementing reform and focus only on the inappropriate implementation of the law in some contexts.

The Brazilian Association of Psychiatry appears to believe that Franco Basaglia is an 'anti-psychiatrist'. But, paradoxically, if he could defend himself, he might consider this Association as an 'anti-psychiatric' community, because it is linked to an ineffective and archaic treatment model (Venturini, 2005). In this case, the key factor is the analysis of the positive results achieved in numerous contexts where the reform law was implemented and psychiatric hospitals were replaced by the new territorial organizations and treatment 'in freedom'. On the other hand, there are a great number of Brazilian psychiatrists who share the Basaglian perspective. These are professionals of notable scientific prestige, such as those who are members of the AMP (the Psychiatry Association of Minas Gerais), who invited Basaglia to their Congress in 1979, which emerged as one of the historical milestones in Brazilian psychiatric reform. Even today, the psychiatrists who are currently members of ABRASME (the Brazilian Association of Mental Health) support Basaglia's ideas with determination.

This analysis leads us to confront the relation between Basaglia's praxis and psychiatric reform law. Brazilian Law 10.216, dating from April 2001, was certainly an important result. It provides for the protection and legal rights of persons with mental disorders, and amends the mental healthcare law. The institutional change was, and still is, one of the most important in the world amongst low- and middle-income countries. It has implemented a 'bold reform' and introduced a new mental health system (Saraceno, 2014, p. 70), involving civil society as well as professionals, users, and families. It could be argued that no other country has made such an effective change from an extremely problematic situation where victims had no legal protection and large economic interests were set against it.

The vast majority of psychiatric hospitals were private and publicly funded, generating great private profits. In the 1990s, the first territorial services of mental health were implemented and, after Brazilian Law 10.216, a huge network of CAPS, inspired by the original model of the Trieste mental health centres (Lancetti and Amarante, 2013), was established. The CAPS are currently distributed throughout the country and the number of beds in a psychiatric hospital has been greatly reduced.

However, it would be a serious mistake to evaluate Basaglia's thoughts from the results of the law that he inspired. In fact, Basaglia himself was critical of the formulation and implementation of Italian law (Venturini, 1979). The implementation of any reform always depends on complex political, social, and financial interactions, together with the flow of historical contingencies. To criticize Basaglia for the limitations in implementing the law would be as absurd as denying the value of the Universal Declaration of Human Rights of 1948 because of situations where these principles have been violated. It is essential, therefore, to distinguish the two arguments: Basaglia's praxis and the results of the reform laws.

This distinction is especially important in a country such as Brazil, where the real opposition is between those who advocate a public, universal, and egalitarian health system (which corresponds to the logic of the Brazilian mental health reform) and those who advocate a substantially private system (which privileges profit and financial efficiency). The reasons for opposition become clearer, however, if we leave the field of psychiatry and explore other areas of clinical practice and understanding. In the publications, articles, and official interventions of social medicine, collective health, and public mental health policies, we find extraordinary and positive references to Basaglia, from the late 1970s onwards. His thoughts appear as an epistemological and historical milestone in the development of health policies. In academic publications (articles, books, as well as theses) in disciplines such as Social Psychology, Sociology, Nursing, Social Work, Occupational Therapy, Anthropology, and Law, the reference to Basaglia's work is noticeable. It is particularly emphasized for its critical value in relation to topics such as the neutrality of science and its application, scientific positivism, and the relations between knowledge and power.

The radicalism of the root

In conclusion, is this psychiatry that Basaglia idealizes and collectively performs considered radical? Amongst the suitable definitions in Portuguese, Italian, and English, we find many possibilities. None of them can, however, encompass the force of the meetings, alliances, and transformations that guided a democratic and fundamentally anti-authoritarian creation.

We can claim the importance nowadays, and the strength of the process of change, originated with the historic meeting between Brazilians and Basaglia. This meeting has had an impact that has echoed for 40 years. Although reformisms and 'replacement ideologies'[6] systematically operate to deplete the strength of this legacy, the current agenda of the Brazilian anti-asylum struggle clearly shows the vital harmony that was established and remained active thanks to the 'Basaglians'. They multiplied in Brazil, establishing alliances, networks, transformations that claim other disciplinary and political leaderships—beyond the academy and the psychiatric corporation. Society without asylums, including the mental ones, acts as an ethical horizon for the Brazilian activism that takes to the streets, rejecting institutions of violence (that have currently, unfortunately, been reinvigorated, threatening and harming the Brazilian mental health network).

The dialectical tension between the pessimism of reason and the optimism of practice, as outlined, projects ever-contradictory alternatives in a permanent process of Brazilian democratic construction. Basaglia's thoughts, work, and philosophy insist and multiply in formal spaces—higher-education centres—and in those which may be called informal and which foster an anti-asylum activist culture. The threats to social and human rights emphasize the essential dimension that Basaglia shared—the risk of psychiatry exerting social control, in coexistence with oppression and violence.

If radical is understood as the root[7] and the ability to subvert the hegemonic order, Basaglia deserves the honour of this term. If it means extremism, we refute this term. The conceptual, technical, and political preciseness of the Basaglian legacy brings us back to the terms of a true 'Democratic Psychiatry' and to the best alternatives, either in dark times or not. The power of democracy vigorously unmasks the rhetoric of social control, which tries to use the medical and psychological sciences as a space of dominance. It silences the virulence of this kind of interpretation of mental suffering, and promotes the necessary mechanisms of resistance in Brazil and beyond.

References

Amarante, P. (1992). A trajetória do pensamento crítico em saúde mental no Brasil: planejamento na desconstrução do aparato manicomial. In: M. Kalil (org.), *Saúde Mental e cidadania no contexto dos sistemas locais de saúde*. São Paulo/ Salvador: Editora Hucitec/ Cooperação Italiana em Saúde, pp. 103–9.

Amarante, P. (1994). Uma aventura no manicômio. A trajetória de Franco Basaglia. *História, Ciências, Saúde-Manguinhos* 1(1):61–77. Available from: http://dx.doi.org/10.1590/S0104-59701994000100006

[6] The term 'replacement ideology' appears in the mid 1970s, in the book *La Maggioranza Deviante* (1971): 'a new ideology of a sociological type which would be placed in such a way as to overlap archaic psychiatric ideologies' (Basaglia, 1982, 157).

[7] The word 'radical' comes from the Latin *radixicis* (root); it is relative to the root, to the intimate essence of something; therefore a 'radical person' is one who is turned to total and substantial change.

Amarante, P. (1995), *Loucos pela Vida—a trajetória da reforma psiquiátrica no Brasil*. Rio de Janeiro: SDE/ENSP.
Amarante, P. (1996). *O homem e a serpente—outras histórias para a loucura e a psiquiatria*. Rio de Janeiro: FIOCRUZ.
Araújo, R. (1976). Basaglia. O Laing Italiano. In: *Opinião* 30 January 1976.
Barros, D.D. (1994). *Jardins de Abel: desconstrução do manicômio de Trieste*. São Paulo: Lemos/EDUSP.
Basaglia, F. (1968). *L'Istituzione Negata*. Torino: Einaudi.
Basaglia, F. (1979). *A Psiquiatria Alternativa—contra o pessimismo da razão, o otimismo da prática. Conferências no Brasil*. São Paulo: Ed. Brasil Debates.
Basaglia, F. (1984). *Conferenze Brasiliane*. Pistoia: Centro di Documentazione di Pistoia.
Basaglia, F. (2000). *Conferenze Brasiliane*. Milano: Raffaello Cortina Editore.
Basaglia, F. (2005). *Escritos selecionados em saúde mental e reforma psiquiátrica*. Rio de Janeiro, Garamond.
Basaglia, F. (2018). *Conferenze Brasiliane—nuova edizione*. Milano: Raffaello Cortina Editore.
Basaglia, F. (ed.) (1967). *Che cos'è la psichiatria?* Milano: Baldini & Castoldi.
Basaglia, F. (ed.) (1982). *Basaglia—Scritti II*. Torino: Einaudi.
Basaglia, F. (ed.) (1985). *A Instituição Negada*. Rio de Janeiro: Graal.
Berlinguer, G. (1969). *Psichiatria e potere*. Roma: Ed. Riuniti.
Colucci, M., and Di Vittorio, P. (2001). *Franco Basaglia*. Milano: Mondadori.
De Oliveira Marques, E.M. (2015). *Vocabulário Basagliano*. Belo Horizonte: s/editor.
De Salvia, D. and Rolfe, A. (1984). Presentazione. In: F. Basaglia (ed.), *Conferenze Brasiliane*. Pistoia: Centro di Documentazione di Pistoia, pp. 5–9.
Foot, J. (2014). Franco Basaglia and the radical psychiatry movement in Italy, 1961–1978. *Critical and Radical Social Work* 2(2):235–49. Available from: https://www.ncbi.nlm.nih.gov/pmc/articles/PMC4430803/
Freire, P. (1971). *La pedagogia degli oppressi*. Milano, Mondadori.
Giannichedda, M.G. (2018). Nota. In: F. Basaglia (ed.), *Conferenze Brasiliane—nuova edizione*. Milano: Raffaello Cortina Editore, pp. IX–XI.
Goulart, M.S.B. (2007). *As raízes Italianas do movimento antimanicomial*. São Paulo: Casa do Psicólogo/Conselho Federal de Psicologia, pp. 205–11.
Goulart, M.S.B. (2010). *Em Nome da Razão: quando a arte faz história*. Revista Brasileira de Crescimento e Desevolvimento Humano, vol. 20, pp. 34–9.
Goulart, M.S.B. (2012). Basaglia: a Franca. In: F. Portugal and A.M. Jacó-Vilela (eds), *Clio Psychè—gênero, psicologia e história*. Rio de Janeiro: NAU, pp. 205–11.
Goulart, M.S.B. (2015). A política de saúde mental mineira: rumo à consolidação. *Gerais: Revista Interinstitucional de Psicologia* 8(2)::194–213.
Goulart, M., et al. (2018). O voluntariado brasileiro em Trieste: a psicologia na desinstitucionalização italiana In: *Clio Psychè—Discursos e práticas na história da psicologia. Volume 1*. Rio de Janeiro: EdUERJ, pp. 265–78.
Goulart, M., Stella. B., Venturini, E., Baliero, H.G., and Chaves, A.L.F. (2015). La presenza storica dei brasiliani nella pratica della salute mentale di Trieste: 'venite a vedere' o fare insieme? *Fogli di Informazione Terza Serie*, 35–36:16–27.
Goulart, M., Stella. B., Venturini, E., Baliero, H.G., and Chaves, A.L.F. (2017). Os brasileiros na prática de saúde mental de Trieste: histórias de laços e de construções In: R. Seabra (ed.), *Boas práticas: caminhos e descaminhos no processo de desinstitucionalização*. São Paulo: Cultura Acadêmica, pp. 267–88.
Kinoshita, R.T. (1987). Uma experiência pioneira. A reforma psiquiátrica italiana. In: R. Marsaglia, D.A. Dallari, J.F. Costa, F.D.M. Moura Neto, R. Kinoshita, and A. Lancetti (eds), *Saúde Mental e Cidadania*. São Paulo: Ed. Mandacaru, pp. 67–83.

Lancetti, A. and Amarante, P. (2013). Saúde mental e saúde coletiva. In: G.W.S. Campos (org.), *Tratado de Saúde Coletiva*. São Paulo: HUCITEC, pp. 661–80.
Liguori, G. and Voza, P. (orgs) (2017). *Dicionário Gramsciano*. São Paulo: Boitempo Editorial.
Moreira, D. (1983). Psiquiatria: controle e repressão social. Petrópolis: Vozes ed.
Nicácio, F., Amarante, P., and Barros, D.D. (2000). I movimenti per la salute mentale in Brasile dagli anni Ottanta. In: F. Basaglia (ed.), *Conferenze Brasiliane*. Milano: Cortina ed., pp. 233–57.
Rotelli, F. and Amarante, P. (1992). Reformas Psiquiátricas na Itália e no Brasil. Aspectos Históricos e Metodológicos. In: B. Bezerra and P. Amarante (org.), *Psiquiatria sem Hospício*. Rio de Janeiro: Relume-Dumará, pp. 41–55.
Saraceno, B. (2014). *Dicorso globale, sofferenze locali. Analii critica del Movimento de Salute Mentale Globale*. Milano: Il Saggitore.
Saraceno, B. (2015). *Conferência de Benedetto Saraceno*. 35 Anos de Basaglia no Brasil. Available from: https://youtu.be/xPjv6Cmk7o?t=1
Schittar, L. (1999). *Franco Basaglia. L'Ippogrifo: atti e documenti*. Pordenone: Associazione Enzo Sarli.
Souza, J. (2017). *A elite do atraso—da escravidão à lava jato*. Rio de Janeiro: LEYA.
Torre, E.H.G. (2018). *Saúde Mental, Loucura e Diversidade Cultural: inovação e ruptura nas experiências de arte-cultura da Reforma Psiquiátrica e do campo da Saúde Mental no Brasil.* Tese de Doutorado. Programa de Pós-Graduação em Saúde Pública. Escola Nacional de Saúde Pública Sergio Arouca. Fundação Oswaldo Cruz. Rio de Janeiro.
Venturini, E. (1979). *Il giardino dei gelsi*. Torino: Giulio Einaudi.
Venturini, E. (2005). Prefácio. In: F. Basaglia (ed.), *Escritos Selecionados*. Organização: Paulo Amarante. Petrópolis: Garamond, pp. 17–21.
Venturini, E. (2009). Le leggi auree. In: P. Lupatelli (cur), *I Basagliati. Percorsi di libertà* Perugia: Ed. Crace, pp. 101-8.
Venturini, E. (2013). L'arte dello spiazzamento. In: P.A. Rovatti (cur.), *Restituire la soggettività, lezioni sul pensiero di Franco Basaglia*. Merano: Edizione alpha beta Verlag, pp. 227–238.
Venturini, E. (2016). *A linha curva*. Rio de Janeiro: Editora Fiocruz, pp. 80–81.

8

From the asylum to community mental health services

The path to human rights

Diana Mauri and Alejandra Barcala

Introduction

Franco Basaglia and his ideas have profoundly impacted on the most progressive actors in the mental health field in Argentina. His reflections and work have become a bulwark in the defence of human rights, and against the disproportionate power of the psychiatric establishment. The initatives undertaken by Basaglia in Trieste in the 1970s remain a point of reference for academics, professionals, trade unions, and movements defending the rights of people with mental suffering in Argentina. Key actors in the deinstitutionalization process have shown a constant commitment by coming regularly to the country in order to discuss their experience. Drawing from Basaglia's legacy, the activity of Franco Rotelli (who directed the Trieste Department of Mental Health after Basaglia's death) was fundamental in fostering these exchanges (De Leonardis et al., 1986, 1995; Evaristo, 2000; Colucci and Di Vittorio, 2006; De Leonardis and Emmenegger, 2011; Rotelli, 2014; Del Giudice, 2017; Mezzina 2017).

In this chapter, we will provide a comprehensive, albeit non-exhaustive, overview of historical events in Argentina which were significantly impacted by Basaglia's ideas. In addition, we will analyse the tensions, contradictions, conflicts, and paradoxes which persist in our mental health policies and practices. In Argentina, different historical periods have seen both advances and setbacks in the State's position over mental health, and the resulting changes in public policies have affected the dynamics between legislation and the main representatives of the field.

It should be remembered that, in the same years when the deinstitutionalization process was taking place in Italy, eventually resulting in the reform law which abolished internment in asylums (Law 180 of 1978), Argentina fell under a military dictatorship (1976–1983). This, among other things, destroyed those professional organizations, welfare institutions, and community health projects that had been doing pioneering work in Latin America. Substantial progress had initiated the transition from traditional psychiatry to a broader concept of the 'mental health' field. The devastating effects of state terrorism impeded the creation of an alternative to the hegemony of the asylum, whose role was actually enhanced during this period

(Chiarvetti, 2008). During the Military Junta, thousands of people disappeared. It is impossible to know how many patients suffered this fate, but available information allows us to estimate that 121 mental health professionals and 267 students disappeared (Carpinterio and Vainer, 2018).

Among the initiatives developed after this period, bearing the mark of Basaglia's thinking, we will highlight three projects. Firstly, the management of the Directorate of Mental Health by Vicente Galli; secondly, the reform in the province of Río Negro; and lastly, the passing of National Mental Health Law 26657 in 2010.

The return of democracy: the management of Vicente Galli, 1983–1989

In 1983, with the return of democracy, mental health policy was defined by the National Government as a priority within healthcare. The legacy of the dictatorship and the genocide (with 30,000 suspected political dissidents having disappeared or been killed) had profound consequences, not only on those directly affected but on social structures as a whole. It also generated a crisis in values, as well as obvious damage to collective mental health and the care and rehabilitation systems. The resulting successful action for transformation was undertaken jointly by the National Directorate for Mental Health and the Provincial Health Ministry (Galli, 2011). The National Directorate for Mental Health, led by Vicente Galli between 1983 and 1989, established links with the protagonists of Italian psychiatric reform, and particularly the progressive experience of Trieste, which Franco Rotelli had been leading since Basaglia's death in 1981. These relations with Italian psychiatry also gave rise to an important international cooperation project between the Italian Ministry of Foreign Affairs and several Argentinian provinces, to supersede internment in asylums.

Silvia Faraone, in her doctoral thesis 'Cartography of Deinstitutionalization in Argentina', documents the influence of Basaglia's thinking in the country. Faraone believes that, within this political context, Italian psychiatric reform was responsible for driving the development of human resources in Argentina, both through its publications and its practical developments. Italian representatives provided advice on the implementation of psychiatric reforms at a national level and, more locally, in the provinces of Córdoba, Río Negro, Mendoza, and Buenos Aires. A significant number of mental health professionals (from senior managers, such as the national director and provincial directors, to heads of services, psychiatrists, psychologists, and mental health residents) visited the Italian services; conversely, several members of the Trieste Department of Mental Health went to Argentina and witnessed the progress of reforms, within international cooperation projects. The links thus established continue to this day, contributing to several national and provincial projects (Faraone, 2012).

Vicente Galli's programme called for important reforms, such as the integration of mental health policies within general health policies, cross-sectoral policy integration, and the expansion of coverage. He envisaged promotion and prevention activities; the participation of users and providers in the definition of requirements, strategies, and resource allocations; the replacement of a hospital–disease model with a community–health model; and a corresponding increase in budget. Lastly, he focused on the transformation of the main public psychiatric hospitals (discouraging private institutions with similar functions) and the conceptual and practical development of a strategy for mental health within primary care.

Central to his programme of deinstitutionalization were the establishment of interdisciplinary mental health residences, ongoing training of new staff, the retraining of existing staff, and the democratization of power. This was achieved through substantial changes in institutional models and progress in legislation regarding hospitalization. In addition, intense activity in the provinces resulted in the recognition of mental health as a pressing problem, and the constitution of a specific team within the Department of Health. An underlying principle was awareness that hospitalization in psychiatric institutions was unjust and ineffective (Chiarvetti, 2008). Various provinces created and reformed programmes and systems for the resocialization of patients. In his analysis of the Trieste experience, Galli states:

> It was from Trieste that the spread started, to the rest of Italy and the western world, of those transformations allowing the transition from the archaic asylum-based psychiatry towards strategies for community, collective mental health—proof of what could be achieved. Trieste remains the benchmark for comparison with other developments. Many who did not include all the components of the reform or trivialized the importance of the change in clinical paradigm on which the Trieste experience is based, failed, without understanding the causes of their own failures. Many failed to close asylums and established community mental health services that function adequately only for a percentage of those they serve, perpetuating processes leading to exclusion and isolation.
>
> **(Galli, 2014, p. 6)**

Basaglia's ideas also influenced the training and development of staff. In 1984, the School of Public Health in Córdoba offered training in the management of mental health systems to provincial policy makers. The objective was to implement the 'Guidelines for a National Mental Health Plan' that the National Directorate of Mental Health had begun to execute (Ferro, 1989). The Master's Degree in Mental Health in Córdoba based its teaching on the Trieste developments by Franco Basaglia and Franco Rotelli, and benefitted from contributions by such key actors as Itzhak Levav and Benedetto Saraceno (Ferro, 2010).

The relationship between psychoanalysts and Basaglia's ideas is a complex one. Psychoanalysts are numerous, and have differing views. The majority agree with Basaglia's progressive ideas, but only a few have been, and are, key actors in the struggle against psychiatric institutionalization. Vicente Galli was a psychoanalyst, as was Emiliano Galende (another central reference in the field of mental health in Argentina), and, in the 1990s, he created both the Master and the Doctorate in Community Mental Health at the University of Lanús. Also, many professionals in charge of community experiences in public institutions and non-governmental organizations, and who favour the National Mental Health Law, are psychoanalysts. In addition, many share Basaglia's drive towards emancipation and the promotion of human rights. Others though, while agreeing with Basaglia's ideas, have avoided any involvement in public institutions and have not gone beyond mere verbal condemnation of the psychiatric establishment, and restricted themselves to their work in their private practices. Vicente Galli's key role is symbolic of the significant presence of psychoanalysis in professional cultures in Argentina. This marks a difference with the reform movement in Italy, which was led by psychiatrists with a non-psychoanalytical background.

Despite these differences, what counts is that you do your job well, as Basaglia said. The very first thing to do is to 'take your coat off', whichever that may be. 'Truth lies in our daily practice, in breaking with prejudices' (Basaglia, 2000, p. 64). This is where 'deinstitutionalization' begins.

The experience of deinstitutionalization in the province of Río Negro

With the return to democracy, the reforms in the province of Río Negro constituted the first experience of deinstitutionalization in Argentina. This is a 203,000-square-kilometre area, with a population of 550,000—located in the Patagonian region in the south of the country—where a new culture in mental healthcare was initiated. Emblematic innovations included the closure of the Hospital Psiquiátrico de Allen in 1988, with the discharge of patients, community-building initiatives, the establishment of mental health professionals in primary healthcare centres, and beds in general hospitals for short-term admissions. Since 1985, these developments have been accompanied by intensive awareness-raising work among local inhabitants, family members, healthcare and other professionals, and political leaders.

An interdisciplinary and cross-sectoral compilation of reflections and lessons learned by the protagonists of the deinstitutionalization in Río Negro (Cohen and Natella, 2007) argues that changes in the field of mental health began in the province in 1983. Hugo Cohen, who was Director of Mental Health, and Graciela Natella, who was chief psychiatrist of the province of Río Negro, were leaders in introducing a new approach to the problem of mental illness and, in turn, a different way to treat people suffering from mental health problems. This in an effort to overcome the traditional view, strongly rooted in society, of the psychiatric patient as a marginalized, different, and maybe dangerous individual (Cohen and Natella, 2007). Their compilation brings together a series of monographs produced for the training course on the practices of deinstitutionalization in 1991–1992. This course was a collaboration between the Directorate of Mental Health of the Nation and the Faculty of Social Sciences and Law of the National University of Comahue in the province of Río Negro, and saw active participation by professionals from Trieste.

> In 1991, Law 2440 for the health and social promotion of people with mental health problems was passed, consolidating this reform and prohibiting hospitalization in asylums and the use of electroshock therapy throughout the province:Law 2440 made legal what had been legitimized by many for several years; now we have to legitimize the law with its daily application. Such application implies an ethical repositioning in the relationship with 'the different'—who is no longer just the mentally ill, or the alcoholic, but also the drug addict, the unemployed person, the battered woman, the pregnant adolescent, the homosexual, the street kid, the AIDS patient, the undernourished, the *Mapuche*, the retiree and any other sector marginalized by our society . . . The work of our mental health teams . . . aims to create a perspective in which the task of rehabilitating the psychiatric patient is no longer limited to a few specialists, but falls on society as a whole.
>
> **(Cohen and Natella, 2007, p. 9)**

The Río Negro experience began before Basaglia's work became known in Argentina. Later encounters with his ideas nourished the experience, particularly during the process of promulgation of the Law.

In a later book, *Deinstitutionalization: Chronicle of the Reform of the Mental Health System of Río Negro*, Cohen and Natella (2013) acknowledged the influence of Basaglia's thinking, particularly the objectivization of people produced by institutionalization (Rotelli, 2015). They argued the need to replace the term 'mentally ill person'— reinforcing prejudices, discrimination, and negative connotations such as dangerousness and chronicity—with 'mental suffering'. This term was taken from 'sofferenza', used by the Italian health services. Its use aimed to create equality around the problem, produce identification and closeness, and prevent fear, as suffering is a part of everybody's experience. From Italian democratic psychiatry, they also took the word 'utente' ('user'), considering it more appropriate than 'patient', which seemed to imply waiting and passivity. They defined users as those who use a service and have citizens' rights and responsibilities that go with the prescriptions they receive.

A further lesson that the reform movement in Río Negro took from Basaglia's psychiatry is the value attributed to work as an option-creating tool for patients, allowing their 'return to life'. Basaglia intended work not as discipline (ergotherapy) or 'entertainment' (the protected laboratory—see Saraceno, 1995). He meant it as participation in a collective enterprise, whereby the quality of work processes and products becomes a springboard for personal emancipation, the promotion of capabilities, and the multiplication of networks of social and economic exchanges (Basaglia, 1973). Basaglia was inspired by the strong Italian cooperative tradition, and its experience of economic democracy. The 'Cooperativa Lavoratori Uniti Franco Basaglia' was the first co-operative, established in 1973 in the Trieste asylum, where psychiatric users had member status, along with operators and other figures. The deinstitutionalization movement, developing in Italy along these lines, led to the law instituting social cooperatives (381/991), in particular those providing work to the 'disadvantaged', such as psychiatric users. The collective work *La Empresa Social* (De Leonardis et al., 1995) recounts experiences deriving from Basaglia's ideas. Today, the Cooperativa Lavoratori Uniti, which has flourished outside the asylum, with as many as 250 members (approximately half of whom are 'disadvantaged') and a turnover of several million Euros, is well integrated within the regional and national cooperative system.

Adapted to the Argentinian context, this idea has inspired a formula in Río Negro whereby social enterprises, within the health system, aim at rehabilitation and social inclusion through work. They function as 'transitional spaces', allowing people to enter the job market, whether formally or informally (in the latter case, through the so-called 'economia popular').

As a variant for the Italian 'deinstitutionalization', the Río Negro Mental Health Directorate, in 1988, coined the term 'desmanicomialización' ('deasylumnization') to signify the mental healthcare transformation process that it was undertaking (Murekian, 2006). This concept refers to the new mental healthcare culture that allows people with mental suffering to live in their communities, and not in psychiatric hospitals or in any form of isolation. They live near their social life, work, home, and opportunities, and have access to effective care. 'Desmanicomialización' was synonymous with 'never again insane asylums' or their equivalent (Cohen and Natella, 2013). The experience implied a change from the asylum culture to a culture of inclusion and the realization of rights; a system of social integration and community care that would completely replace institutions of confinement.

The adoption of a 'protagonist role' by the recipients of psychiatric intervention created the need for mental health professionals to undergo a process of learning that was to completely redefine their competences. Neither Basaglia's 'deinstitutionalization' nor the 'desmanicomialización' in Río Negro could stay confined to the world of psychiatry. As highlighted by Basaglia, those promoting this change in Argentina were well aware that the transformation would impact the legal and health systems as a whole, the concepts of health and illness, as well as social care, in order to reach other vulnerable groups exposed to institutional stigma and consequent marginalization (Goffman, 1963).

Whilst in Basaglia's reform, psychiatry, after leaving the asylum, has developed into a rich network of community services in the local area, in Río Negro it remains centred in the general hospital. This follows the recommendations and earliest experiences of Mauricio Goldenberg and Valentín Baremblit, two important Argentinian psychiatrists and psychoanalysts committed to community care. In Río Negro, an important role is also played by the 'agentes sanitarios', essential figures of South American primary care, who guarantee active assistance in the whole of the Province.

In the 1980s and 1990s, the international organizations WHO and PAHO were just beginning to direct strategies towards the human rights of psychiatric users and models of community care. The historic Caracas Conference in 1990, framed within a regional and global process, allowed the Río Negro reform to emerge from the isolation in which official Argentinian psychiatry wanted it kept. It became recognized as a leading experience in the continent, as far as an internment-free mental health system is concerned (Saraceno, 2014).

The Río Negro developments were alternatively characterized by tensions, contradictions, difficulties, and achievements. These depended on changes in the political orientation of the provincial governments, with different degrees of commitment to reform (Murekian, 2013; Baffo et al., 2018). However, this pioneering experience gave rise to multiple models and local innovations in mental health policies throughout Argentina. It allowed the five provinces of Patagonia to declare themselves 'asylum free'.

The 1990s: until the passing of the National Mental Health Law

The neoliberal policies of 1990s generated profound socioeconomic and cultural transformations that disadvantaged numerous groups due to growing poverty and unemployment. The withdrawal of the State from many areas of social policy (health, education, social aid) led to social fragmentation and disintegration. The precariousness of employment and the inadequacy of traditional safety nets excluded more and more individuals (Castel, 1986). The absence of the State was compounded by the fragility of social support networks. The implementation of market-oriented reforms set back the development of equity, accentuating existing social inequalities (Svampa, 2008). Mental health disappeared from the State's agenda, as shown by the downgrading of the Directorate of Mental Health to an executive unit of the Ministry of Health.

In this period, key figures in mental health in Argentina depicted Basaglia's ideas and the Trieste experience in their scientific production (Galende, 1990; Saidon and Troianoski, 1994), and the *Zona Erógena* magazine (1993) held a permanent debate on deinstitutionalization. The principles of Italian reform were also adopted for institutional transformation in the legislative reforms tackled in different provinces. These included Cordoba, Buenos Aires, Entre Ríos (Chiarvetti, 2008; Sava, 2009), San Luis (Pellegrini, 2009), and Santa Fe (Faraone and Valero, 2013). However, political, financial, and ideological shortcomings prevented any comprehensive change, although significant reforming proposals emerged in such cities as Buenos Aires and La Plata (Sava, 2009; Barcala and Torricelli, 2013).

Active dialogue with key figures of Italian reform renewed and broadened discussion within the movement of professionals and users, despite its fragmentation (Alberdi, 2012). Basaglia's influence in Argentina spread thanks to the work of Franco Rotelli, who directed Mental Health Services in Trieste after Basaglia's death. As the leader of the implementation of Italian reform, he has, since 1990, coordinated several international cooperation projects with Argentina. Rotations of young professionals were formalized along these lines, allowing them to visit Trieste and observe the deinstitutionalization process within the framework of a complex, articulated system of public health and social services. Upon their return, they presented their experiences in workshops and published them in the mental health residents' journals (Garcia and Torricelli, 1996; Sturla et al., 2009). Throughout these years, many residents travelled to learn about Italian reform, and collaborative projects were consolidated. Several training experiences are still ongoing; promoted by the Department of Mental Health, they have been coordinated by Roberto Colapietro.

Since 2002, the Universidad Popular de las Madres de la Plaza de Mayo has organized an annual Mental Health and Human Rights Conference, with the aim to legitimize the struggle against asylums, promote the rights of people with mental suffering, and allow exchange between innovative community practices. In 2007, *Vidas Arrasadas: The Ssegregation of People in the Argentine Psychiatric Asylums. A Report on Human Rights and Mental Health in Argentina* (MDRI/CELS, 2007) was published. This documented human rights violations against 25,000 people who in 2004 were sectioned in Argentinian psychiatric institutions. The report generated indignation and forced the issue of mental health back onto the State's agenda.

The National Mental Health Law

> National Mental Health Law 26657 was passed in December 2010 and its regulatory decree was promulgated in 2013. Laws 180 (Italy) and 2440 (Río Negro) were central to its drafting. Many of its principles were inspired by collective and community mental health practices in Latin America, such as those in Río Negro and Brazil (Amarante, 2009; Nicasio, 1999), but especially by the ones in Italy and Trieste. These experiences showed that insane asylums could be entirely replaced by a community mental health system:The impossible has become possible. Ten, fifteen, twenty years ago, it was unthinkable that an asylum could be destroyed. Asylums may revert to their closed state, even more so than before, I do not know, but anyway we have shown that the mentally ill can be treated in a different way, and that testimony is fundamental. I do not believe that the fact that an action can be recreated in different contexts necessarily means victory. What counts, however, is that now we know what can be done.
>
> **(Basaglia, 2000, p. 57)**

Law 26657 ordered all psychiatric institutions to be closed by the year 2020, prohibited the creation of new public or private ones, and promoted the construction of an integrated community care model. The Law was a clean break with the traditional paradigm in mental health, recognizing mental patients as individuals with rights, regardless of their age or diagnosis.

The adaptation of regulations to international human rights guidelines aims to effect and consolidate a paradigm shift in the field of mental health in our country, in order to establish political and social responsibilities promoting effective access to the exercise of rights. Therefore, it fosters new practices and models in mental health-care: the improvement of local care; the creation of community services; interdisciplinary work; the involvement of the community, families, and users in the care process; and the integration of mental health within general healthcare. Lastly, but fundamentally, it sets a date for the definitive closure of psychiatric institutions. However, as Basaglia pointed out 40 years ago: 'The law on psychiatry is a very difficult one to apply because prejudice against the mentally ill is long standing and cannot be eliminated by law, just as a law cannot eliminate mental illness' (Basaglia, 2000, p. 70). In this respect, the Mental Health Law triggered intense debate between important figures with different political, ideological, and economic positions.

In the psychiatric world, Law 26657 represented a clear stance in favour of the reforming attitudes advocated by the emerging paradigms of social and community psychiatry, versus the traditional, positivist, medical/clinical approach. As opposed to treatment models based on forced and prolonged hospitalization, the Law ratifies the choice of a health-promotion perspective, which considers the individual as a whole, seen in the context of his/her life circumstances. It also employs psychotherapeutic, social, rehabilitative, and preventive tools, capitalizing on social bonds to support people and integrate them into their communities. It gives therapeutic relevance to the participation of users and their families in the care process, where the user's consent to his/her treatment is paramount (Galende, 1997).

The Law adopts this perspective in designing a mental health system which entirely replaces the mental hospital. Not only is the 'right to mental health' being established, but it is also complemented with the person's rights, as a citizen, in his/her relationship with the mental health system. Thus, the Law acknowledges and regulates the right to health in general, to dignity and autonomy, to legal capacity, to freedom, to personal integrity, to equality and non-discrimination, to information, to privacy, to identity, and to community integration. Accordingly, the rights recognized in the Law must be read as the concrete application of general human rights instruments to any particularly vulnerable population, in this case users of mental health services (Barcala and Laufer, 2015).

The approval of Law 26657 and its theoretical, disciplinary, institutional, and professional implications generated tensions. On its side were the legal and human rights sectors, as well as professionals' and users' movements and associations. These had fought for four years in its favour with such a broad consensus that—worthy of notice—the law was unanimously approved by Parliament. On the other hand, as might be expected, strong resistance emerged from many psychiatrists, especially the official National Association of Psychiatry (APSA), who felt their power threatened. These tensions were concentrated on the law's implementation, which, in public debate, represented a fundamental opportunity to radically rethink the social function of psychiatry. This included its modus operandi, its constituent knowledge, and its epistemological foundations, as Rotelli stated recalling Basaglia's political and ethical positions (Rotelli, 2014).

Three points created the fiercest debates. The first regards the central role of interdisciplinary work and the consequent redistribution of power among different professionals. Psychologists and social workers are now entitled to direct mental health services and even make decisions regarding hospitalization. This redistribution was clearly consistent with the Law's general orientation towards the psychosocial paradigm. It was opposed by the psychiatric establishment represented by APSA who, reaffirming the medical/clinical character of mental pathologies, claimed the primacy of its own competences and of medical/hospital facilities. The traditional competences and techniques of normalization through the control of the body, dealt with by Foucault (2002), also benefitted from the growing influence of the biomedical paradigm in predicting human behaviour. In the event, it is the closure of psychiatric hospitals that encountered the most resistance.

The second conflict was of a symbolic nature and concerned the definition of the problem. As in the Río Negro reform, the Law adopts the term 'mental suffering' ('sufrimiento mental') instead of 'mental illness'. This choice is aimed at reducing the risk of stigma, notoriously associated with psychiatric diagnoses. It is a clear limitation of psychiatrists' (and thus psychiatric power's) role in legimitizing internment and forced treatment. As such, it has been a central target of criticism by the psychiatric establishment.

The third conflict surrounded the creation of two organizations for the protection of human rights and monitoring of the implementation of the Law. The Mental Health National Monitoring Body and Legal Unit No. 22 of the National Public Defender Office both limited the power of psychiatrists to detain patients, breaking with psychiatric hegemony. The Body's function is to verify compliance with the Law and guarantee the respect of human rights in the mental health system. It also monitors conditions of hospitalization and evaluates treatments and the need for involuntary hospitalization. In 2015, it took a stand in the defence of the Mental Health Law against attempts to repeal articles resulting from changes in the government. The Unit of Public Defenders has jurisdiction in the City of Buenos Aires and provides legal assistance for people institutionalized in mental health settings. It both guarantees free, universal, and equal treatment and rehabilitation in health services, and protects the right of people with mental suffering to be heard, thus contributing to their release from hospital and to community integration. Both agencies guard against abusive practices that still exist in certain institutions. These include seclusion, prolonged physical restraint, involuntary treatment, involuntary medication or electroshock therapy, indefinite hospitalization, and segregation from family and the community.

That conflict triggered by the reform law revolves around the aforementioned three points is not accidental. They represent the Law's intent to question the centrality of the asylum, in the technical/professional, symbolic, and legal fields respectively. As such, they attract the most resistance from traditional psychiatry, eager to defend its power of internment and hospital treatment.

Mental health in Argentina today: tensions, paradoxes, antagonisms, and obstacles

The National Mental Health Law of 2010 guarantees the abstract right, but not its active exercise, which also depends on extra-legal factors of which the two most important are the political will to execute stated principles through appropriate regulatory systems, and the intent to practice them in the relationship between professionals and users. This is a crucial combination, as maintained by Basaglia on the subject of Italy. However, in our case, both these elements are weak and there remains a wide gap between principles and practice.

Since the passing of the Law, and particularly in the Macri government, whose neoliberal orientation tends to sacrifice the rights and needs of the weakest in the name of 'growth', few investments have been made in its implementation. Action for the practical realization of its principles has been taken mainly in the legal field by human rights movements. In Argentina, these are the protagonists in the struggle for a more just, equal, and inclusive society. The services, however, have been far less responsive, and initiatives for implementation have developed only in a few local contexts. Overall, there has been no real deinstitutionalization, whereby resources and competences should be transferred, along with users, from psychiatric hospitals to the community. Little has been done to create services in the community such as apartments for users, beds for acute crisis management in general hospitals, job placement schemes, and the like. In other words, the infrastructure of community services and practices, necessary in order to really supersede the asylum model, remains very weak. Conversely, as we have seen, survival of the latter is backed by traditional psychiatry.

So, contradictory practices and models coexist, psychosocial conceptions coexist with the persistent presence of the asylum, still exerting its charm. The presence of community-based services does not really interrupt the vicious circle between the psychiatric focus on controlling behaviours, the label of dangerousness on mental suffering, and the related treatment in terms of internment. Rights are still frequently violated, and routine forms of institutional violence on people's dignity and bodies are repeated. Moreover, despite advances in the active presence of users' associations, users do not have a leading role, nor are their voices heard loudly in society or within health services.

A comparison with Italian reform, driven by Basaglia's ideas, which, as we have seen, has profoundly impacted the mental health law in Argentina, shows that some major obstacles to implementing the latter seem to be connected to a few differences between the two. The first one lies in the different role attributed to the general hospital. In Italy, this only provides crisis units supporting a community-based mental health system centred around mental health centres. These centres, well integrated within urban contexts and open 24/7 (as happens in Trieste), are responsible for coordinating the whole of the system's resources (including social cooperatives) and those of the social and health services in the territory. They handle all problem situations affecting people's health and ensure continuity of care (although not all Italian regions have such a comprehensive system). This is consistent with Basaglia's recommendations on the importance of making the community-based system entirely fit to replace hospitalization (De Leonardis and Emmenegger, 2011).

In Argentina, on the other hand, the system is centred around the general hospital, which is in charge of providing hospitalization (the alternative to the asylum), and of promoting and coordinating community-based agencies. This choice, implied in the term 'desmanicomialización' in the Río Negro experience, aims at a medical normalization of psychiatry. This, however, has the perverse effect of medicalizing situations of mental suffering. It is well recognized how reluctant medicine is to abandon the logic of hospitalization and open up to social reality, particularly where the biomedical paradigm plays a hegemonic role (Rotelli, 1999; Saraceno, 2017). Therefore, there is little impulse to the development of community-based agencies and little action can be taken to overcome the fragmentation of the health system, which facilitates exclusion. The disarticulation between the different national, local, and municipal jurisdictions limits the opportunities to establish new ways of treating mental suffering. The persistent compartmentalization between policy sectors makes it difficult to pursue the integrated perspective which is possible in Italian mental health centres in the community.

Secondly, the different experience of professionals in the two cases should be considered. The Italian reform process was characterized by the strong and widespread engagement of professionals, whatever their competences and their levels in the hierarchy. 'Psichiatria Democratica' (and now 'Forum Salute Mentale') were, and are, veritable national movements. In Argentina, on the other hand, activism by professionals was, and is, limited and fragmented. There is little attention to their involvement and training in the new care paradigm.

These issues have triggered discussion and fostered local projects and associative actions. Among these, the Basaglia Argentina Conference, established in 2012 and included in the Permanent Conference for Mental Health in the World (COPERSAMM), serves as an important base for dealing with these matters and illustrating Italy's psychiatric thinking and experience. Training programmes, backing of local projects for services' reorganization, promotion of public debates (all coordinated by Giovanna del Giudice) are still being launched with the financial and technical support of Regione Friuli Venezia Giulia and the Trieste Department of Mental Health, and with the cooperation of groups and associations (inside and outside the realm of psychiatry) actively engaged in the defence of human rights.

Conclusions

The first thing to highlight when summing up the influence of Basaglia's thought and practice in Argentina is its durability. It began to make itself felt at the end of the dictatorship, through the participation of a few prominent innovating professionals—Vicente Galli on the one hand, and the protagonists of the Río Negro reform, Graciela Natela and Hugo Cohen, on the other—in the network of international exchanges that developed around Basaglia and other leaders of the Italian experience. Basaglia's influence was felt in local experiences, provincial reforms, and interventions on national regulations, until the passing of Reform Law 26657, which, in its aim to supersede the asylum, adopted Basaglia's underlying perspective. Therefore, it had an impact at policy-making level and on national political choices. To this day, in the slow and troubled implementation of the reform, associations and projects continue to be inspired by the Italian reform process. They continue to cultivate relations and exchanges with the experience in Trieste, where Franco Rotelli and his collaborators have been fundamental in giving practical shape to Basaglia's ideas. The publication in Argentina of books and articles on Italian reform and the Trieste reality also bears testimony to this interest (Rotelli, 2014; Del Giudice, 2017; Mezzina, 2017; De Leonardis et al., 1995; De Leonardis and Emmenegger, 2011).

Even the difficulties, obstacles, and fragilities that affect the implementation tell us something about this influence, and especially about its potential for innovation, where people are treated within their social contexts and these contexts, in turn, become a treatment resource.

In the capital city alone, four public asylums are still working, two of which have more than 600 people hospitalized, and one of which is for children. Not only is the process of reform slow but also, in relation to asylum closure, a more general, more radical game is being played—a change which goes beyond psychiatry. The large numbers we are still facing remind us of the asylum's historical function, so well recounted by historial-critical literature (starting from Foucault, 1998), and which has acted as a benchmark for Basaglia's challenge of deinstitutionalization. In Basaglia's words, what is needed is:

> The analysis of a series of problems, which are not specific psychiatric problems, to show how action—laden with contradictions—is possible within an *institution of violence*, and how this action reflects the global violence of our social system ... Our anti-institutional, anti-psychiatric discourse cannot be limited to the specific terrain of our field of action. Confrontation with the institutional system goes beyond the psychiatric sphere to enter the domain of the social structures that support it and forces us into a critique of scientific neutrality, acting in favour of dominant values—and must eventually turn into political critique and action.
>
> **(Basaglia, 1968, pp. 7–9).**

These numbers tell us that the function of segregation and neutralization of life forms clashing with the social order is operating still. It excludes human suffering caused by margination, poverty, and solitude, by maladjustment to or expulsion from the labour market, and by the lack of social protection. The label 'social dangerousness' attributed to human suffering, as claimed by Basaglia, is due to its embodying the contradictions of the capitalist social order, the destructive potential of which originates from its subjection to economic imperatives. This is all the more so in the current neo-liberal regime.

This 'denial of contradiction' finds its archaic form in the asylum. Currently, however, more modern techniques of segregation, 'expulsion', silencing are widespread (Sassen, 2014). In Italy, asylums may be closed but techniques to deny the problem—the unacceptability of (mental) suffering—are multiplying, especially against migrants. The persistence (in Argentina and elsewhere) of the asylum model is only one piece of this varied puzzle of exclusion. Old and new 'walls' coexist (De Leonardis, 2013).

But this persistence also highlights the continuing complicity of psychiatry with the violence thus exerted, as denounced by Basaglia. This is the revolutionary basis of his political thought. A very interesting development is the encounter between Basaglia's heritage and the heritage of human rights struggles, of which Argentina is a significant example. It is an example of where two perspectives (from the North and the South) can be combined, and which is worth monitoring, by investigating the common projects we have mentioned.

The strong support given to anti-asylum drives by movements and institutions for the defence of human rights means that a strong synergy exists against old and new forms of institutional violence. These manifest, in the North and the South alike, in removing, denying, and silencing suffering inflicted by an unjust system. This system seems to have itself silenced and expunged the issue of social justice. This encounter could bear additional fruit. Despite differences between the legal frame of 'social rights' (including the right to health) and that of 'human rights' (including the right to services and advocacy), a point of convergence can be found.

The core of Basaglia's programme was, what he called, 'patients' protagonism' or, as Amartya Sen would say, 'the capability for voice" of the most disadvantaged (Sen, 1999). Sen's thinking and approach serve as a good bridge between the two perspectives. Basaglia's objective to reverse 'people's invalidation' processes by giving them a say on what directly concerns them means cultivating their 'capability for voice', even in the face of obstacles and denial.

Acknowledgement

The authors wish to express their gratitude to the translator, Chiara Arnone, for her extensive work in making this chapter possible.

References

Alberdi, J.M. (2012). Desafíos políticos y asistenciales de la nueva ley de salud mental. El caso de la provincia de Santa Fé [Political and welfare challenges of the new mental health law. The case of the province of Santa Fé]. *Revista Debate Público, Reflexión de Trabajo Social* 2(4):93–107.

Amarante, P. (2009). *Superar el manicomio. Salud mental y atención psicosocial* [*Beyond the Asylum: Mental Health and Psychosocial Care*]. Buenos Aires: Editorial Topía.

Baffo, C, Paulin, M, and Onocko, R. (2018). *Perspectivas de la Desmanicomialización* [*Perspectives of Desmanicomialización*]. Buenos Aires: Editorial Kuruf.

Basaglia, F. (1968). *L'Istituzione Negata* [*The Institution Denied*]. Torino: Einaudi.

Basaglia, F. (1973). *Che cos'è la psichiatria?* [*What is psychiatry?*]. Torino: Einaudi.

Basaglia, F. (1973). Il lavoro rende liberi? [Does work make free?] In: *Che cosa è la psichiatria?* Torino: Einaudi, pp. 69–151.

Basaglia, F. and Ongaro Basaglia, F. (1975). *Crimini di pace: Ricerche sugli intellettuali e sui tecnici come addetti all'oppressione* [*The Crimes of Peace: Research on Intellectuals and Technicians as Agents of Oppression*]. Milano: Baldini Castoldi Dalai.

Basaglia, F. (1977). *La utopía de la realidad* [*The Utopia of Reality*]. Trieste: Departamento de Salud Mental de Trieste. Available at: http://www.triestesalutementale.it/spagnolo/basaglia_1972_lautopiadelarealidad.pdf

Basaglia, F. (2000). *Conferenze Brasiliane* [*Brazilian Conferences*]. Milano: Raffaello Cortina.

Barcala, A. and Laufer, M. (2015). La Ley Nacional de Salud Mental y su enfoque de derechos humanos: la interdisciplina y el nuevo rol de la defensa pública [The National Mental Health Law and its human rights approach: interdisciplinarity and the new role of public defense]. In: S. Faraone, E. Banchi, and S. Giraldez (eds), *Determinantes de la salud mental en Ciencias Sociales.* Buenos Aires: Departamento de publicaciones de la Facultad de Derecho y Ciencias Sociales de la Universidad de Buenos Aires, pp. 79–90.

Barcala, A. and Torricelli, F. (2013). Ampliando los márgenes de la clínica. Trayectoria de un Programa de Salud Mental Comunitaria para niños, niñas y adolescentes desde una perspectiva de derechos en la Ciudad de Buenos Aires [Expanding the margins of the clinic. Trajectory of a community mental health programme for children and adolescents from a perspective of rights in the City of Buenos Aires]. *VERTEX, Revista Argentina de Psiquiatría* 24:67–75.

Castel, R. (1986). *Las Metamorfosis de la Cuestión Social?* [*The Metamorphoses of the Social Question*]. Buenos Aires: Paidos.

Carpintero, E. and Vainer, A. (2018). *Las huellas de la memoria II: psicoanálisis y salud mental en la argentina de los '60 y '70: tomo II* [*The Traces of Memory II: Psychoanalysis and Mental Health in Argentina in the '60s and' 70s*]. Buenos Aires: Editorial Topía.

Cohen, H. and Natella, G. (2007). *Trabajar en salud mental: la desmanicomialización en Río Negro* [*Working in Mental Health: Desmanicomialización in Río Negro*]. Buenos Aires: Editorial Lugar.

Cohen. H. and Natella, G. (2013). *La desmanicomialización: crónica de la reforma de salud mental en Río Negro* [*Desmanicomialización: A Chronicle of Mental Health Reform in Río Negro*]. Buenos Aires: Editorial Lugar.

Colucci, M. and Di Vittorio, P. (2006). *Franco Basaglia.* Buenos Aires: Ediciones Nueva Visión.

Chiarvetti, S. (2008). La reforma en salud mental en la Argentina: una asignatura pendiente [The mental health reform in Argentina: a pending issue]. *Revista Argentina de Clínica Psicológica* 17:173–82.

De Leonardis, O. (2013). Altrove. Sulla configurazione spaziale dell'alterità e della resistenza [Elsewhere. On the spatial configuration of alterity and resistance]. *Rassegna Italiana di Sociologia* LIV(1):21–43.

De Leonardis, O. and Emmenegger, T. (2011). La desinstitucionalización italiana: pistas y desafío [Italian deinstitutionalization: clues and challenge]. *Revista Argentina de Psiquiatría* 22(95):31–44.

De Leonardis, O., Mauri, D., and Rotelli, F. (1986). Deinstitutionalisation another way: the Italian mental health reform. *Journal of Health Promotion* 2:84–98.

De Leonardis, O., Mauri, D., and Rotelli, F. (1995). *La empresa social* [*The Social Enterprise*]. Buenos Aires: Edición Nueva Visión.
Del Giudice, G. (2017). La contención mecánica: ¿tratamiento sanitario o violación de derechos humanos? [Mechanical containment: sanitary treatment or violation of human rights?] In: *Derechos de las Personas con Discapacidad*. Buenos Aires: Ministerio Público de la Defensa, pp. 65–74. Available at: https://www.mpd.gov.ar/pdf/publicaciones/biblioteca/Libro%20discapacidad%20con%20ISBN.pdf
Evaristo, P. (2000). *Psiquiatría y Salud Mental* [*Psychiatry and Mental Health*]. Trieste: Asterios Editore.
Faraone, S. (2012). 'Cartografía Sobre la Desinstitucionalización en Argentina' ['Cartography on the Deinstitutionalization in Argentina']. PhD Thesis. Buenos Aires: Universidad de Buenos Aires, Facultad de Ciencias Sociales.
Faraone, S. and Valero, A. (2013). *Dilemas en Salud Mental: sustitución de las lógicas manicomiales. Resultados de una investigación en torno a las instituciones totales* [*Mental Health Dilemmas: Replacing the Asylum Logic. Results of an Investigation into Total Institutions.*]. Buenos Aires: Editorial Madres de Plaza de Mayo.
Ferro, R. (1989). *Análisis y Evaluación del Desarrollo de Recursos Humanos para la Salud Mental en Argentina 1983–1989* [*Analysis and Evaluation of the Development of Human Resources for Mental Health in Argentina 1983–1989*]. Buenos Aires: OPS/OMS-Dirección Nacional de Salud Mental.
Ferro, R. (2010). Salud Mental y Poder. Un abordaje estratégico de las acciones en salud mental en la comunidad [Mental health and power. A strategic approach to actions in mental health in the community]. *Revista de Salud Pública* 14(2):47–62.
Foucault, M. (2002). *Vigilar y castigar* [*Discipline and Punish*]. Buenos Aires: Editorial Siglo XXI.
Foucault, M. (1998). *Storia della follia nell'età classica* [*Madness and Civilization: A History of Insanity in the Age of Reason*]. Milano: Rizzoli.
Galende, E. (1990). *Psicoanalisis y salud mental* [*Psychoanalysis and mental health*]. Buenos Aires: Editorial Paidós.
Galende, E. (1997). *Un horizonte incierto. Psicoanálisis y salud mental en la sociedad actual* [*An uncertain Horizon. Psychoanalysis and Mental Health in Today's Society*]. Buenos Aires: Paidós
Galli, V. (2011). Problemática de la salud mental en Argentina [Mental health issues in Argentina]. *Voces en el Fénix* 4(7). Available at: www.vocesenelfenix.com
Galli, V. (2014). Introducción [Introduction]. In: F. Rotelli (ed.), *Vivir sin manicomios: la experiencia de Trieste*. Buenos Aires: Editorial Topía, p. 6.
Garcia, M. and Torricelli, F. (1996). Dispositivos de una red sanitaria europea [Strategies for a European health network]. *Revista Clepios* 1(2):16–20. Available at: http://www.editorialpolemos.com.ar/docs/clepios/clepios3.pdf
Goffman, E. (1963). *Stigma: The Deteriorated Identity*. Buenos Aires: Amorrortu Editors.
Mezzina, R. (2017). Servicios comunitarios de salud mental con puertas abiertas y sin restricciones en Trieste, Italia [Mental health community services with open doors and without restrictions in Trieste, Italy]. *Revista Topía*. Available at: https://www.topia.com.ar/articulos/servicios-comunitarios-salud-mental-puertas-abiertas-y-restricciones-trieste-italia
Mental Disability Rights International (MDRI) and Centro de Estudios Legales y Sociales (CELS) (2007). *Vidas arrasadas: la segregación de las personas en los asilos psiquiátricos argentinos* [*Destroyed Lives: Segregation of people in Argentina's Psychiatric Asylums*]. Buenos Aires: Siglo XXI Editores.
Murekian, N.G. (2006). 'Salud mental y representaciones sociales: estructuras, procesos y contextos. De la desmanicomialización y sus impactos representacionales en población

adulta y en grupos de expertos, Ciudad de Viedma y Ciudad de Buenos Aires' ['Mental health and social representations: structures, processes and contexts. Desmanicomialización and its representational impacts in adult population and in groups of experts, City of Viedma and City of Buenos Aires]. PhD Thesis. Buenos Aires: Universidad de Buenos Aires, Facultad de Psicología.

Murekian, N. (2013). La desmanicomialización como objeto de estudio [Desmanicomialización as an object of study]. In: H. Cohen and G. Natella (eds), *La desmanicomialización: crónica de la reforma de salud mental en Río Negro*. Buenos Aires: Lugar Editorial, pp. 359–90.

Nicasio, F. (1999). Proyectos de inserción en el trabajo. Producción de autonomía, itinerarios de ciudadanía [Work placement schemes: production of autonomy, itineraries of citizenship]. *Materia Prima* 11:23–32.

Pellegrini, J. (2009). *Salud ES sin encierros* [*Health IS without Closures*]. Buenos Aires: Editorial Polemos.

Rotelli, F. (1999). *Per la normalità* [*For Normality*]. Trieste: Asterios Editore.

Rotelli, F. (2014). *Vivir sin manicomios: la experiencia de Trieste* [*Living Without Asylums: The Experience of Trieste*]. Buenos Aires: Editorial Topía.

Rotelli, F. (2015). *L'istituzione inventata* [*The Invented Institution*] *Almanacco Trieste 1971–2010*. Merano: AlphaBeta Verlag.

Saidon, O. and Troianovski, P. (1994). *Políticas en Salud Mental* [*Policies in Mental Health*]. Buenos Aires: Editorial Lugar.

Saraceno, B. 1995). *La fine dell'intrattenimento* [*The End of Entertainment*]. Milano: Ethas Compass.g

Saraceno, B. (2014). Prólogo [Preface]. In: H. Cohen and G. Natella (eds), *La desmanicomialización: crónica de la reforma de salud mental en Río*. Buenos Aires: Lugar Editorial, pp. 9–12.

Saraceno, B. (2017). *Sulla povertà della psichiatria* [*On the Poverty of Psychiatry*]. Milano: Derive e Approdi.

Sassen, S. (2014). *Expulsions: Brutality and Complexity in the Global Economy*. Boston: Harvard University Press.

Sava, A. (2009). Una experiencia desmanicomializadora [An Experience of Desmanicomialización]. *Diario Página* 12. Available at: https://www.pagina12.com.ar/diario/psicologia/9-120171-2009-02-19.html.

Sen, A. (1999). *Development as Freedom*. Oxford: Oxford University Press.

Svampa, M. (2008). *Cambio de epoca. Movimientos sociales y poder politico* [*Change of Time. Social Movements and Political Power]*. Buenos Aires: Siglo XXI.

Sturla, S., Cocciaglia, N., and Bistuer, J. (2009). Testimonio de lo posible, Trieste [Testimony of the possible, Trieste]. *Revista Topía*. Available at: https://www.topia.com.ar/articulos/testimonio-de-lo-posible-trieste

9
Spain

The critical movements and the influence of Franco Basaglia and 'Democratic Psychiatry'

Victor Aparicio Basauri

> It is proper for the critical spirit not to accept any assertion without prior investigation of its validity and meaning, either from the perspective of its content, or from its origin.
>
> **(Muñoz, 2003, p. 123)**

Introduction

The critical movements in the field of Spanish psychiatry arise in the context of the 'tardofranquismo'—the final period of the dictatorship of General Franco. It was a period when the decline of the regime coincided with the twilight of the dictator (Sánchez Recio, 2015).[1] This period stretches from 1969, when Franco appointed the future King Juan Carlos as his successor, until his death in 1975.

In the tardofranquismo, the opposition movements and resistance to the regime were increasingly active and increasingly represented the majority of the population. Universities played a key role after May 1968. Together with demonstrations and demands for the establishment of a democratic regime, the universities encouraged critical thinking about social and political reality. The environment was filled with hope and a thirst for change. A number of student leaders emerged who would subsequently play a fundamental role in the various areas of social and political life in the country. From these student movements—especially from the Universities of Madrid, Barcelona, Valladolid, Salamanca, Seville, Barcelona, Zaragoza, and Valencia—a group of young psychiatrists emerged who would later frame the psychiatric response movements that began in 1971.

[1] From 1960, Franco suffered from Parkinson's disease.

'The Psychiatric Coordinator' (1971–1975)

Origin

In September 1971, during the Eleventh Congress of the Spanish Association of Neuropsychiatry[2] in Malaga, the clandestine organization called 'The Psychiatric Coordinator' was created (González de Chávez, 2003). This was formed mainly of young psychiatrists and trainee doctors specializing in psychiatry, many of them with experience in the universities' radical movements. This organization was to be the engine of the critical movements in psychiatric care in the country, and operated between 1971 and 1975.

During this period, the mental healthcare model continued to be institutional, based on poorly equipped mental hospitals that depended mostly on provincial administrations (González Duro, 1975). The total number of psychiatric beds, provided by public administrations and religious orders, reached 42,751 in 1970, for a population of just over 34 million (Arroyo Pérez, 2003)— a bed rate of 126 per 100,000 population. In 1973, there were 24,312 beds for psychiatric patients (González Duro, 1980), but the needs of psychiatric care had been growing for years. The central government economic development plans of 1968 and 1971 included the construction of new mental hospitals, consolidating the dominance of the institutional model. In this context, a few provincial administrations (provincial councils)[3] began to modernize their mental hospitals, providing them with more staff and more resources. This was the case in Asturias (Oviedo Mental Hospital), La Coruña (Conxo Hospital), Vizcaya (several hospitals), Pontevedra, Huelva, and others. In the process of modernization, some of the most paradigmatic and influential psychiatric conflicts of the time arose.

The first two conflicts that contributed to the creation of the Psychiatric Coordinator related to the Mental Hospital of Oviedo and the Psychiatric Clinics of Ibiza, dependent on the Francisco Franco Provincial Health City in Madrid.[4] The Mental Hospital of Oviedo served Asturias and, in 1964, housed more than 1,300 patients. The reform process began in 1965 and was based on community psychiatry principles. A central idea of this process was to consider the asylum 'as an inadequate and ineffective place for the treatment of the mentally ill' (García González, 1980). Although initially, elements were taken from Anglo-American community psychiatry, in the end, the organization of care was based on the psychiatry of the French sector (García González, 1980).[5]

2 It is the first association of psychiatrists in Spain and was founded in 1924, in Barcelona, in the presence of E. Kraepelin (Aparicio Basauri, 1993). In 1932, it had 200 members.

3 A decree law of 1925 reinforced the role of the provincial councils as managers of assistance to the insane and indicated that, as a minimum obligation, they had to support a house of imprisonment for the demented poor (Defensor del Pueblo, 1991).

4 Francisco Franco Provincial Health City is now called General University Hospital 'Gregorio Marañón'.

5 The Mental Hospital of Oviedo opted for a deinstitutionalizing model following the experience of Basaglia in Trieste during the second psychiatric reform initiated in 1982.

The first crisis arose in May and June of 1971, after the struggle of the trainee doctors—referred to in Spain as internal and resident doctors (MIR)—over working conditions, with the aim of democratizing the management of the hospital. The initial response was dismissal of the MIRs and the Director. However, this sparked a movement of national solidarity which was remarkable for the time. With 25 hospitals and more than 2,000 doctors protesting, the Provincial Council acceded and reinstated the MIRs and the Director. In the second crisis of 1972, the emphasis was on democratic participation by hospital management. On this occasion, the administration decided to end Oviedo's deinstitutionalizing experiment, and dismissed 86 professionals. Thus ended the first great community experiment in Spain. Also, in August and September of 1971, conflicts arose in the Psychiatric Clinics of Ibiza in the Francisco Franco Provincial Health City. Here, the administration had decided, in an arbitrary manner, to reduce the number of beds. The sequence of the Oviedo conflict was repeated: dismissal of professionals, a solidarity protest in other hospitals, followed by reinstatement of the professionals. In addition, public administration committed to negotiate any future change with the staff (Rivas Padilla, 1980).

The experiment in the Mental Hospital of Oviedo (Asturias) was to be repeated in the Conxo Psychiatric Sanatorium (Santiago de Compostela-La Coruña). Here, the dismissed Director of the Mental Hospital of Oviedo arrived with a group of dismissed professionals. Conxo was a custodial and dehumanized institution with 1,502 patients when the reform began in 1972. The reform included organization into sectors, plus a therapeutic community model[6] within the institution, with participatory engagement in daily management (García González, 1980). The experiment in the Conxo Psychiatric Sanatorium ended in September 1975, after the dismissal of 16 professionals (García, 1979). Solidarity came from different parts of Spain, as well as from the 'International Network of Alternatives to Psychiatry' (known as 'Reseau') and from 'Psichiatria Democrática' (García Gonzalez, 1980).

Catalonia's institutions and Basaglia's influence

An experiment which was to have a special significance in this period took place in the Mental Institute of the Holy Cross (1972–1973) attached to the Hospital de la Santa Pau in Barcelona. This development was marked by a more anti-institutional character, with a practice that proposed 'the liberation of the most clearly oppressed group (the insane there)' (García, 1979). In January 1973, the group most active in anti-institutional practice was dismissed (21 professionals). This crisis had a great impact in the media and professional circles. Its echo reached international groups critical of official psychiatry. Even the Spanish Association of Neuropsychiatry, in

[6] The therapeutic community model implied that inpatients would participate in the life of the hospital, making decisions in assemblies and therapeutic group activities.

an agreement in January 1974, declared its criticism of the medical direction of the Mental Institute of the Holy Cross (García, 1979). Franco Basaglia's team from Trieste in Italy also sympathized with the dismissed staff (Sánchez Clemente and Infante, 1975). The leader of this development, Ramón García, had met Franco Basaglia between 1969 and 1970, in Barcelona, at a lecture by Basaglia at the Academy of Medical Sciences. From that moment on, the relationship was maintained, and members of Ramón's team learned about the experience of the Psychiatric Hospital of Trieste.

Ramón García, with Ana Serós and Luis Torrent, contributed the foreword to the Spanish version of *The Denied Institution* that was published in 1972 and became a reference book for Spanish radical movements. That same year, Ramón García promoted three other publications in Spanish by Franco Basaglia (García, 1972). The first was *Notes of Institutional Psychiatry. Psychiatric Care as an Anti-institutional Problem*; the second was *I Think of the Crazy People*; and the third, co-written with Franca Ongaro Basaglia, was *The Disease and its Double*. From his relationship with Basaglia arose Ramón's collaboration in the 'map of the shame'. This project had the objective of giving an account of the situation regarding psychiatric care in various parts of Europe (France, Germany, Italy, Spain, and England). Although the project was never completed, it formed 'an active group of international solidarity and support for the movements of rupture with the asylum' (García, 1979). It was also important as the antecedent of the birth of 'Réseau' in Brussels, in 1975 (Elkaïm, 1979).

The critical movements that worked in the psychiatric hospitals of Catalonia were propelled by the experience of the Mental Institute of the Holy Cross. The protest was kept up by the Psychiatric Coordinator in Catalonia. Together with the Psychiatry MIRs, they maintained continuous activity between 1973 and 1975 in three of the four provinces of Catalonia (Barcelona, Gerona, and Tarragona). Every Friday, meetings were held at the College of Physicians of Barcelona, where the situation in each psychiatric hospital and the strategies to be followed were analysed. The fruit of this activity was the success of the complaint about degrading conditions in the Psychiatric Hospital of Salt (Gerona), which three MIRs of that hospital presented in 1974. With the collaboration of the Psychiatric Coordinator of Catalonia, they presented it to the College of Technical Architects of Catalonia in Barcelona.[7] The complaint cited the living conditions of the 860 patients, focusing on the 'monotony, poor hygienic conditions, prohibitions such as not being able to talk between men and women or women not being allowed to smoke or wear pants' (Aparicio Basauri, 1980). The situation was a perfect example of what Goffman (1961) called a 'total institution'. Along with this, there was talk of a lack of human resources and funding, of overcrowding, and of the use of punishment measures (cells, chains). The denunciation had its effect and the Provincial Council of Girona began a reform process with increased funding and staffing and the start of a sector organization with social reintegration policies.

[7] The conference was entitled 'Psychiatric care, a problem for everyone' and doctors Víctor Aparicio (from Salt Hospital), Luis Cabrero, and Luis Isern participated.

In the period from 1971 to 1975, more conflict situations arose in other mental hospitals with similarly limited resources. However, demands for improvements in care and the defence of human rights of the patients were now being raised. Crises arose when hospitals moved their care practices towards community models and also when they promoted more democratic management processes. The Dictatorship in this period was showing signs of weakness in the face of these various periodic conflicts. It made some concessions, but when the processes of change and criticism were sustained, the response was forceful: enforced lay offs of staff and an end to the developments.

In this tumultuous period, conservative psychiatry initially viewed the movement created by the Psychiatric Coordinator as transient and easily controllable. This judgement echoed the overestimated view of the Dictatorship that everything was under control. Attempts to modify the established order were repressed. However, little by little, the discourse of conservative psychiatry began to criticize the young psychiatrists in the critical movements. For instance, Professor López Ibor of the Complutense University of Madrid said, in 1972:

> Antipsychiatry, in reality, has to do with the ignorance of some people who believe themselves to be psychiatrists. Many new psychiatrists have come out lately who, if not immature, are certainly utopian and would surely do more to benefit psychiatry by working on and applying themselves to constructive things rather than disturbing it.
>
> **(Cited in Fábregas and Calafat, 1976)**

Similarly, the young Professor Valdés argued, in 1974, for the suppression of antipsychiatry and, in 2016, at the end of his career, he returned to the subject:

> As a consequence of this furious criticism, psychiatry foresaw danger in that cultural intelligence would end up dynamiting its conceptual foundations, burying psychiatrists and patients under the rubble. They had spent nineteen centuries trying to convert asylum inhabitants into patients and insane asylums into hospitals, and when psychopharmaceuticals allowed them to see the light, intellectuals would come with their pitchforks to threaten them with ostracism.
>
> **(Valdés, 2016)**

Conservative psychiatry moved away from mental hospitals to Chairs of Psychiatry of Medicine schools. It remained centred on the Spanish Society of Psychiatry, an association created during the dictatorship and with a marked biological emphasis.

Objectives and organization

The genesis of the 'Psychiatric Coordinator' is found in the environment created by these psychiatric conflicts. It was organized around groups of psychiatrists from these hospitals and others where there was interest in modifying care. Its operational framework was simple, especially since it was a clandestine organization. There was only one secretary to coordinate the actions of the organization and spread information from the different groups in the hospitals involved. The headquarters of the secretariat was located in one of the hospitals attached to the coordinator and, for security reasons, every so often was transferred to another hospital. The first secretariat was in the Clinics of Ibiza of the Francisco Provincial Health City of Madrid in 1971. It then moved to the Mental Hospital of Huelva (1972–1973), the Mental Hospital of Salt (Gerona) (1973–1974), and, finally, the Neuropsychiatric Center of Martorell (Barcelona) (1974–1975).[8]

The objectives of the Psychiatric Coordinator were to maintain coordination between the groups working for transformation in different mental hospitals across the country. It promoted actions of solidarity when conflicts with the public administration arose, providing analysis of the situation and proposals for strategies of change. It also acquired influence on the decisions of the Spanish Association of Neuropsychiatry, which was the most sensitive issue for the hospitals. The Psychiatric Coordinator was most active in the hospitals of Oviedo and Conxo in the north zone, in the hospitals of Seville and Huelva in the south zone, in the hospitals of Valencia and Castellón in the east zone, and in the hospitals of Madrid and Catalonia (Aparicio Basauri, 1993).

Between 1971 and 1975, 10 national meetings of the Psychiatric Coordinator were held (González de Chávez, 2003). The first was in September 1971 during the Eleventh Congress of the Spanish Association of Neuropsychiatry. Here, the Association was able to agree to defend the democratic management of psychiatric centres after the first conflicts that had arisen in some hospitals. The Sixth Congress had a special meaning and was held in October 1973 at the Medicina School of Valladolid University on the occasion of the XII Congress of the Spanish Association of Neuropsychiatry.[9] During the inauguration, the organization of the Congress was requested to read a written document signed by 109 professionals. This asked Congress to address the issues of deficient mental healthcare in the country, plus the serious conflict in the Mental Health Institute of the Holy Cross of Barcelona. The organization of the Congress rejected the request and, as a consequence, the dissenting professionals organized a parallel Congress, the working groups of which looked at: (1) the study of psychiatric conflicts; (2) the Spanish Association of Neuropsychiatry; (3) the problems of mental health workers; (4) the rights of the mentally ill; and (5) alternatives to psychiatric care (González de Chavez, 2003).

The last meeting of the Psychiatric Coordinator was in 1975 in La Coruña, as an act of solidarity with those dismissed from the Mental Hospital of Conxo.[10] It was marked

[8] This Center belongs to the religious order of the Sisters Hospitallers and today is called Sacred Heart Hospital.

[9] The majority of the professionals who participated in the Psychiatric Coordinator were members of the Spanish Association of Neuropsychiatry.

[10] F. Guattari attended this meeting.

with an air of pessimism following the Conxo crisis, earlier that year, and the dismissal of MIRs in several mental hospitals (e.g. Salt, Albacete) after the national MIR strike of that summer (Sánchez Clemente and Infante, 1975). At the meeting, various proposals were raised about the future of the Psychiatric Coordinator, including its attitude towards the Spanish Association of Neuropsychiatry. The lack of agreement led me not to attend the XIII Congress of the Spanish Association of Neuropsychiatry in Mérida. Two months later, the political context changed radically with the death of the Dictator in November 1975.

The Psychiatric Coordinator maintained the close relationship with the Movement of the MIR Coordinator as this extended throughout the country, coordinating the MIRs of all medical specialties. This MIR Coordinator was very active in the defence of the labour rights of the MIR and in the improvement of the teaching system. Its most important activity was a strike, in the summer of 1975, about employment contracts. However, its consequence was the dismissal of numerous MIRs in several progressive mental hospitals, including the Mental Hospitals of Salt (Gerona) and Albacete.

Two years after the creation of the Psychiatric Coordinator, in October 1973, 'Democratic Psychiatry' was founded in Bologna (Basaglia et al., 1976), promoted by Franco Basaglia. From that moment, the relationship between the two organizations was continuous, with frequent exchanges and shows of support and solidarity in the most difficult moments. Table 9.1 shows the characteristics of each organization.

Table 9.1 Characteristics of the 'Psychiatric Coordinator' (Spain) and 'Democratic Psychiatry' (Italy)

	'Psychiatric Coordinator' (Spain)	'Democratic Psychiatry' (Italy)
Year/Place	1971 (Málaga)	1973 (Bolonia)
Status	Clandestine	Legal
Promote	Psychiatric reform (1985)	Law 180 of 1978 that promotes the closure of psychiatric hospitals
Current situation	Dissolved in 1975. Its ex-members elected to the Board of Directors of the Spanish Association of Neuropsychiatry in 1977, and transformed it into an association of mental health professionals.	Remains
Objectives	• Analysis of the situation of psychiatric care • Support and solidarity in conflict situations • Share information • Coordinate the different centres	• Continue the fight against the asylum • Continue the fight against exclusion • Underline the dangers of reproducing the excluding mechanisms

This generation of psychiatrists, who fought, through the Psychiatric Coordinator, for dissolution of the places of exclusion and for the human rights of those interned in mental hospitals, was called 'the generation of Democracy' by Gonzalez de Chavez (2003). Aparicio Basauri (1991) called it 'the generation of 72'—the year that Basaglia's *The Denied Institution* appeared in Spanish and supported the nascent Spanish anti-institutional movement (see Figure 9.1). It was also the year of the great crisis that ended with the first experiment in community psychiatry at the Mental Hospital of Oviedo.

In this period 1971–1975, other influential books, in addition to those of Franco Basaglia, were translated into Spanish. The most influential was the *History of Madness in the Classical Era* by Michel Foucault, which came out in Spanish in 1967.

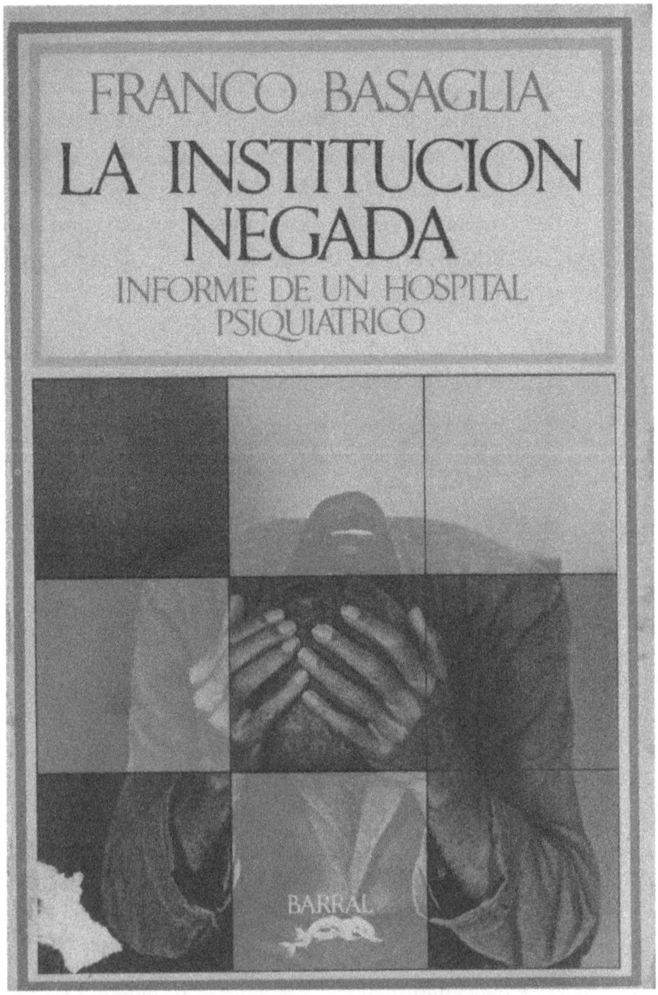

Figure 9.1 Cover of the first Spanish edition of *L'Istituzione Negata*, published in 1972.
Reproduced from *L'Istituzione Negata*. Translated by Seix Barral, 1972.

Erving Goffman's *Asylums*, much loved by Franco Basaglia, was published in Spanish in 1970. Finally, David Cooper's *Psychiatry and Antipsychiatry* appeared in Spanish in the same year as *The Denied Institution*, in 1972. Foucault (1973) was, for the Spanish critical movements, the first introduction of critical thinking about the place of psychiatry in relation to power. Foucault understood anti-psychiatry as 'everything that calls back into question the role of the psychiatrist formerly charged with *producing the truth of illness in the hospital space*' (Foucault, 2013, p. 37). Goffman's book (1961) clarified what a 'total institution', with its practices of 'mortification of the self', was in the Spanish institutional context. He defined it as 'a place of residence and work, where a large number of individuals in the same situation, isolated from society for an appreciable period of time, share in their confinement a daily routine, formally administered' (Goffman, 1970, p. 13). Basaglia's *La Institución Negada* [*The Denied Institution*] (1972) meant recognizing that it was possible to change psychiatric institutions.

The transition to psychiatric reform (1975–1982)

This period of transition took place in the context of political change after the death of the Dictator, with a new era marked by the approval of the democratic Constitution in 1978. A first qualitative change was the creation, in 1977, of the Ministry of Health. Before 1977, the authority of the Spanish state regarding health issues (which were then within the scope of the Home Office under a General Directorate of Health) had a lower administrative rank. Another of the changes to have repercussions in health was the administrative organization of the state into 17 autonomous communities, a federal formula very similar to that in Germany. Little by little, the governments of these autonomous communities assumed a range of responsibilities, among them health. However, this was not to be until 1982, when the socialist party won the elections, returning a state government without ties to the dictatorship. This produced a new sociopolitical context that provided a boost to the processes of psychiatric reform.

At the end of the period of the Psychiatric Coordinator (1975), the various conflicts had caused a diaspora of many of its members who had lost their jobs. Also, in this new period of political transition, remaining clandestine ceased to make sense, and so the Psychiatric Coordinator dissolved after the death of Franco. This did not prevent professionals critical of the country's healthcare situation, who longed for radical changes in this field, to continue contacts in an informal manner until 1977. In 1977, a fundamental change took place, influencing the changes to come in the following years. Ex-members of the Psychiatric Coordinator won the elections to the Board of Directors of the Spanish Association of Neuropsychiatry. From that year on, this Association led the anti-institutional movement and worked for psychiatric reform in the country. During this period, contacts and exchanges with Franco Basaglia and Democratic Psychiatry intensified.

In 1977, Franco Basaglia clarified his concept of anti-psychiatry in the Spanish magazine *El Viejo Topo*. He wrote:

> From time to time a certain misunderstanding about antipsychiatry is confirmed by understanding it as a 'new specialized technique' of psychiatric science. Antipsychiatry (I would like to clarify my opinion on this issue since the movement that I represent in Italy can be defined as anti-institutional or anti-psychiatric) is not a technique, nor a new methodology to be included within the psychiatric field, but a movement of denial and transformation that tends to put into discussion the schemes and parameters that are considered absolute values. It is, therefore, a critical movement that goes further away from the simple specialized problem facing a science that has become metaphysical, dogmatic, and that does not respond on a practical level to the patient and his illness, but is limited to the separation of the healthy and of the patient and, consequently, to the codification of the disease following established schemes as immutable.
>
> **(Basaglia, 1977, p. 35)**

Franco Basaglia, in his frequent contacts with the Spanish critical movements, was expressing his revolutionary ideas through lectures and interviews. The issue was increasingly taking a more important role in the media. In 1978, the year of Law 180, a debate programme on Spanish Television was entitled 'Are there crazy people?'. This debate included Basaglia, with the conservative psychiatrist Juan José López Ibor Jr., plus the newly appointed President of the Spanish Association of Neuropsychiatry, the progressive Valentin Corcés. In February of the same year, Basaglia held another debate at the Hospital of the Red Cross in Madrid, which was reported in the newspaper *El País* (García Pérez, 1978), in which he said that 'under all mental illness there is a social conflict'. Basaglia also held a critical discourse on Laing's position:

> Laing abandoned institutional psychiatry to go and create new institutions. The situation in the United Kingdom explains the appearance of an antipsychiatry alongside socialized medicine which is also repressive. The term antipsychiatry does not make sense. Laing is on the way to turning his activity into something intellectualistic ... He, in his criticism of psychiatric institutions, does not ask how and why what happens in the asylums happens.
>
> **(García Pérez, 1978)**

During this period, in addition to the relationship with Basaglia, links were established with other Italian professionals in Democratic Psychiatry. For the first time, a work appeared in Spanish on the characteristics and functioning of Democratic Psychiatry. This was produced by González de Chávez (1978) on the occasion of the screening of the movie *Locos de desatar*, produced in Parma and highlighting Democratic Psychiatry (Sáez Buenaventura, 1978). Basaglia's last intervention in Spain was at a conference of the Spanish Association of Neuropsychiatry in Gerona in 1980. The title of his conference paper was ' Legislation of commitment in Italy'; in the same meeting, his successor in Trieste, Franco Rotelli, made a presentation entitled 'The experience of Trieste'.[11] During those days, there were very intense debates. Among other things Basaglia commented that 'we have given the Word to the patient, giving the Word to the patient means changing the relationship with him'. Also, in replying to Carlos Castilla del Pino's presentation about the problems of psychosis psychotherapy, Basaglia told him that 'until I know what I can do with the asylum I can not know what to do with the psychotic' (Cascante et al., 1981).

This period was very dynamic, with the emergence of innovative developments in established psychiatric institutions, such as those of the Mental Hospitals of Málaga, Jaén, Sevilla, and Almería, directed by professionals who came from the Psychiatric Coordinator. Other changes occurred outside the institutions, such as the creation of community teams (Social Center of Ferrol-Coruña, Center for Mental Hygiene of Cornellá- Barcelona) and development of a day hospital under the principles of the therapeutic community in Madrid. Community work in Talavera de la Reina (Toledo) utilized a sectorization model and a psychiatric unit in a general hospital. The Spanish Neuropsychiatry Association underwent important changes when it approved new statutes to become a multidisciplinary association in 1980. At the same time, it promoted the development of associations in the autonomous communities, of which the Andalusian Association of Neuropsychiatry was the first in 1982. From 1977, the Spanish Association of Neuropsychiatry took a very active role in psychiatric care, promoting the abolition of asylums. It also promoted reform of the laws on hospitalization, seeking greater protection of patients' rights. At the same time, it acted where conflicts arose by sending a commission of experts who prepared a report with conclusions and operational recommendations.

Consolidation of the psychiatric reform project (1982–1986)

The victory of the Socialist Party in 1982 marked the beginning of social and political changes to strengthen the welfare state and democracy. During this period, there were significant changes in health and, more specifically, in mental health. A priority issue was to bring psychiatric commitment in line with the new Constitution of 1978. So, in 1983, the civil code on guardianship was amended to introduce judicial authorization of commitment (Article 211 of Law 13/1983 passed on 24 October), which presupposes a greater guarantee of patients' rights. The second important step was to approve the general framework for a reform of mental healthcare. After hard work in April 1985, the Ministry of Health and Consumer Affairs issued a *Report of the Ministerial*

[11] The 1979 *Bulletin of the Spanish Association of Neuropsychiatry* (2(2):10) shows the programme for those days.

Commission for Psychiatric Reform. In this, it indicated the need for 'specific plans for psychiatric hospitals, aimed at their transformation and progressive improvement'. The last great step was, in 1986, to approve the General Health Law that dedicates Article 18 to mental health. This requires that mental health 'will be carried out in the community sphere' and that 'the hospitalization of acute patients who require treatment

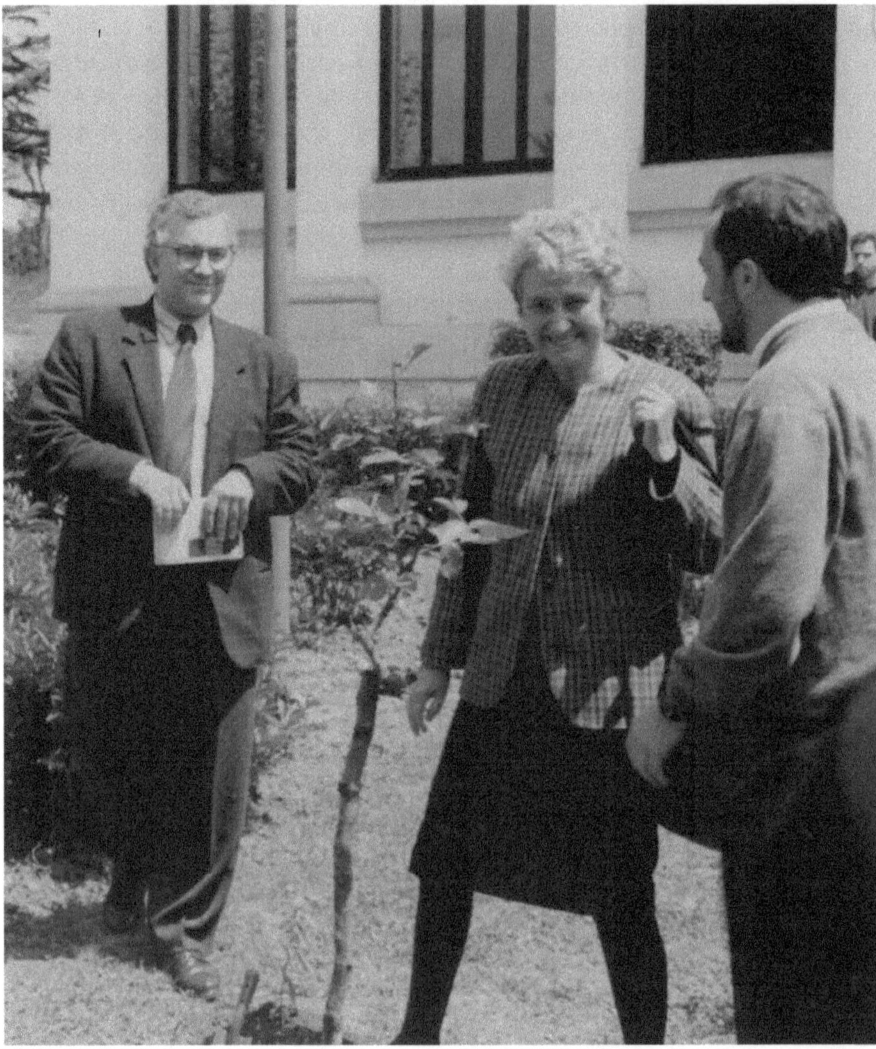

Figure 9.2 Franca Ongaro Basaglia (centre) at the unveiling of a plaque dedicated to her husband, Franco Basaglia, outside the Psychiatric Hospital in Oviedo in Spain. The other people in the photo are (left) Víctor Aparicio Basauri (the former Mental Health Director in Asturias) and (right) Javier Montejo (the former Director of the Mental Hospital of Oviedo).
Courtesy of Víctor Aparicio Basauri

under internment will be carried out in the psychiatric units of the general hospitals'. Both the report on psychiatric reform and the General Health Law are less explicit than the Italian Law 180 of 1978 that closed psychiatric hospitals. One reason may be that Italy, before the Law, had already accumulated experience of deinstitutionalization processes, while in Spain there was no such experience (see Figure 9.2).

The Law did, however, allow deinstitutionalization processes. An example is the reform in Asturias that created a network of community services for one million inhabitants, with the elimination of the Mental Hospital of the Oviedo, which in 1983 had housed more than 1,000 patients. The experience of Asturias was followed by that of other autonomous communities. The reform, however, has not been homogeneous throughout the country, and psychiatric hospitals still remain in some autonomous communities.

Conclusions

There is a certain parallel between the experiences of Italy and Spain—countries with very close cultures and languages, and both starting from an institutional model. Franco Basaglia and his team in the psychiatric hospitals of Gorizia and Trieste proposed a revolutionary change in the understanding of the processes of deinstitutionalization. Basaglia's thoughts had an important echo in the Spanish critical movements, and his relationship with Spain was intense and continuous, including participation in multiple acts and conferences. There was a striking harmony, collaboration, and parallelism between the two organizations that led the critical movements in both countries—the Psychiatric Coordinator in Spain and Democratic Psychiatry in Italy.

References

Aparicio Basauri, V. (1980). Análisis de la transformación del Hospital Psiquiátrico de Salt. In: M. González de Chávez (ed.), *La transformación de la asistencia psiquiátrica.* Madrid: Asociación Española de Neuropsiquiatría, pp. 553–65.

Aparicio Basauri, V. (1991). La generación del 72 ante el homenaje. *Anthropos* 121:21.

Aparicio Basauri, V. (1993). La Reforma Psiquiátrica de 1985. In: V. Aparicio Basauri (ed.), *Evaluación de Servicios de Salud Mental.* Madrid: AEN, pp. 127–82.

Arroyo Perez, A. (ed.). (2003). *Tendencias demográficas durante el siglo XX en España.* Madrid: INE.

Basaglia, F. (1972). *La institución negada.* Barcelona: Barral.

Basaglia, F. (1977). Anti-psiquiatría y 'Nuevas Técnicas'. *El Viejo Topo* 4: p. 35.

Basaglia, F., et al. (1976). Psiquiatría Democrática. In: A. Bauleo (comp.), *Los síntomas de la salud. Psiquiatría social y Psico-higiene.* Buenos Aires: Cuarto Mundo, pp. 35–9.

Cascante, C., et al. (1981). Los efectos de la institucionalización. *Revista de la Asociación Española de Neuropsiquiatría* 1:86–96.

Defensor del Pueblo (1991). *Situación jurídica y asistencial del enfermo mental en España. Informes, estudios y documentos.* Madrid: Defensor del Pueblo.

Elkaïm, M. (comp.) (1979). *Réseau Internacional, Alternativa a la psiquiatría.* Barcelona: Appiani Editora.
Fabregas, J.L. and Calafat, A. (1976). *Política de la Psiquiatría (Charlando con Laing).* Bilbao: Zero.
Foucault, M. (2013). Historia de la locura y antipsiquiatría. In: V. Galván (ed.), *El evangelio del diablo. Foucault y la Historia de la locura.* Madrid: Biblioteca Nueva, pp. 27–42.
García, R. (comp.) (1972). *¿Psiquiatría o ideología de la locura? Cuadernos Anagrama, Volume33.* Barcelona: Anagrama.
García, R. (1979). *¡Abajo la autoridad¡. Ciencia, manicomio y muerte.* Barcelona: Anagrama.
García Gonzalez, J. (1980). Una década de asistencia psiquiátrica (1965–1975) y dos intentos de psiquiatría comunitaria: el H.P. de Oviedo y el Sanatorio Psiquiátrico de Conxo. In: M. González de Chavez (ed.), *La transformación de la asistencia psiquiátrica.* Madrid: Asociación Española de Neuropsiquiatría, pp. 411–56.
García Perez, A. (1978). Franco Basaglia: 'Debajo de toda enfermedad psíquica hay un conflicto social'. *El País* 2 May 1978.
Goffman, E. (1961). *Asylums. Essays on the Social Situation of Mental Patients and Other Inmates.* New York: Anchor Books.
Goffman, E. (1970). *Internados. Ensayo sobre la situación social de los enfermos mentales.* Buenos Aires: Amorrortu.
Gonzalez de Chavez, M. (1978). Psiquiatría democrática. In: S. Agosti, et al. (eds), *Locos de desatar.* Barcelona: Anagrama, pp. 123–201.
Gonzalez de Chavez, M. (2003). La generación de la democracia: de la coordinadora psiquiátrica a la Asociación Española de Neuropsiquiatría. *Frenia* III(1):87–114.
Gonzalez Duro, E. (1975). *La asistencia psiquiátrica en España.* Madrid: Castellote Editor.
Gonzalez Duro, E. (1980). Historia reciente de la asistencia psiquiátrica en España. In: M. González de Chavez (ed.), *La transformación de la asistencia psiquiátrica.* Madrid: Asociación Española de Neuropsiquiatría, pp. 117–29.
Ministerio de Sanidad y Consumo [Ministry of Health and Consumer Affairs] (1985). *Informe de la Comisión Ministerial para la Reforma Psiquiátrica.* Madrid.
Muñoz, J. (2003). *Diccionario Espasa de Filosofía.* Pozuelo de Alarcón: Espasa Calpe.
Rivas Padilla, E. (1980). Análisis de la experiencia de cambio en las Clínicas Psiquiátricas de la Ciudad Sanitaria provincial de Madrid. In: M. González de Chávez (ed.), *La transformación de la asistencia psiquiátrica.* Madrid: Asociación Española de Neuropsiquiatría, pp. 457–502.
Saez Buenaventura, C. (1978). Comentario a 'Locos de desatar'. In: S. Agosti, et al. (eds), *Locos de desatar.* Barcelona: Anagrama, pp. 101–21.
Sanchez Clemente, M. and Infante, A. (1975). Los movimientos de masa del sector. In: A. Infante (ed.), *Cambio social y crisis sanitaria.* Madrid: Editorial Ayuso, pp. 247–78.
Sanchez Recio, G. (2015). *El tardofranquismo (1969-1975). El crepúsculo del dictador y el declive de la dictadura. Hispania Nova: Revista de Historia Contemporánea.* Número 1 Extraordinario: 329–48.
Valdés Miyar, M. (2016). *La arquitectura de la psiquiatría.* Barcelona: Plataforma Editorial.

10
Franco Basaglia's influence on the Greek mental health system

Theodoros Megaloeconomou

Introduction

The discussion of Basaglia's influence, on the fortieth anniversary of Law 180/78, has a crucial significance for the present, described by some as the 'dying of today', (Barker, 2008), with a deep economic, social, and political crisis across Europe. Currently, this is without any perspective of relief, and brings a diffused xenophobia and racism, and the rise of far-right populism. This does not leave psychiatry, mental health systems, and the rights of users unaffected. The Italian far right Interior Minister Matteo Salvini —relentless prosecutor of refugees, immigrants, and Roma —did not take long to attack those with mental health problems as responsible for an 'explosion of aggressive acts' in Italy. He specifically criticized Law 180/78 and the closure of the forensic mental hospitals: 'We are working for a better Italy. I am thinking of this absurd reform that has left in miserable conditions thousands of families, with mentally ill relatives' (Salvini at Pontida-Bergamo on 1 July 2018).

It is necessary to return to the conditions (the complexity of conditions) that made the establishment of Law 180 possible. First, the alternative psychiatric 'culture and practice', that contested, simultaneously, the dominant psychiatric 'circuit of control' and the dominant social norms, towards a system of services 'beyond all kinds of walls' (in and out of the total institution). A return to the practice that was the motive force, that made the establishment of this Law possible, re-examining, also, its actual implementation in those places where the practice already existed. A return also to the emancipative imperatives of that epoch—May 1968 in Europe and the 1970s in Italy—which made possible this deinstitutionalization movement and Democratic Psychiatry.

Can we conceive the establishment of Law 180/78 without the radical social and political movements during the 1970s in Italy? These movements contested the dominant social norms with their constituent micro-powers, as outlined by Michel Foucault. Such a return is indicated, as prevailing policies lead to ongoing dismantling (underfinancing, understaffing, etc.) of mental health systems. Orthodox psychiatry, with its commitment to social control and manipulated by big pharma, responds by the adaptation of its 'culture and practice' towards more repressive and controlling practices. In all countries, repressive practices, restraints, seclusion, revolving door, abandonment, and the like have risen to unprecedented levels.

Looking for alternatives to 'institutional walls'

In Greece, Franco Basaglia's influence began during the 1980s, with minority groups searching for an alternative to the dominant psychiatric paradigm. This was the period when the 'scandal of Leros' had broken out, and external pressure was being put on Greece to reform its obsolete institutional mental health system.

In psychiatry, as in many other sectors, Greece operated as a country 'importing models' from advanced countries. Given the nature of such international interaction, it was common that the imitation (or transcription) of such imported theories and practices was simple mechanical reproduction. One of the problems with this process is that it treats the various international practices as prototypes with a universal, absolute, and sometimes eternal validity. This can fail to consider the logic and methodology followed in creating them, and the unique, concrete reality that stimulated them.

Psychiatry in Greece was always (until recently) determined by the import not simply of these foreign models, but of their *crises*. They arrived when their limits and inadequacies were already obvious, both in their capacity to answer to the real needs of the users and in their ideological function in the renewal of social control mechanisms. One example is the French 'Secteur'. Not only were the inherent inadequacies of the original 'model' (its administrative characteristics, etc.) inflated, but its fundamental goal of ensuring 'continuity of care', from asylum to community, totally neglected. What was established was a 'triadic system' (mental health centre, general hospital, mental hospital), with inherent therapeutic fragmentation, instead of continuity of care.

The 'psychiatric reform' which started in Greece in 1984, with special financing from the EU (Regulation 815/84) because of the 'scandal of Leros', followed this process. The first years were characterized by a mixture of ignorance, perplexity, and bureaucratic impasses, but also by feverish discussions, searches, arguments, enthusiasm, and hopes. Social psychiatry, psychotherapeutic approaches, and deinstitutionalization efforts in the mental hospitals generated a small front against biological psychiatry and institutionalism. During this period, the demand (and promise) for developing a 'welfare state' was defeated as a consequence of the austerity measures required for Greece to join the EU.

The bulk of Greek psychiatry, the universities, the training of new psychiatrists, and the operation of the services, had remained committed to a traditional psychiatric paradigm. This transmutes *mental suffering* (the *experience* of the subject) and institutionalizes it in *disease*, in the sterilized abstraction of a *diagnostic category*. Its reaction to the revelations of the miserable conditions produced in Leros by such psychiatric practice fluctuated. It varied between superficial and limited engagement, at the level of 'image changing', and open opposition to any alternative approach. This included both biological and psychoanalytical schools.

All attempts towards real reform, on the basis of radical challenge to the dominant psychiatry (almost always through 'bottom–up' initiatives rather than official policy), were generally influenced by Franco Basaglia's thinking and the Italian deinstitutionalization camp. These attempts, although defeated by the system that they did not manage, in the end, to change, nevertheless left an indelible mark.

The emphasis was on the need for a practical approach which focused on the primacy of 'the person and not the illness'. The struggle against the psychiatric institution was a struggle against all institutions (including social,), knowledge, and practices that, instead of curing, suppress; against institutions that respond not to the needs of the person, but of the institution itself and the broader social order. To put 'the patient at the centre' and 'the illness in parentheses', Basaglia wrote that:

> The situation of the psychiatrist in our society which is more obvious from others, in the sense that his immediate contact with the visible condition of violence, of abuses and arbitrariness, requests the violence against the system which produces and permits them: either we become accomplices, or we react and destroy it.
>
> **(Basaglia, 1968)**

A crucial dimension of Basaglia's approach was that what we call a 'therapeutic dimension' has a *technical* and a *political* element. We should seek neither a techno-scientific reductionism nor an abstract politicization of mental illness or psychiatry. What matters is to find, in everyday practice, the political dimension of the contradiction which is obscured by the dominant psychiatric model.

> If the patient, is the only reality, to which we refer, both aspects of which this reality is constituted have to be faced: that he/she is a patient, with a problem of psychopathology (dialectical and not ideological) and that he/she is excluded, socially stigmatized.
>
> **(Basaglia, 1982)**

Consequently, the question is not the mere recognition of the complexity of the existential, social, and political dimensions of mental suffering, as something that gives an account of it from outside. We need, at the same time, for these dimensions to enter into *everyday therapeutic practice*. Real transformation in mental health is not just dissemination of so-called good practice, as our experience was in Greece all these years. The absorption of the political element by the technical one leads to an atrophy of the critical aspect, and to an undermining of the therapeutic dynamic. It reproduces the old 'paradigm' in a new form, serving the system for social control in new social conditions.

Basaglia goes on to demonstrate what he considered the meaning of *therapeutic*. This considers not only the mental hospital, but also community services, which may likewise become mechanisms for social control if they lose what Basaglia called the 'margin of freedom and of practical invention in a process of transformation'. (Basaglia, 1982). It is this 'margin of freedom' that constitutes the crucial point of the therapeutic dynamic of a real transformation. This is based on the theoretical and practical critique of the existing situation, and contests the function of psychiatry as an institution of control and assimilation. It is this critical/practical procedure, in which all parts participate and in which everything (the relations between all participants, roles, power relations, culture) is transformed, and not just transmuted.

First efforts during the 1980s

In line with this thinking, important developments took place in Greece in the 1980s. The Mental Hospital of Thessaloniki is a good example. Tens of inmates went out of the asylum into small group apartments, and most of them found paid work in co-operatives, created in the context of deinstitutionalization. Despite the positive results of this project, confirmed in successive reports of a special committee of the EU, this project was abandoned. Its 'sudden death' in the prevailing Greek situation was unavoidable. The attitude of the psychiatric community of the Mental Hospital had fluctuated from total opposition at the beginning to an, at most, lukewarm tolerance. This was, in part, because the project had been proposed by a university psychologist (Kostas Bairaktaris). He was scientifically responsible for it, had formulated its plan, and was leading the team that was implementing it. When the government changed, the administration of the Mental Hospital also changed (as is the case in the Greek public sector). A new orthodox university psychiatrist was appointed as head, who, through several subversive interventions, forced the leader to resign. The transformation had started in some long-stay wards but had not yet managed to influence the admission wards. So, some of the successful results of this attempt persisted, at least humanizing the hospital practice. The hospital's key position in the psychiatric system was not contested.

During this period, a first attempt was made at direct, official collaboration with Trieste. The move came from in the largest Greek mental hospital, the Psychiatric Hospital of Attica (PHA), once the largest in the Balkans. During the turbulent situation created by the international denouncements about Leros, there were moves by some psychiatrists and nurses to change the unbearable institutional conditions, particularly in the overcrowded long-term wards. The worst ward (for those one hundred judged 'irresponsible because of insanity') with extremely repressive conditions was abolished. With no proper provision for such patients, either in the traditional custodial form of a forensic hospital or in the direction of an alternative approach (beyond the concept of the absolute irresponsibility and the resulting indefinite detainment), they were transferred to the admission wards, where they remain today.

In parallel to these moves and demands from staff, there was a response from the Hospital's administration. Contact was made with Trieste, which was seeking acceptance by the Greek authorities for a programme of international intervention in Leros. It was agreed that a team of five mental health professionals would come from Trieste to work in the PHA, introducing an alternative paradigm for transcending the mental hospital. A feverish and subversive intervention was undertaken which lasted the agreed one year. This was perhaps too ambitious given the conditions. The whole venture failed to convince or take root. The hostile atmosphere in the psychiatric community and in the department in which the programme was implemented did not permit the changes proposed. The end of this programme meant also the end of any collaboration/interaction with Trieste and Basaglia practice for many years. The so-called reform in PHA was focused on developments, sometimes significant, but always partial, in the context of the enhancement of an institution that was never questioned as such.

At the same period, in Dromokaiteion, Athens' second mental hospital, attempts took place to oppose repressive practices and for the creation of cooperatives with paid work. One significant aspect of the intervention here was the move from the inside to abolish two so-called punitive wards (one male and one female), to which patients judged as 'undisciplined', were transferred. They remained for weeks, months, years, or, more often, permanently. These locked and extremely repressive wards were finally abolished by intervention from inside. However, this move had no effect on hospital functioning. The hopes and expectations generated from the successful experiences of paid work and for the creation of cooperatives, ended as simply occupational therapy, with, at most, some pocket money for a very few.

The situation had also changed significantly regarding rehabilitation, showing, in a concrete and material way, the possibility of going beyond the mental hospital. But as all these attempts were islands in a hostile environment, and constantly undermined, a comprehensive implementation was not possible. It could not be extended to the admission wards or the function of the psychiatric system in its totality. Although very significant, these experiences only partially challenged the mental hospital. The state and psychiatric community either remained indifferent to what was introduced or, through its incorporation into the system, transformed it into an image of modernization, obscuring its real message.

Leros: where 'the impossible became possible'

Confronted by the most complicated and difficult problems, Leros, in the 1990s, adapted an approach that acknowledged the complexity of whole problem of the planning and practice for real deinstitutionalization. This approach and practice —to make 'possible' what was considered 'impossible'—received substantial involvement from Trieste, in its methodology, culture, and practical delivery. The Leros experience is critically important not just because of its international dimensions but also for showing how Franco Basaglia's thinking and practice formed the axis for the whole work of transformation and for its successful results.

The Mental Hospital in Leros, officially called the 'Leros Colony of Mental Patients', was established in 1957, in the post-war and post-civil-war period in Greece. At that time, there was tremendous overcrowding in all mental hospitals and the only 'solution' found was the transfer of 'redundant patients' to new institutions, which would be created for this purpose. One of these institutions was created in the empty barracks left in Leros after the end of the Italian occupation in 1947. This was destined to shape the subsequent history of psychiatry in Greece. It had already been used (and continued to be used after the 1960s) for the internment of 'unwanted groups' (political prisoners, etc.).

From 1958 to 1982 (when transfers were stopped) about 4,000 mental patients, from mental hospitals across Greece, were transferred to Leros. The main criterion for transfer was the absence of any visit from a family member for a period of two years, later reduced to one year. Inevitably, the first to be transferred were those considered 'undisciplined'. The number of patients peaked at 2,700 at the beginning of the 1980s. Packed together, in squalid conditions, they experienced an enormously high death rate. When we went to Leros in 1990 to implement the reform programmes, the number of patients was 1,100. Patients had total institutional stays ranging from 30 to 50 years, Institutionalization, in its severest form, due to deprivation of the most elementary basics for a human life, was their main disease. There were only one or two psychiatrists and a completely untrained custodial staff, recruited from the local residents. This provided full employment on the island and created an economy that was entirely dependent on the institution (an 'institutional economy').

This situation was brought to light at the beginning of the 1980s, by a group of young doctors undertaking their Greek specialization training requirement (to work for one year in a rural health service) in Leros. After photographers and film-makers had visited and produced documentaries, the 'Leros situation' took on an international dimension and was discussed in various conferences. There was a public outcry and a demand from all over Europe for immediate change. This triggered an EU intervention (Greece had just become an EU member), which resulted in a decision to finance Greek psychiatric reform. This reform would focus on the 'Leros problem' but be implemented in all services across Greece.

At the time, there was no real enthusiasm on the part of official Greek psychiatry or universities to become involved in Leros. However, there were various international groups keen to engage. After a complex and risky process, involving protracted pressures and negations, a programme, comprising two parts, was formulated and finally approved in 1990 (this was a period of political instability in Greece). The first part of the programme was to be implemented by 10 Greek mental health NGOs. This provided for a two-month intervention by each NGO in order to select the most high-functioning patients and transfer them to hostels in mainland Greece. This part of the programme reflected the prevailing idea that the solution to the 'Leros problem' was its closure, by transferring the internees to other units in Greece. The second part of the programme provided for work 'from inside' towards the radical transformation and deinstitutionalization of the mental hospital.

It was this second part of the programme that benefitted from the participation of a group from Trieste (five persons—psychiatrists, psychologists, nurses) and a group from the Mental Hospital of Maastricht in Holland (five persons, all nurses). These collaborated with the Greek team, restricting themselves to the one part of the hospital where the responsible psychiatrists had formulated the programme. The two groups, from Trieste and Holland, had an 'advisor role through practical participation'. After two years, the programme was renewed and extended to all departments of the hospital, but without participation of the foreign teams. The programme was co-financed by the EU and the Greek State, with much greater funding of the NGOs' intervention than the internal transformation intervention.

The Trieste group took, in an unofficial way, a determining and leading role, through its strict collaboration with the two Greek psychiatrists (oriented towards the Basaglia approach). These had undertaken the initiative to form the second part of the programme, which involved an intense struggle for its approval with the Ministry of Health. Formation of the programme followed Franco Rotelli's proposals, after his visit to Leros in 1989. His proposal was not for abolishing, but for transforming and deinstitutionalizing the hospital, creating an 'International Rehabilitation Centre'. Members of the European Social Fund, which was to finance the programme, contributed to the international participation, as well as to its approval. The Greek team was composed mainly of young psychologists, just graduated from the Psychology Department of the Thessaloniki University (under Professor Bairaktaris), social workers, nurses, and occupational therapists. There were no new psychiatrists, except for the two already responsible for the programme. This team initially comprised about 30 individuals and grew to about 200 towards the end of the programme, with the addition of non-specialized personnel (carers, etc.).

'Leros' remains, in Greece, a term for what cannot be described, cannot be conceived; a kind of concentration camp or, even, a death camp. The miserable situations in any institution are often conveyed, in Greece, by the word 'Leros'. Today, we might use this term with a diametrically different meaning: meaning how people with severe mental health problems, handicaps, learning difficulties, or behaviour disorders were able, in Leros (though not only there), to be reintegrated into the community and to live a more or less autonomous life. How people previously considered as 'incurable' by their therapists, and unwanted by society and by their families, have reacquired a voice and social visibility, exercising and claiming their citizenship rights.

The term 'incurable' is usually attributed to people with severe mental health problems who, often, do not respond to the established treatments. They fall short of the therapist's expectations and, hence, are abandoned. People with such severe and complex problems are not usually selected to participate in rehabilitation and deinstitutionalization programmes. They constitute the usual excuse for insisting on the necessity for psychiatric hospitals. However, in mental illness, severity, as with chronicity, is not an exclusive, inherent element of mental illness. It depends on and is determined by the interactions of the subject with the totality of his/her social relations and social institutions. Among these, the psychiatric institution is not insignificant. It is mainly this institution that is responsible for institutionalization, chronicity, regression, and desocialization.

Basaglia referred to these questions in a discussion between the members of the team, in 1967, in Gorizia, about opening the last locked ward door. They discussed the relation between overthrowing the institution (the dismantlement of the mental hospital) and the overthrow of psychiatry. Does the latter come after the former? Basaglia says: 'We do it simultaneously, breaking (overthrow) of the wards and the breaking (overthrow) of Psychiatry... it is probable ... that modern psychiatry, is nothing less than a perfection of old psychiatry' (Basaglia, 1968). The programme that had to be formulated in Leros could not have been an a priori construction, but had to come into being through practical intervention. By understanding and responding to the needs of each person, they acquire the capacity and are given the opportunity to unfold their own life plan. Instead of the institution's power, we tried to establish a relationship through negotiation; a contractual relationship where all possibilities, all eventualities, were open.

In Leros, there was scarcely the possibility, even if one wanted otherwise, to select patients with higher functional ability and who promised the most likely positive outcome. This is because the internees in Leros had already been selected, before being transferred there, in the 1960s and 1970s. They were amongst the severest cases from the rest of the Greek psychiatric hospitals, who had been completely abandoned by their families.

The first challenge was to avoid the temptation (which might seem legitimate considering the appalling conditions in the hospital) to limit our action to a simple improvement of the patients' living conditions. We thought that the fact itself of responding to mental illness with internment in the hospital, irrespective of the conditions (albeit of considerable importance), constituted a simplified, one-dimensional answer to the complexity of their needs. It is this simplification that constitutes the essence of the total institution's violence.

Consequently, we saw the issue of humanization of the living conditions not as a question of merely upgrading the buildings and the facilities. We saw it also as a matter of transformation of the overall established, institutional relationship, that serves to objectify the patient. The question became one of how the suffering subject's complexity is restored. How the subject, with his/her own particular needs and wishes, comes to be the centre of attention, beyond diagnostic categories and prefabricated scientific aphorisms. How the institution's apparatus ceases to operate with the aim of its own propagation, but is gradually destructured and dismantled, to meet the subject's needs. In the place of the institution's power, we tried to establish a relationship through negotiation, a contractual relationship, where all possibilities, all eventualities, were open.

The intervention started from inside the institution, from within the psychiatric wards. To establish, firstly on a practical level, a new policy of mental health, from the bottom up, and driven by internees, mental health professionals, and other staff. To be established initially was the importance and immediacy of the personal relationship between staff and internees, for whom the primary concern was to secure the basic conditions of human dignity. Those who have worked this way, inside a psychiatric ward, can easily understand which new contradictions, which new forces, are set in motion. Such institutional changes reveal patients' basic needs (e.g. to get his own shoes, his own clothes, his personal space).

The slogan 'Freedom is therapeutic' in practice

In the beginning, some practical steps were implemented—simple things that are of great strategic significance. These not only met patients' needs but also transformed staff attitudes towards mental illness and the mental patient. The practice of restraints and seclusion were eliminated, emphasizing the establishment of personal relationships. This demonstrated, in a practical way, the principle *freedom is therapeutic*, not as an ideology, but as a therapeutic principle. We tried to organize, together with the staff, the answer to all the new contradictions that its implementation inevitably provoked.

Locked doors were unlocked and opened. The patient was helped to renew the relationship with his body. He was restored the right, the capacity, and the opportunity to acquire and use personal possessions; and also the right and the capacity to have a voice, so as to express emotions, needs, and wishes. We tried to foster the production of new relations, of new spaces for expression, and new topics of interest for discussion and exchange. There was the effort to create conditions and opportunities for freeing emotions, and for eliminating oppression and the practice of imposing a style of behaviour, a way of life, and such like. Practical steps were taken, together with the staff, in the direction of demystifying the mental patient's 'dangerousness'. This is a foggy concept, in need of clarification and a deeper analysis, around which the whole of the institution was organized, as is the overall social and scientific answer to madness. Strenuous efforts were made to obtain personal income (pensions, etc.), necessary for the material base for participation and access to social exchange. We also tried hard to limit, and then eliminate, 'black labour' within the psychiatric wards and the practice of simple occupational therapy, by introducing paid work. This soon resulted in the creation of the first informal cooperative activities.

We used the same means, the same resources, the same personnel that, until then, had been used for operating a closed, anti-therapeutic, and oppressive institution, to create the bridges, the means, and the resources towards autonomy and social integration. What we changed was the system of interaction within which these factors were operating, Our aim was to change the staff's attitude towards the mental patient. Consequently, we did not begin by creating structures alongside the institution, independent from the processes occurring within. Instead, the new structures arose as a result of the patients' new needs and wishes, as a product of the internal transformation of the mental hospital and of a new culture (or mentality) of the workers within it. In short, these structures came as an answer to the new needs which the institution could not satisfy.

It was through these processes that the creation of group apartments, outside of the hospital and within the community of Leros, began in December 1991. In the period, up until 1995, 20 community-group apartments were established within the local community, accommodating a total of 106 residents. This often-contested process brought about a change in the attitudes and the culture of local society. These developments required inclusion of provisions for their inevitable interactions with an alternative evolution of the local economy. This made clear the multidimensional character of the deinstitutionalization process: in addition to its therapeutic/scientific aspects, it has social, economic, political, and cultural aspects, and none of them can be treated separated from the others.

The logic behind the planning for the interior area of the mental hospital retains its significance, independent of the concrete reasons that necessitated it in Leros. It could be implemented wherever, in the deinstitutionalization process, there remained a number of patients who cannot or do not want to leave the premises. At the same time, a huge facility, with empty rundown buildings, was left in decline. Such buildings may also be threatening—reminiscent of internment, but also attracting some new kind of internment (which began, in 2015, with the creation of a camp for hundreds of refugees). The plan—more a "dream" than a "written programme"—was to transform the area of the hospital, including the new residential units, into an integral part of the urban development plan for the island. The aim was that by eliminating the walls, by transferring productive, cultural, and educational activities into the ex-psychiatric hospital, to give the old buildings a new use. However, this never happened.

The changes that took place in Leros State Mental Hospital did not create an ideal, non-contradictory situation. On the contrary, every new stage in the establishment of patients' rights meant resolving a contradiction by creating a new one; a lot of the old problems were maintained, together with new ones which arose from the emergence of patients' new needs. Patients started to have plans, hopes, and perspectives for the future. The most prominent new contradiction was between the new level of needs (e.g. a return to place of origin, more personal income, improved social and emotional relations), achieved through the deinstitutionalization process, and our now limited resources to respond. The institutional apparatus is not always able or willing to understand and respond to these emerging new needs from patients or services.

We cannot speak of a completed or finished situation. We must see deinstitutionalization as a continuous process that does not stop with the move of the patient outside the institution. Deinstitutionalization continues in community services and within social institutions, with the constant threat of a modernized (new) institutionalization. It asks for a simultaneous essential change in the provision of material resources, in legislative/institutional regulations, and in social attitudes and relations.

The demystification of the incurability concept

An indisputable result of our experience (which, of course, did not emerge only in Leros) is the demystification of the incurability concept. We saw the very real possibility of people with very severe mental health problems, through individualized support and protection, being able to recover. They developed the capacity for performing, the ability to access, and the subjective consciousness for claiming their citizenship rights. Finally, this experience exposes existing social racism, and the pseudo-scientifically anchored racism of psychiatric practice. It also makes explicit the anti-therapeutic, oppressive, and inhuman anachronism of the mental institution, whether low-, medium-, or high-security.

Leros, in the end, could not escape what usually (or always) happens in Greece when a deeply transformative attempt is completed. When the radical transformation wiped out the shame of the international scandal, the state authorities and psychiatric community (which had abstained from any participation in the intervention) considered that abnormal episode in Greek psychiatry to have ended. With the period of shame ended, we could pass on to the next stage with an unaltered traditional psychiatric paradigm, namely that which had created 'Leros'. Consequently, psychiatric reform in Greece, after Leros, is governed by theories and practices diametrically opposed to those that made radical transformation possible. Abruptly, in the middle of 1995, the EU proceeded to end financing of the programme. The Greek State did not provide support, and the process of transformation stopped, uncompleted. The partly transformed mental hospital was left to waste away. The evacuated buildings, for which proposals had already been made (creation of an international rehabilitation centre, a museum of psychiatric history, a museum of political history, etc.), were left to collapse. As predicted, we were left with an abandoned set of buildings, 'reminding and attracting some new kind of internment'. Such a new internment restarted in the creationin 2015 of a camp for hundreds of refugees.

Admission units with 'open doors and no restraints': neither illusion, nor utopia

Two further developments deserve to be considered. In 2006, the Chania Mental Hospital in Crete was closed. This was a small mental hospital. In accordance with the directives of the programme for psychiatric reform (still co-financed with the EU), it was due to close that year, together with four other small mental hospitals around Greece. On the initiative of a psychiatrist, practices of 'going beyond' the mental hospital were adopted and implemented. Chania Hospital was replaced by a comprehensive network of community services (e.g. a mental health centre, a mobile unit, cooperatives, community hostels), without leaving even the smallest gap that would open the way for the introduction of private psychiatric clinics, as had happened elsewhere when mental hospitals had closed down.

In the Psychiatric Hospital of Attica (PHA), in 1999, a new attempt was made, in one of its nine departments, to operate a mental health centre (MHC) to serve a defined catchment area (sector). This decision was made and implemented in a Greek context, where there is not (even today) any sectorization of services. The admission ward of this department started to work, from the beginning, with open doors and no restraints or seclusion. All this took place despite an extremely hostile reaction from the Ministry of Health and the Administration, and also from the majority of the hospital's psychiatrists, staff, and trade unions. The establishment of the mental health center MHC (Aghii Anargiri) resulted from a process of deinstitutionalization from inside the hospital. First, a long-term ward was closed (through the discharge of inmates to community hostels and group apartments), and then the admission unit was established in 2004.

A constituent element of the approach was the destructuring, in practice, of internment, initially in its more visible and restrictive forms (e.g. locked doors, restraints, seclusions). According to Basaglia, the practice of internment comprises a nucleus centred around the concept of protection, and delivered mainly in the form of custody, and therapy that is usually interwoven with deprivation of freedom. Open doors, with no repressive practices, operate as both symbolic and material expressions of an alternative approach, in the direction of a dialogue (real and not ostensible) and negotiation. This contrasts with various restrictive/repressive practices, direct or indirect, open or hidden, visible or invisible. The psychiatric asylum (either as a mental hospital or psychiatric clinic within the general hospital), being an anti-therapeutic institution, embodies a contradiction. It contains the element of protection, but in the form of objectification and reification of the person, so that this protection finally exists as 'cancelled protection'. In any process of a real (not simply cosmetic) transformation of the asylum, the element of protection has to be maintained, but not connected with repression, and under radically different conditions. It has to be provided in connection with the subject's freedom—a freedom that does not become equivalent to abandonment, but includes all-sided support of the person in the community. Ignoring the element of protection means practices of dehospitalization and of not going beyond the institution towards an alternative and comprehensive, community-based system of services. If these elements are not taken into consideration, then the culture and practice of internment are transferred, unaltered, into the psychiatric clinics of the general hospitals, as we have seen in Greece and in much of Europe.

The attempts in the PHA (Dafni), which functioned successfully for many years, had reached their limits when, for administrative reasons, the composition of the team was changed. The whole effort, under constant pressure from the hostile environment, came to an end through an inevitable implosion.

For all the reasons outlined here, Basaglia's influence in Greece did not take root. With the more conservative shift in economic, social, political, and cultural spheres, plus the monolithic rigidity of the psychiatric community, it did not manage to influence the system of services, or their culture and practice. The mental health system in Greece has proceeded in a modernized, neo-institutional direction, without transcending its repressive, hospital-based structure and operation. It is a system that is guided and determined by the dominant biological psychiatry, in close collaboration with (and manipulation by) the pharmaceutical industries. It has a high percentage of involuntary hospitalizations (around 65%), all executed by the police. The very few, understaffed MHCs function just as outpatient clinics (ambulatories). In addition, the greater number of all neo-institutional units (various types of hostels, with locked doors and sometimes restraints, and mobile units) are operated by NGOs as complementary elements to the dominant institutional structure-and several have been accused of corruption. All admission units, either in mental hospitals or in general hospitals, are constantly overcrowded. Wards with a capacity of 20–25 beds usually house 30–50 patients, packed into the corridors, or wherever space can be found. In most cases, locked doors are usual, as is the use of restraints (even for voluntary patients) In most admission units restraints for many patients, last for days, weeks, or even months.

The prevailing psychiatric culture and practice has responded to the high percentage of involuntary hospitalizations, by the introduction and implementation of compulsory community treatment orders, presented as the answer to the problem. The declared aim is to diminish these hospitalizations, without questioning the system that produces them; it is also to reduce the number of 'revolving door' patients. In both respects, it has been a complete failure.

The present significance of Basaglia's theory and practice

We need to be conscious that the current conditions (economic, social, political) are very different from those which anchored the movements for deinstitutionalization, for an alternative psychiatry, for anti-psychiatry. We know that, as with all dimensions of social life, mental health has a concrete, historically-shaped relation with the social organization, inside which it emerges. Franco Basaglia's remarks seem apposite to the current situation:

> The problem of the rehabilitation of mental patients—with the corresponding problem of the opening, or of the closing of the asylums and, because of this, of the grade of suppression or tolerance with which their management is taking place—is not connected directly so much with the presence or the absence of the pathological factor, as with the bigger or smaller need for disposable labor reserves necessitated by production, that is, the bigger or smaller demand by the market. As far as the economic criteria do not exist for absorbing the marginal minorities, the intervention of the experts of Psychiatry will remain a possibility unrealizable on the practical level. And then, the limits of normality will remain immovable in a way that exclusion and rehabilitation coincide simultaneously and in an equivalent way ... The rehabilitation of the patients in countries where the problem of full employment has not been

> resolved is an illusion of the experts, simultaneous with restriction of the norm (and as a result, of the exclusion of the deviants to the outmost ...) ... Those who are rehabilitated our society does not know what to do with them. Neither does it know what to do with all the individuals that are marginated as surplus of the concrete mode of production. Which means that the technical-therapeutic action, which seems capable to rehabilitate the mental patient ... cannot become acceptable and practically materialized by our present economic situation.
>
> **(Basaglia, 1982, pp. 105–25)**

For this reason, as he underlined elsewhere:

> If the reciprocity of the relation between the therapeutic place and the external society is not given, we will never be sure that walls, the cancels, the violence will not come back in order to be re-proposed, even under different forms, confirming the impossibility of a real rehabilitation.
>
> **(Basaglia, 1982, pp. 71–9)**

And, in conclusion:

> What is important is that we demonstrated that the impossible can become possible. Ten, fifteen, twenty years earlier it was inconceivable that the mental hospital could be destroyed ... Besides, it can happen that mental hospitals will be again closed and even more closed than before, I don't know that. But in many ways we proved that we can encounter the mad in a different way and this testimony is fundamental.
>
> **(Basaglia, 2000, p. 142)**

References

Barker, H. (2008). The dying of today. In: *Plays Four*. London: Oberon Books London.

Basaglia, F. (1968). Presentazione. In: *L' istituzione negata. Rapporto da un'ospedale psichiatrico.* Turin: Einaudi, p. 269.

Basaglia, F. (ed.) (1968). *L' istituzione negata. Rapporto da un'ospedale psichiatrico.* Turin: EinaudiTurin.

Basaglia, F. (1982a). Le istituzioni della violenza. In: F. *Scritti I*. Turin: Einaudi, Turin: pp. 497.

Basaglia, F. (1982b). Riabiliazione e controllo sociale. Presentation at the International Committee against Mental Illness, Helsinki. In: F. *Scritti II*. Turin: Einaudi,Turin

Basaglia, F. (1982c). Introduction to Maxwell Jones. Ideology and practice of social psychiatry. In: *Scritti II*. Turin: EinaudiTurin.

Basaglia, F. (2000). *Conferenze Braziliane*. Milan: Raffaello Cortina Editore.

Basaglia, F. and Ongaro Basaglia, F. (1969). Introduzione. In: *Morire di classe*. Turin: Einaudi, p. 78.

11
The United Kingdom's rejection of Basaglia

Tom Burns

Introduction

Franco Basaglia's influence beyond his native Italy is extensive, as this book confirms. In Mediterranean Europe and in South America he is a towering figure in the reform of mental healthcare, responsible for the movement to abolish mental hospitals and for a long-overdue focus on the human rights of the mentally ill. The fortieth anniversary of Italy's Law 180 ('Basaglia's Law') has been rightly celebrated in several countries, and there are established institutions in Brazil, Argentina, and Italy to honour his name and to perpetuate and develop his teaching. The World Health Organization has promoted his approach to psychiatry as a blueprint for development internationally, and his model service in Trieste has long served as a teaching and demonstration site. Despite this, it would not be unfair to say that his work has had limited attention, and negligible impact on clinical practice, in Northern Europe and North America.

The UK reception (or, more correctly, rejection) of Basaglia's reforms are probably the best documented, and so may serve to tease out some of these issues and throw light on his neglect in the anglophone literature. Basaglia's message and his Italian reforms were actively rejected in the UK—they were not simply overlooked or ignored. While similar processes occurred in other Northern European countries (including that from Germany which was, if anything, even more forceful), it was the UK rejection that appears to have been felt most strongly.

The UK's dismissal of Basaglia stems, at least in part, from some shared similarities—siblings are often the keenest critics. Both countries have centralized, tax-funded National Health Services (established in the UK in 1948 and in Italy in 1978, at the same time as Law 180). Such monolithic and centrally directed health services remain a minority, internationally, compared to the more common approach of mental health provision which is through a range of service providers responding to locally configured, insurance-based funding systems. It is, therefore, possible to talk of a 'British Health Service' and an 'Italian Health Service' in a way that it is perhaps not so meaningful to talk of a 'German Health Service' or a 'French Health Service'. Consequently, there was a distinctly 'British take' on Basaglia, as well as a range of individual opinions. This structural similarity between British and

Italian mental healthcare provision throws the issues into sharp relief, but also limits the generalizability of any conclusions to other countries. They do not transfer at all to the USA with its federal, fragmented, and commercially dominated healthcare system.

This analysis of British resistance to Basaglia will concentrate on clinical rather than sociological assessments or cultural receptions, and will consequently focus predominantly on publications in scientific journals. Ready access to anglophone scientific journals is probably one factor for the UK's high profile in this debate, crystallized in two high-profile articles in the *British Journal of Psychiatry*. The UK's established expertise in social and community psychiatry and in rehabilitation in the 1960s and 1970s, plus its maturing deinstitutionalization process, ensured an informed assessment of Basaglia's work. Visits by Basaglia and a number of his team to Dingleton Hospital in Scotland, in 1963, with his early incorporation (and subsequent rejection) of some of its pioneering principles, lent an extra local dimension.

Three sources of resistance

The UK's rejection of Basaglia can be broadly attributed to three sources. The most important of these was a belief that the claims for the Italian reforms were exaggerated, and possibly even misleading. The UK's own 'move into the community' had been underway for some years; psychiatrists were only too well aware of how difficult it was to provide, effectively and humanely, for patients discharged after long periods in mental hospitals. So some scepticism was inevitable given the dramatic nature of the Italian claims.

There was also a sense at that time that UK community services, which had been spurred into action by the 1959 Mental Health Act, were generally more advanced and more established than those in Italy, and so there might not be that much to learn. There was a belief that the UK was in the vanguard in this area, with its early open-door policies and its establishment of day hospitals, therapeutic communities, and district general hospital units. It had also fully engaged in programmes of gradual deinstitutionalization, and counted amongst its own influential social psychiatrists such figures as Joshua Bierer and Maxwell Jones.

Lastly, and perhaps less definable, there is a long tradition of pragmatism and a suspicion of grand theories. Basaglia's ideological and political language was alien to UK psychiatric discourse and was initially equated with the writings of the anti-psychiatrists. Indeed, the first mention of Basaglia in the anglophone psychiatric literature was in Sir Martin Roth's presidential address to the Canadian Psychiatric Association in 1972, where Roth simply lumps Basaglia in with 'the other anti-psychiatrists' (Roth, 1972). Roth was to return to his attack on Basaglia in 1986, still casting him in the role of an anti-psychiatrist who denied the existence of mental illness (Roth and Kroll, 1986).

Rhetoric and reality

The UK's rejection of the Basaglia message can be traced to two highly influential (or notorious, depending on your position) articles in the *British Journal of Psychiatry* in 1985 and 1986, by Kathleen Jones and Alison Poletti. Theirs were not, however, the first articles published in the English literature about the Italian reforms. Loren Mosher, an American psychiatrist, had spent seven months in Italy in 1980 studying the reforms (Mosher, 1982). Mosher concluded that 'the new Italian law mandating the phasing down and out of large mental hospitals is being successfully implemented, albeit to varying degrees and at varying rates in different sections of the country' (Mosher, 1982, p. 203). He noted, in contrast to the USA, the absence of any wholesale discharges, with many long-stay patients staying put and simply being recategorized as 'guests'. Mosher was concerned about the dropping of dangerousness as a necessary criterion for compulsory admission and feared it might lead to an increase in coercion. His final conclusion was that 'only time will tell the direction . . . and ultimate fate of this radical change' (Mosher, 1982, p. 203).

While Mosher's is the only significant psychiatric publication in English about the Italian reforms before Jones and Poletti, there were a number of highly positive, descriptive articles in nursing and social work journals (Hanvey, 1978; Heptinstall, 1984; Ramon, 1983; Daniels, 1983), and one soon after, by a medical student, in the *Lancet* (Lovestone, 1986). Heptinstall's article advertised a series of exhibitions, to be held in England in the spring of 1984, which included staff from Trieste, sponsored by the leading mental health charity MIND. These comprised a number of film shows and exhibitions in London at the King's Fund and London School of Economics, followed by exhibitions in Manchester and Sheffield. The exhibitions led Ron Lacey, MIND's deputy director, to write in the *Guardian* that 'Trieste and other places like it have shown that it is possible to provide a credible service for mentally disordered people without mental hospitals. In this, Italy is at least ten years ahead of Britain' (Lacey, 1984).

Jones and Poletti: 1985

Kathleen Jones was a historian of mental healthcare and professor of social policy at York University, a department which she had personally founded. She was a formidable, independent-minded, and self-made individual. Her very broad interest in society's marginalized groups had come, over time, to focus increasingly on mental health. She was not only a widely travelled academic, but also the senior Mental Health Act Commissioner responsible for investigating psychiatric practice for the north of England, with a track record of challenging poor care and exposing gaps between policy and practice. From her many contacts, she knew that there were differences of opinion in Italy about the success of the implementation of Law 180. She recognized that the available statistics were of little value, being both dated and unreliable, so decided that the only course was to go and see for herself. Her interest lay in practical implementation, not theory. For that reason she, along with an Italian graduate student, Alison Poletti, travelled the 800 miles from north to south visiting Como, Milan, Pavia, Pisa, Lucca, Florence, Salerno, and Reggio di Calabria, taking in a wide range of services, including both enthusiasts and sceptics (Jones and Poletti, 1985).

Although primarily interested in the pragmatic implementation of Law 180, the first article gives a succinct outline of Basaglia's theoretical foundations. It also offers some observations on the special nature of Italian society which they believed were relevant to understanding the Italian reforms. They cite three specifically Italian concerns as essential for anglophone readers to understand. *Anti-emarginazione* is the concern that no individual should be marginalized or treated as second class. This is central to Basaglia's thesis that liberating patients is the single most important objective in Psichiatria Democratica. *Pluralismo* represents a reluctance to rely on monolithic state provision and a decided preference for a mixed system. This they attributed to a reaction to experiences under the recent Fascist regime and the influence of the Catholic Church, but also perhaps to a frustration with inefficient bureaucracies. Lastly, *gattopardismo* is the term they used for the Italian identification with very specific localities, your own village and ways of doing things, rather than with a region or country. The term is very dated and comes from the famous novel and film *Il Gattopardo* (*The Leopard*) set in Sicily. This habit of preferring your local habits and produce ('Our Lake Garda olives are less salty and *much* better than those from Genoa') is familiar to any visitor to Italy. However, it is more likely now to be referred to as *campanilismo*—preferring the sound of your own village's church bells. Certainly, the Italian mental health system is very highly devolved, down to individual Unità Socio-Sanitaria Locale (USSL).

Jones and Poletti devoted part of their 1985 article to reporting objections to Law 180 that they heard from its opponents. They commented on its rushed transit through the legislative process in just 23 days. They also reported on the risks from patients discharged to families unable to cope with them, on those ending up in prison, and even anecdotal reports of individual tragedies of suicide and neglect. It is disappointing that Jones allows herself to report such lurid anecdotes when she must have been equally familiar with them much nearer home, as a Mental Health Commissioner. Such tragedies are, after all, experienced by even the very best mental health services and are unlikely to have had a major impact on psychiatrists, familiar with such occurrences. In the event, they were not the source of the outcry from Italy.

The most stinging observation in this article was that mental hospitals in Italy were simply not closed at all. Jones and Poletti report finding long-stay patients, in significant numbers, still living in wards in every one of the services they visited. These wards were often labelled as something else and the patients simply re-designated as 'guests' (*ospiti*): 'We saw "alternative structures"—"family homes" or "villas"—and often did not realize what they were at the time because they looked like ordinary mental hospital wards' (Jones and Poletti, 1985, p. 345). The conditions for these long-stay patients were, if anything, even poorer than they had been before Law 180 because repairs and maintenance of the wards were no longer being carried out, and there were fewer staff. They report wards with up to 60 deteriorated patients, with only two or three untrained nurses. They also describe many of these wards being locked and patients often heavily medicated and some subject to mechanical restraint. There were no structured day programmes (logical if the patients were no longer patients) and no support staff such as occupational therapists or social workers. Jones was clearly incensed that specialist training for psychiatric nursing had been abandoned in 1975.

They were also critical of the Diagnosis and Cure Units. They reported these as generally bleak and crowded, with overworked staff caring for a variety of confused and disturbed patients who often stayed for extended periods. Psycho-Social Centres varied, but many seemed not that different from routine outpatient clinics. They observed that the further south they travelled, 'the provision became less and the problems greater'.

The last part of the article is concerned with 'Proposals for changing the Law' and 'Lessons for Britain?'. However their central conclusion, and the thrust of their article, comes earlier: 'the general standard of provision was desperately low. If the old system was regimented and repressive, laissez-faire merely substituted a chaotic poverty of provision' (Jones and Poletti, 1985, p. 346).

Italian outrage and the response: 1986

The 1985 article generated a rapid and vigorous response from Italy. Jones and Poletti were accused of 'being in favour of mental hospitals' (Tansella, 1985), giving an inaccurate picture of Trieste (Ramon, 1985), and even predicting 'the certainty of catastrophe for any country if mental hospitals are abolished' (De Girolamo, 1985). These specific criticisms were easy to deal with. They had never visited Trieste, so had given no account of it, nor had they predicted catastrophe, and Jones had been a long-term critic of mental hospital care. There were also a number of rather technical criticisms, which they address in their 1986 paper. However, there are two overarching criticisms that they felt needed a fuller response. The first was that they presented impressionistic judgements without providing the evidence on which they based them. The second was that by failing to visit the centres of excellence, Trieste in particular, they could not fully understand the nature of Psichiatria Democratica.

They point out, in their defence of the first criticism, that they had referenced an earlier paper, 'The mirage of reform' (Jones and Poletti, 1984), which provided the detailed descriptive data for their conclusions. In many ways, it may have been a blessing that Tansella and his colleagues had not read this paper in *New Society* as it is even more hard-hitting than the 1985 paper. It contains verbatim extracts from their visit notes:

> The male open ward is frankly a doss-house: a large, completely bare room with a stone floor. The men sit around and play cards and smoke—there is nothing else to do. The only treatment is by heavy doses of psychotropic drugs, plus basic physical care, of which de-lousing forms an important part ... Some of the guests are in straitjackets or arm-muffs, one guest is strapped to his bed. Technically they can leave if they apply in writing ... The male locked ward ... has frosted glass panes so that the guests cannot look out.
>
> **(Jones and Poletti, 1984, p. 344)**

There is more along the same vein that hardly needs further reporting. Jones would undoubtedly have experienced unacceptable neglect in many of the English mental hospitals she visited. However, she clearly found some of the conditions in Italy to be utterly inexcusable. She certainly would have been shocked by the use of physical restraints, something she would never have encountered in the UK.

In response to the Italian criticisms, Jones and Poletti undertook a second study visit and, in the three weeks, they visited Trieste, Rome, Ferrara, and Bologna. They are very positive in commending their Italian hosts who, despite the acknowledged differences of opinion, were hospitable and friendly and allowed free access. They took time to list the achievements they observed in Trieste and described the services in some detail. They praised the optimistic, informal, and warm atmosphere achieved in these services and noted that the use of medication was lower than they had observed elsewhere. Despite these positive experiences, they retained four major reservations.

First, the Trieste hospital, San Giovanni, was decidedly not closed in any meaningful sense. Learning from the response to their first article, Jones and Poletti gave the figures to justify this conclusion, as they did in the subsequent site visits. In addition to the various other activities on site, San Giovanni housed:

- '.over 200 patients who "just happened" to be there when the reforms took place and could not find outside accommodation' (*Ospiti*);
- a 'particularly restrictive and unsuitable' locked ward for 48 senile dementia patients;
- 15 beds in an alcoholic unit; and
- 20 beds for severely mentally handicapped young people.

Second, they were struck by the focus on young disturbed patients and the risk that the rehabilitation and care needs of less demanding patients might be overlooked. Their third concern was about the elderly mentally ill, particularly those with dementia. They questioned whether simply redesignating them as a medical rather than a psychiatric problem was in their best interests. Lastly, their attention was drawn to what was *not* being provided. For ideological reasons, psychotherapy was not much in evidence (psychoanalysis being considered bourgeois, group-work manipulation). Nor was there much in terms of structured activity for patients, as any form of work therapy was tainted with echoes of exploitation.

The other three sites (Ferrara, Rome, and Bologna) are dealt with in less detail, but the variations between them are noted. Ferrara's psychoanalytical flavour is reported, as is the presence of some high-quality training courses in Rome. Jones and Poletti reported that they 'never doubted [the] good faith or complete sincerity' of the staff they met, 'despite our ideological differences'. However, they

> remained mystified by the insistence of Psichiatria Democratica on 'closing the mental hospital' when it was patently obvious that mental hospitals were not being closed ... The distinction is not a particularly subtle one, but it has led to massive misunderstandings. When the Trieste team say 'We closed the mental hospital' they do not mean 'We closed the mental hospital'. They mean 'We broke the power of the mental hospital over the patients.'
>
> **(Jones and Poletti, 1986, p. 149)**

Reading these two papers after an interval of over 30 years, it is easy to see how they would have had a decisive impact on British psychiatrists' judgements of Basaglia's claims. The anti-psychiatrists (Laing, Goffman, Foucault, and Szasz) had, in the 1960s, mounted a searing critique of psychiatry and the legitimacy of diagnosis. Throughout the 1970s, Ronald Laing had remained a prominent figure in British cultural life. His eloquent attacks had sensitized the profession; indeed, had incensed and traumatized some of its senior members. Psychiatrists had struggled (often clumsily and ineffectually) to counter the view that mental illness was in some way purely a social or political construct, with the implication that simply acknowledging this would somehow automatically dispel the associated disability and suffering. For veterans of this struggle, Basaglia's insistence on the political nature of diagnosis and the crucial role of marginalization, with the slogan 'La libertà è terapeutica', struck a familiar chord. Many saw it as another example of what Andrew Scull termed 'word magic' (1977).

What is less easy to understand is why the Italian responses failed to engage more fully with the sources of the criticisms and so generate a productive dialogue. Jones and Poletti are accused of missing the point and being ungenerous. There is some justification for this accusation in the first paper, but certainly not in the second. In their 1986 paper, Jones and Poletti are quick to praise their Italian hosts and acknowledge the very real conceptual differences, but return to the source of the 'misunderstanding'. In part, the mismatch of the criticism and response may reflect the value sets of the two sides. Jones and Poletti are making an entirely rational set of observations (e.g. the hospitals are simply not closed, the level of care is well below what should be expected in Europe). Their respondents are making a more ideological and emotional point. The destructive framework of traditional psychiatry and its unjustified power imbalance have been disrupted, the plight of patients has been identified with and solidarity shown. Jones and Poletti are making a narrow clinical case, whereas their Italian respondents are making a broader, sociopolitical one. This failure to engage more fully resulted in mutual withdrawal, with both sides going their own ways. Although there were continued visits to Trieste from the UK, and some centres of enthusiasm such as Alec Jenner's unit in Sheffield, Basaglia and the Italian reforms effectively disappear from mainstream anglophone psychiatric literature by the end of the 1980s.

Psychiatry in the United Kingdom in the 1980s

The second source of UK resistance to the Italian reforms stems from the perceived differences in quality of the respective psychiatric services and practice at the time. This is not actively specified, but is implicit in Jones and Poletti's criticisms.

The UK in the period after the Second World War had a strong tradition of social psychiatry and liberal practice. Physical restraints had been entirely abolished across the UK a whole century earlier, in 1845, as a consequence of John Conolly's successful non-restraint movement. The open-door movement was also well established. Dingleton Hospital in Melrose, Scotland, which Basaglia visited in 1963, started to open its doors in 1943, and its last locked door was removed in 1948, and it remained open until the hospital itself closed in 1981. Warlingham Park Hospital in Croydon was not far behind: under the direction of T.P. Rees, a home-visiting service by nurses had been introduced for psychotic patients in 1953. Day hospitals and patients' social clubs had begun to be established and written about in the late 1940s and early 1950s. Maxwell Jones had developed the therapeutic community from his experiences treating traumatized soldiers during the Second World War, and had gone on to apply the principles to general psychiatry in Dingleton in the 1960s. Dingleton Hospital was a small mental hospital serving all the needs of a mainly rural population of 125,000 from three or four small towns.

Russel Barton had published his book *Institutional Neurosis* in 1959. This proposed that much of the 'deficit' state observed in long-stay patients was a result of a stultifying environment rather than an illness process. This stimulated the growth of rehabilitation psychiatry. The downsizing of hospitals was already well underway by the early 1960s, accelerated by Goffman's book *Asylums* (1960). The 1959 Mental Health Act fostered this approach by providing a rigorous structure for protecting and monitoring patients' rights. It also mandated close working between health and social services, laying the framework for multidisciplinary teams and the same geographically defined community psychiatry structure as in the French *secteur* system.

In 1973, I worked as a junior doctor in Dingleton. At that time, there were only 11 acute beds for the population of 125,000 (the same level of 15 beds for 150,000 recommended in Law 180). Inpatient numbers had more than halved and there were no locked doors. We worked closely with local general practitioners, and all referrals were assessed and usually treated in their own homes by a doctor and either a nurse or social worker—there were no outpatient clinics. Like Trieste, everyone was on first-name terms (patients and staff), we all ate in the same dining room, and we attended the regular community meetings. The hospital had the same bohemian atmosphere that Jones and Poletti described in Trieste in 1985, with young volunteers, mainly from Scandinavia and South America, and constant visitors from around the globe.

In short, UK psychiatrists considered their training and services to be pretty good at this time. There may, as has been suggested, have been a degree of smugness or arrogance in their response to the Italian claims. There certainly was envy of the glamour, flair, and self-confidence displayed by the Italians. But there was also extensive experience of just how difficult it was to reform mental healthcare, and particularly how difficult it was to provide adequate community care. As the Social Services Committee commented in 1985: 'Any fool can close a long-stay hospital: it takes more time and trouble to do it properly and compassionately'. So it is no surprise that there was scepticism within the profession, and it is not helpful to simply dismiss this as medical conservatism or self-interest.

Grand theory

British culture is traditionally very sceptical of grand theories; indeed, it has been criticized for its distrust of intellectualism altogether. Unlike Continental Europe and the USA, it has no written constitution, nor does it have a Napoleonic legal code. Constitution and legal practice are based on common law and precedent. Pragmatism takes the place of ideology. Even in its schools of philosophy, the UK's analytical and 'realist' approach has been contrasted, for the last century or so, with 'Continental idealism' and what Foucault referred to as the European 'totalizing' endeavour. So Basaglia may have also met resistance because he was viewed as too ideologically driven.

Basaglia claimed, influenced by writers such as Michel Foucault and Franz Fanon, that psychiatric diagnosis was primarily a political act used deliberately to marginalize and disempower unwelcome voices. In his paper to the Fourth International Congress on Law and Psychiatry in Oxford in 1979, he stated:

> Madness . . . .slowly begins to take its various shapes in that vast and varied social terrain which makes up both a nation's wealth . . . and its poverty . . . The task of the productive organization is to force this wretchedness to fit into pre-ordained structures . . . so that it produces the wealth required by the new society . . . That which society defines as sick is, in fact, that which the social set-up defines as dangerous for its equilibrium . . . to be identified, isolated and sterilized within the social vacuum of the asylum.
>
> **(Basaglia, 1980, p. 17)**

Basaglia's focus was on removing the power of the mental hospital. This could be experienced as having a greater concern with destroying the edifice than in providing alternatives. It undoubtedly would be a source of disquiet for British psychiatrists. This is not to say that there was no recognition of these malign processes in the UK, but they were more likely to be expressed in dry public health measures to reduce inequalities. The contrast between Russell Barton's explanation of institutionalization and that proposed by Goffman vividly demonstrates the clinical versus political mindset. The difference between Basaglia and his British critics is more one of *passion* and *motivation* than any lack of specific awareness or concern.

Focusing entirely on liberty as the absence of oppression may also have been viewed with some scepticism. Isaiah Berlin was that rare phenomenon, a UK public intellectual, during this period. A Latvian Jew, who went on to establish Oxford's first new college in the twentieth century, his inaugural lecture 'Two concepts of liberty' was widely read (Berlin, 1958). Essentially, Berlin distinguished between 'freedom from' and 'freedom to', and argued that simply freeing people from oppression was not enough if they were still, through infirmity or want, unable to exercise agency. He wrote that the boundary of liberty is:

> a matter of argument, indeed of haggling. Men are largely interdependent, and no man's activity is so completely private as never to obstruct the lives of others in any way . . . It is true that to offer political rights, or safeguards against intervention by the state to men who are half naked, illiterate, underfed and diseased is to mock their condition . . . First things come first—there are times when boots are superior to Pushkin.
>
> **(Berlin, 1958, p. 26)**

Berlin, like several thinkers to follow, such as Nussbaum and Amartya Sen, recognized that true agency requires attention to the individual's personal resources and aspirations, rather than simply an absence of direct oppression. More recently, this has been discussed in terms of 'positive' and 'negative' freedoms. To be genuinely free, patients need to be able to engage with the world and exert agency, and to do this they may need active involvement in alleviating their illnesses. American critics of deinstitutionalization have expressed this exclusive attention to restricting compulsion, without provision for homeless and neglected psychotic patients, as 'dying with their rights on'.

This difference of emphasis between theory and pragmatism was evident in the broad sweep of Psichiatrica Democratica encapsulated in Trieste with the slogan 'la libertà è terapeutica', but also evident in day-to-day practice. The blanket abandonment of electroconvulsive therapy (ECT) after Law 180 is a striking example of this dismissal of clinical reality in the service of theory—or even of image. ECT (ironically an Italian discovery) has had an undoubtedly torrid history of excessive and indiscriminate use. By the mid 1970s, however, its place as an effective (in some cases the only effective) treatment for some severe and resistant depressions was established, and its application had become more consistent and judicious. The Italian dismissal of this often life-saving treatment because of its poor public reputation would appear, to experienced UK psychiatrists, as a self-indulgent act of ideology or even intellectual vanity.

Basaglia's attitude to community meetings—a core feature of therapeutic communities—is perhaps a more revealing illustration. When Basaglia visited Dingleton in 1963, he was impressed by the daily community meetings. In these, patients and staff talked through the current issues, large and small, affecting life in the hospital. Sometimes these meetings were unruly and difficult, sometimes just boring, but they were usually well attended and valued as an essential part of the culture of the institution. The introduction of such community meetings into a wide range of different institutions (mental hospitals, prisons, schools, etc.) across the world, since, has usually led to more humane relationships, resulting in fewer misunderstandings and disturbances. Basaglia introduced such community meetings in Gorizia and Trieste in the early years. Eventually, he concluded that they were not effective as they did not adequately empower patients. He complained that the patients did not grasp their power firmly enough and vote down unpopular practices, and so he abandoned this 'gilded cage' approach.

Basaglia clearly valued the community group as a platform for political empowerment of patients, and the vote as a vital, symbolic act in challenging power. Maxwell Jones, on the other hand, always insisted that there should *never* be a vote in a community meeting. As far as he was concerned, the purpose of these meetings was as 'living–learning' situations in which demoralized and disillusioned patients could recover their self-respect and competence by engaging in the decision-making process. For Maxwell Jones, it was the patient's personal experience, not the specific decisions, which mattered. It is likely that Basaglia would have agreed with this, but he clearly saw it overwhelmingly in terms of only one aspect of personal experience—political empowerment. Maxwell Jones allowed a multiplicity of valuable experiences—being assertive, learning how to listen, learning how to compromise, recognizing communality, recognizing differences, perhaps just sitting quietly with others and not being frightened.

What has been gained and what has been lost?

The results of anglophone psychiatry's rejection of Basaglia's message have been mixed and they have been enduring. Because the literature on the topic ceased so abruptly, such conclusions can only be impressionistic—there is no public record to draw upon. I will suggest two possible major benefits and two major losses from this stand-off. This separation is relatively artificial. The two gains and the two losses can be seen as two sides of the same coin. Indeed, there are some downsides to the gains, although I cannot discern upsides to the losses. However, I will present them individually to try and draw out the issues. As in any generalization about complex social systems, these are *generalizations*—there are always exceptions to the rule.

A vibrant research culture and evidence-based practice

The continuing emphasis on pragmatism in anglophone psychiatry has underpinned a highly successful research culture. The evidence-based medicine (EBM) movement has been particularly strong in the UK, where the monolithic and cash-strapped NHS provides a perfect home. The Cochrane Collaboration and the National Institute of Health and Care Excellence (NICE) effectively regulate which treatments are available on the NHS. These use highly sophisticated quantitative algorithms, and are prominent markers of this rational approach. UK psychiatry has also embraced EBM and, since the mid 1980s, this has included mental health services themselves. This dates from Stein and Test's landmark study of assertive community treatment (1980). Since then, mental health service structures and team configurations have become the object of high-quality research with international reach. The UK has carved out a prominent role for itself in this area, and has probably been the major European (if not world) player. In the late 1990s, Michele Tansella in Verona bemoaned the fact that he was the only clearly identified professor of social and community psychiatry in Italy, despite their international reputation and flair, whereas at that time the UK had over half a dozen, all research-active.

Specialist rehabilitation services

The gradualist approach to deinstitutionalization and the closure of mental hospitals in the UK led to a rapid growth in psychiatrists tasked with overseeing this process. The scale of the challenge had been long acknowledged. As far back as in 1961, the then Health Secretary made his iconic 'water tower' speech to the annual conference of social workers, credited with setting in motion the UK's drive to community care. In this, he declared that there was no future for the asylums, and predicted that the intellectual and philosophical challenges of closing them would be as great as the physical and financial challenges. A specific subspecialty of rehabilitation psychiatry was formally established, requiring defined and rigorous training. Several research programmes were undertaken into the reprovision of care for long-stay patients. Of these, the Team for the Assessment of Psychiatric Services (TAPS) project in north London became the most extensive and productive (Leff et al., 2000).

Whether this careful research did or did not result in better-quality reprovision for patients it did, at least, ensure that there was reliable information about the process. It helped refine the high-risk and dependent groups, helped classify needs, and established the merits or otherwise of different forms of group living. The careful monitoring of discharged patients also helped to challenge media stories of homelessness and criminality. The establishment of a rehabilitation subspecialty also went some way to addressing Jones and Poletti's concerns (1986) that the chronically disabled might be overlooked.

The UK emphasis on EBM and the development of expertise in rehabilitation teams (and subsequently other specialized teams) are presented here as positive outcomes of rejecting the Basaglian model. Such specialized teams have permitted more sophisticated and targeted treatments, allowing staff to increase skill levels. They have gone a long way to addressing what Jones and Poletti identified as unskilled practice. However, this highly rational approach has brought with it considerable fragmentation of services. Instead of the single, generic community mental health team (CMHT) that characterized 1980s' British psychiatry (and still dominates Basaglian practice and Italy in general), referrers and patients are now faced with a complex, and often bewildering, range of services. More importantly, continuity of care has been lost and, with it, the focus on the centrality of the therapeutic relationship.

Societal engagement with mental health

Rejecting the Basaglian approach was a massive missed opportunity for UK psychiatry's image and its engagement with public opinion and wider cultural life. Basaglia's eloquence, vitality, and flair—quite apart from the warmth and optimism of his movement—provided a once-in-a-generation opportunity to reconfigure psychiatry's relationship with society, and for society to engage creatively and generously with the issues of mental illness.

Basaglia was always outward-looking—not surprising as he considered it his aim to change society as much as to change mental healthcare. His approach to deinstitutionalization was marked as much by its theatricality as by its politics. When the steel gates of Trieste were finally to be removed, he made sure that patients and local residents were involved in their dismantling and that the press were there to report the whole performance (as performance it was). An enormous, blue, papier maché statue of a horse (Marco Cavallo, named after the horse who regularly dragged the laundry cart out of the hospital) was constructed in the hospital. Its procession through the town in 1973, to celebrate the new freedoms of the patients, was a stroke of genius. Widely photographed and reported, Basaglia even made a point of having to 'break down' the doors of the ward (although not necessary). Perhaps the most strikingly successful publicity for his movement was a television programme featuring the regime in Gorizia: *I Giardini di Abele* (*The Gardens of Abel*). This was produced by Sergio Zavoli and broadcast in 1969 on prime-time television to an estimated nine million Italians. Zavoli's message was that Gorizia and mental illness were everybody's problem, not just psychiatry's.

Basaglia and the Basaglians were what we now would call 'media savvy', and this tradition has continued in Italy. The contrast between the UK and Italy in public engagement events and programmes to celebrate mental health could not be more striking. Italian events are much more ambitious. They are joyful and lively, and much more professional, with extensive contributions from high-profile artists and cultural figures. South American Basaglians are, if anything, even more exuberant. UK initiatives are generally very worthy but, in truth, often quite dull. Why did UK psychiatry not recognize the value of this celebratory and outward-looking approach?

There is, of course, a fundamental difference in culture. Italy, as Kathleen Jones acknowledged in her infamous articles, is a more demonstrative and romantic, a more theatrical culture. My memory of this time is that the more puritanical UK position was exaggerated by two extra factors. Firstly, as previously mentioned, was a resentment that local achievements were being so overshadowed by what was seen as exaggerated and simplified stories coming from Italy. UK psychiatrists were jealous and knew that they could not compete with the glamour and flair of the Basaglians. Secondly, they had spent much of the preceding decade fighting off the attacks from equally glamorous anti-psychiatrists—Laing, Cooper, Esterson—and unthinkingly treated Basaglia in a similar manner (Roth, 1972; Roth and Kroll, 1986). This was a profound mistake. Although Basaglia did have much in common with the anti-psychiatrists, he differed by offering a possible alternative to an old system, not just a critique.

Recruitment and morale in psychiatry

Linked to Basaglia's impact on society's image of mental illness is, inevitably, society's image of psychiatrists and other mental health staff, and linked with this, mental health staff's image of itself. Basaglian psychiatry has succeeded in presenting a humane, optimistic image of psychiatry; one that is coherent and attractive. For many reasons, the UK has struggled to maintain a coherent and attractive image of the profession. There are a number of reasons for this, including an increasingly risk-averse society and chronic underfunding, but undoubtedly the profession's image of itself has contributed. A lack of self-confidence within UK psychiatry shows itself in a wide range of ways. It shows itself in a failure to respond openly and actively to the media criticisms that public mental health services inevitably attract. Rarely, if ever, does a psychiatrist appear in the media to defend what was done and explain the realistic limits of what can be achieved. Similarly, the profession has passively tolerated the increasing fragmentation of services imposed on it by an excessively prescriptive and top–down managerial culture. It has also passively tolerated a return to more oppressive practices such as higher rates of compulsion and locked doors.

The last 30 years in the UK has seen an increasingly strident campaign to identify psychiatry entirely with medicine, denying its unique human and interpersonal dimensions. This ultra-rational, biological, and technological approach was hoped to reduce stigma for patients and make the profession attractive to new doctors. In both, it appears to have failed: stigma stubbornly persists for patients, and recruitment of staff remains a constant challenge.

Lessons from the United Kingdom clash with Basaglia

Franco Basaglia undoubtedly warrants a very special place in psychiatry's history. The dominant feature of the second half of twentieth-century mental healthcare is the move from the asylum to the community. This was an international movement reflecting the mood of the time. It arose in many parts of the world simultaneously, rather than from one place or the ideas of any one individual, and it took many forms. Basaglia's aim was to 'abolish the asylum', not to reform it or downsize it. His achievements in regard to this aim were very considerable, but neither as complete nor as straightforward as often presented, and they remain controversial.

Exploring the clash between UK psychiatry and Basaglia's reforms may help highlight some of the contextual aspects of his successes that might otherwise be overlooked. His reforms took root most strongly in countries which had strikingly underdeveloped services and were emerging from periods of repressive, often military, rule (Italy, Spain, Brazil, Argentina). Not surprising then that the message of liberty was so attractive. However, his message arrived at the UK at just the time when its psychiatrists were having to revise their own overoptimistic expectations of deinstitutionalization. Despite the writings of Goffman and Barton, 'institutionalization' did not evaporate with discharge. They were 10 years into their programme of deinstitutionalization, and the brutal reality of the persistence of severe disabilities was having to be faced. Liberty may be therapeutic but it certainly is not necessarily curative.

A less nationalistic and defensive revisiting of this clash, with its failure to understand on both sides, could be highly productive. A more reflective and analytical approach could provide new perspectives and improved practice all round.

Although the UK 'rejection' of Basaglia's reforms is unusually well documented, the UK was not alone in deciding not to incorporate them, as this book testifies. Services and deinstitutionalization were farther advanced in several countries: the German 'Psychiatrie-Enquête' was published, after years of preparation, in 1975; and radical alternatives to mental hospitals existed, in the 1970s, in a number of countries, and those in the Netherlands and Scandinavia, though short-lived and localized, were well known. Psychiatrists in a number of these countries might argue that they did as well, perhaps in some respects better, by their patients during this period without all the upheaval of Law 180.

But maybe that is the point about Basaglia—not so much that he was ahead of the game in any psychiatric sense, but that he captured and harnessed the 'spirit of 1968' for psychiatry. Good psychiatry may need evidence-based practice, rigorous research, and thorough training, but it also needs passion and commitment. It needs society to engage with it and support it. Basaglia and his team certainly achieved that, and in a vibrant, enduring form.

The UK medical student who wrote so positively in the *Lancet* of his time in Trieste is now a distinguished professor of psychiatry and knight of the realm (Lovestone,

1986). His judgement on Basaglia to me, looking back after three decades, is that 'Basaglia did not close the mental hospital. Basaglia's genius was that he *opened* the mental hospital'.

References

Basaglia, F. (1980). Problems of law and psychiatry: the Italian experience. Report of the Fourth International Congress on Law and Psychiatry. *International Journal of Law and Psychiatry* 3:17.

Berlin, I. (1958). *Two Concepts of Liberty*. Oxford: Clarendon Press.

Daniels, G. (1983). One nurse's week. *Nursing Mirror* 40.

De Girolamo, D. (1985). Misunderstanding the Italian Experience. *British Journal of Psychiatry* 147:451–2.

Goffman, I. (1960). *Asylums: Essays on the Social Situation of Mental Patients and Other Inmates*. Harmondsworth, Middlesex: Penguin Books.

Hanvey, C. (1978). Italy and the rise of democratic psychiatry. *Community Care* 25 October 1978:22–4.

Heptinstall, D. (1984). Psichiatria Democratica. *Community Care* 1 March 1984:17–19.

Jones, K. and Poletti, A. (1984). The mirage of a reform. *New Society* 70(1137):341–7.

Jones, K. and Poletti, A. (1985). Understanding the Italian Experience. *British Journal of Psychiatry* 146:341–7.

Jones, K. and Poletti, A. (1986). The Italian experience in mental health care. *Hospital & Community Psychiatry* 37:795–802.

Lacey, R. (1984). Where have all the patients gone? *Guardian* 4 July 1984.

Leff, J., Trieman, N., Knapp, M., and Hallam, A. (2000). The TAPS Project: a report on 13 years of research, 1985–1998. *Psychiatric Bulletin* 24:165–8.

Lovestone, S. (1986). The Trieste experience. *Lancet* 2:1025–8.

Mosher, L.R. (1982). Italy's revolutionary mental health law: an assessment. *American Journal of Psychiatry* 139:199–203.

Ramon, S. (1983). Psichiatria democratica: a case study of an Italian community mental health service. *International Journal of Health Services* 13:307–24.

Ramon, S. (1985). Misunderstanding the Italian Experience. *British Journal of Psychiatry* 146:208–9.

Roth, M. (1972). Presidential address: 'Psychiatry and its critics'. *Canadian Journal of Psychiatry* 17:343–50.

Roth, M. and Kroll, J. (1986). *The Reality of Mental Illness*. Cambridge: Cambridge University Press.

Scull, A. (1977). *Decarceration*. New Jersey: Prentice Hall.

Social Services Committee (1985). *Community Care*. London: House of Commons.

Stein, L.I. and Test, M.A. (1980). Alternative to mental hospital treatment. I. Conceptual model, treatment program, and clinical evaluation. *Archives of General Psychiatry* 37:392–7.

Tansella, M. (1985). Misunderstanding the Italian Experience. *British Journal of Psychiatry* 147:450.

12
Franco Basaglia

Another conspicuous non-event in the history of psychiatry in Ireland?

Brendan D. Kelly

Introduction

Franco Basaglia was one of the most interesting, original, and provocative psychiatrists and thinkers of the twentieth century (Foot, 2015). He belongs to a small group of psychiatrists who not only developed new ideas about psychiatry and society but also acted on those ideas to bring about radical change. But while Basaglia's work, and that of his colleagues, had significant public impact in several countries around the world, it had virtually no apparent or direct effect in others. Ireland belongs in the latter group.

Ireland has always been wary of radical social change, and the history of psychiatry in Ireland can be usefully read as a story of sustained resistance to change in relation to the mentally ill (Kelly, 2016a). More precisely, perhaps, the history of psychiatry in Ireland is largely a history of institutions—their emergence, their remarkable durability, and their slow decline as result of a broader process of social change rather than as a result of demands for a more democratic psychiatry (Leane and Sapouna, 1998; Sapouna, 2006).

This chapter explores this story in greater detail, seeking to establish why Basaglia had so little apparent public or professional influence in Ireland, and to unearth any evidence that his work might have had some covert effects behind the scenes. More specifically, this chapter:

1. provides a background to the local context of psychiatry in Ireland in the 1900s, leading up to the time of Basaglia;
2. explores other key actors and developments that, like Basaglia, did not seem directly to affect Irish psychiatry over this period, despite reasonable expectations that they might do so (e.g. the Roman Catholic Church, psychoanalysis);
3. searches in vain for public signs of Basaglian influence within Irish psychiatry, especially in light of lively discussions of Basaglia's work in psychiatric publications from the United Kingdom; and, finally,
4. searches, with more success, for evidence that Basaglian thought had (and possibly still has) some influence behind the scenes in shaping the ideas of certain influential psychiatrists in Ireland.

Irish psychiatry in the 1900s

In the mid 1900s, Ireland had more asylum beds per head of population than any other country in the world (Brennan, 2014). Why? Did Ireland have an especially high rate of mental illness? Or were the asylums filled with people other than the mentally ill: the intellectually disabled, the homeless, the eccentric, anyone who did not fit in?

The history of psychiatry in Ireland is a complicated and fascinating one (Kelly, 2016a). Thousands of asylum beds were opened in Ireland during the 1800s as part of a transnational wave of institutionalization of the mentally ill, and also in response to Ireland's tragically ill-advised Dangerous Lunatic Act (1838) and the voracious needs of a society hungry for custody and control. This extraordinary mass institutionalization was ostensibly underpinned by concern for the destitute mentally ill who were increasingly visible as they lived lives of vagrancy or languished in Irish prisons. But conditions in the resultant asylums deteriorated rapidly. The new institutions were immediately overcrowded, and emphasis moved swiftly from care and cure to custody and control.

In 1817, a House of Commons Select Committee on the Lunatic Poor in Ireland heard a first-hand account of conditions at the 'Lunatic Asylum of Limerick, where the accommodation afforded to the insane' was 'such as we should not appropriate for our dog-kennels':

> Two, and sometimes, I believe, three of the insane have been condemned to lie together in one of those cells, the dimensions of which are six feet by ten feet seven inches; some of them in a state of furious insanity. In order to protect them from the obvious results, the usual mode of restraint was by passing their hands under their knees, fastening them with manacles, fastening bolts about their ankles, and passing a chain over all, and then fastening them to a bed ... They have so far lost the use of their limbs, that they are utterly incapable of rising.
>
> **(Select Committee on the Lunatic Poor in Ireland, 1817, pp. 14–15)**

In 1843, another Select Committee heard similarly disturbing evidence from Francis White, Inspector General of Prisons, who reported that:

> The state of the Wexford lunatics in the local asylum is most disgraceful ... The cells were the worst I ever saw. There were two patients under restraint, one of whom was chained to a wall. When I went to his cell, with the keeper and the medical officer, I asked to go in. The keeper said it would be dangerous and frightful to go in. However, we went in. He was naked, with a parcel of loose straw around him. He darted forward at me, and were it not that he was checked by a chain which went round his leg, and was fastened by a hook to the wall, he would have caught hold of me, and probably used violence ... I could not describe the horror which seized me.
>
> **(Select Committee of the House of Lords, 1843, p. vii)**

But the government's belief in asylums was unshakeable. In 1858, the Lunatic Asylums, Ireland, Commission remained steadfast, affirming that 'it is of the utmost importance that cases of insanity should as speedily as possible be removed to an asylum' (p. 12). This belief persisted as an article of faith well into the twentieth century.

As a result, the Irish asylum system expanded faster than those in other countries during the 1800s, and was much slower to decline in the 1900s. It is now clear, however, that Ireland suffered from an epidemic of mental hospitals and not an epidemic of mental illness. The institutions were fundamentally driven by unmet social need, poor legislation, and a desire by communities to find places for the mentally ill, intellectually disabled, and people who did not fit in. Families often had limited resources to care for such persons at home; the only solution offered by the state was an institutional one; and vociferous objections by asylum doctors fell on deaf ears, creating a sense of defeatism all round.

This trend persisted well into the 1900s, with the local asylum dominating many provincial towns right up until the era of Basaglia. In 1951, for example, the town of Ballinasloe in the west of Ireland had a population of 5,596 people, of whom no fewer than 2,078 were patients in the mental hospital (Walsh, 2006). As a result, virtually everyone in the locality was a stakeholder in the institution in one way or another (patient, relative of patient, worker, supplier), and there were powerful economic, social, and community interests in maintaining the hospital's enormous size. Local politics sustained the local institutions.

There were other factors at play too. The Great Irish Famine (1845–1852) magnified social need; the mentally ill in workhouses increased pressure on asylum beds in the early 1900s; catastrophic governmental neglect of the intellectually disabled was a constant feature; and free-floating public and professional hysteria about the apparent 'increase of insanity in Ireland' fuelled the general panic. All of these factors created and sustained the gargantuan Irish asylum system, compounded by the emergence of clinical professions keen for recognition and respect, especially in the early 1900s.

Reform, when it eventually arrived, stemmed from the (belated) Mental Treatment Act 1945, the 1966 governmental Commission of Inquiry on Mental Illness, and the emergence of new treatments in the 1950s and 1960s (e.g. antipsychotic medications). These trends were critically underpinned by broader changes in Irish society, characterized by diminished tolerance for all kinds of institutions. It was, however, the 1966 *Report of the Commission of Inquiry on Mental Illness* that acted as the greatest catalyst for change.

The 1966 Commission recommended 'radical and widespread changes' including a move away from 'barrack-like structures characterised by large wards, gloomy corridors and stone stairways', and its report displayed a curious mixture of bright-eyed enthusiasm about 1960s' psychiatry and resigned institutional defeatism:

> The capacity of modern psychiatry to give good results with intensive and comprehensive in-patient treatment in a great number of cases, together with the desirability of providing such treatment within the ambit of general medicine, has

> led the Commission to recommend the setting up of short-term residential units in, or in association with, general hospitals. Such units would require to be adequately staffed and equipped, to be associated with the community services of a particular area, to be ready to treat all types of mental illness requiring short-term in-patient care, and to work in close conjunction with the other psychiatric services and with the general hospital ... For the patient requiring long-term treatment, the Commission recommends the development of long-term hospitals fulfilling a positive and creative role. The aim will be to provide active treatment as well as residential care, to rehabilitate and restore to the community as many patients as possible, and to provide for all patients lives as full and happy as their disabilities permit.
>
> **(Commission of Inquiry on Mental Illness, 1966, p. xv)**

Overall, the Commission aimed 'to reduce the present estimated total of 10,000 long-stay places to approximately 5,000 over the next 15 years'.

These proposals, which emanated primarily from government rather than professional groups, charted a long-overdue pathway to reform for a mental health system that was still essentially based in institutions. The history of that system was remarkable not only on account of its size and durability but also its uncanny resistance to outside influences. Two of these outside influences, the Roman Catholic Church and psychoanalysis, merit particular mention in order to set the scene for the system's eventual, inevitable resistance to Basaglia too.

The missing actors: the Roman Catholic Church, psychoanalysis ... and Basaglia?

In Ireland, the Roman Catholic Church was deeply involved in education, general healthcare, orphanages, and politics over a sustained period of time (Kelly, 2017a). The Church founded and operated primary and secondary schools, established and ran hospitals, influenced and shaped any number of other institutions, and exerted direct and indirect influence on voters and politicians on virtually all issues of significance in Ireland. Ultimately, the Church single-handedly dominated many areas of Irish life for much of the nineteenth and twentieth centuries. Even so, however, the Church did not develop formal, systematic involvement in mental healthcare over this period. Given the general dominance of the Church in Ireland, this is perhaps unexpected—but there are some possible explanations.

Firstly, with its multiple involvements in other areas, the Church in Ireland possibly never focused explicitly on the asylum system because it had so many other things to concentrate on. By focusing its efforts elsewhere, it maximized impact. Secondly, the Irish public asylum system evolved largely from the prison system (in which the Church was not deeply involved), rather than the health system (in which the Church played a central role). The ideas of the 'deserving' and 'undeserving' poor might also have been relevant, at least in the minds of some. Thirdly, prominent figures from religious traditions other than the Roman Catholic Church were involved in the early phases of mental healthcare in Ireland. In 1731, novelist Jonathan Swift, an ordained priest in the Established Church of Ireland and Dean of St. Patrick's Cathedral in Dublin from 1713 to 1745, decided to bequeath his entire estate to establish a hospital for 'idiots and lunaticks' in Dublin. Following Swift's death in 1745, a royal charter was granted to St. Patrick's by King George II in 1746, and it became the first psychiatric hospital in Ireland. There was also early Quaker involvement in mental healthcare, with the establishment of two asylums in Dublin.

For these reasons and possibly others, the Roman Catholic Church was not directly involved in establishing or running the Irish asylums. While it is likely that certain people with psychological problems sought individual guidance from Roman Catholic priests or other religious figures, the Church itself still did not become systematically involved in formal mental healthcare, with the result that the Irish asylums of the 1800s and 1900s were very much state creations rather than Church ones.

One area where the Church might, however, have played an indirect role was in shaping the intellectual atmosphere of Irish psychiatry in the 1900s, not only through its general emphasis on custody and institutional control but also through its opposition to Sigmund Freud and his developing ideas about psychoanalysis. This hostility towards external ideas such as psychoanalysis is directly relevant to Basaglia's lack of impact in Ireland.

In the early twentieth century, psychoanalysis was the pre-eminent intellectual movement of the day and its influence was felt in many countries, in many spheres of life: psychiatry, psychology, literature, drama, and even, arguably, politics. Freud's creation, however, conspicuously failed to grab the imagination of psychiatrists in Ireland, with just some very limited impact in Belfast (Kelly, 2016a). In 1920, Jonathan Hanaghan (1887–1967)—poet, writer, and psychoanalyst—began psychoanalytical practice in Ireland and, in 1942, founded the Irish Psycho-Analytical Association. Even so, Hanaghan did not belong to the medical establishment, and psychoanalysis did not have an enormous impact on Irish psychiatry, possibly owing to Ireland's peripheral location, the absence of a pre-eminent *medical* professional keen to take the lead in the early days (Fitzgerald, 2003), or the Roman Catholic Church's general disapproval.

In 1963, the Archbishop of Dublin and Primate of Ireland, the Most Reverend John C. McQuaid (arguably the single most powerful figure in Irish public life) wrote an introduction to a remarkable, generally progressive book entitled *The Priest and Mental Health*. In his introduction, McQuaid stated that Freud had not discovered reality but attempted to construct it (McQuaid, 1963). This was plainly intolerable to the Church. In that year, the Irish Psycho-Analytical Association had just five practicing psychoanalyst members—and the Church was determined to keep it that way, ensuring that psychoanalysis, like communism, gained no significant foothold in Ireland (Kelly, 2017a).

Both of these non-events—the non-involvement of the Roman Catholic Church and the failure of psychoanalysis to have an impact—meant that Irish mental hospitals continued to operate during the early and mid 1900s in much the same way as they had in the 1800s: continually expanding, offering asylum to some but simple custody and control to most; and filling complex social roles that often had minimal connection with mental illness or the psychological needs of the patients confined within them. This resistance to change, that saw off both the Church and psychoanalysis, also accounts, in significant part, for Basaglia's lack of impact. The Irish mental hospitals simply could not be stopped by anything or anybody during this period in their history. New movements in psychiatry across Europe were essentially irrelevant. Not even psychoanalysis gained a foothold and, for most psychiatrists, Basaglia never even registered.

Searching for Basaglia in twentieth-century Ireland

The propagation of Basaglian thought in Ireland, if it had occurred (which it did not), would likely have been mediated through professional journals such as the *British Journal of Psychiatry*, the most widely read psychiatry journal in Ireland in the late 1900s. Ireland did not have its own journal in this field until 1982, when the *Irish Journal of Psychiatry* was founded by Dermot Walsh (1931–2017) and published by the Irish Institute of Psychiatry, and the *Irish Journal of Psychological Medicine* was founded by Mark Hartman (1942–1994) and later became the research journal of the College of Psychiatrists of Ireland (Kelly, 2012, 2016b). The former journal (now defunct) does not have an online archive or cumulative index, and a search for 'Basaglia' in the online archive of the latter journal yields no results.

In the *British Journal of Psychiatry*, Katherine Jones and Alison Poletti published an influential paper in 1985 aimed at 'understanding the Italian experience' and the impact of Basaglia in Italy (Jones and Poletti, 1985). They reviewed the relevant literature and went on a study tour of the country in April 1984. They concluded that, contrary (they said) to supporters of the Italian reforms, mental hospitals could not be abolished by legislative change and good intentions alone (arguing that the hospitals simply reappeared in disguise); patients do not automatically improve if discharged (arguing that they still need care); and abandoning professional roles is not a substitute for good training programmes (which, they argued, were still needed). Above all, Jones and Poletti formed the view that political groups such as that in Italy could not substitute for well-informed mental health movements. They concluded that the reported success of the Italian movement was a myth and that community care structures in the UK, although admittedly inadequate, at least provided a framework for future development. In short, they were not at all impressed with the Italian experiment and concluded, flatly, that it had failed. There was nothing to learn from Italy, it seemed.

Jones and Poletti were taken soundly to task by several respondents to their paper. Michele Tansella in Verona argued that they had not engaged sufficiently with the scientific literature on this topic (Tansella, 1985). Giovanni De Girolamo in Cremona felt that their arguments were untrue, incomplete, and lacked objectivity [De Girolamo, 1985]. Harold Bourne at the Hammersmith Child Guidance Unit in London struggled to believe that the Italians could have *absolutely nothing* to teach the British (Bourne, 1985). Shulamit Ramon at the London School of Economics and Political Science pointed to several alleged omissions and misreadings by Jones and Poletti and argued that, contrary to their conclusions, the Italian experience demonstrated that it *is* possible to dismantle psychiatric hospitals and provide good community care (Ramon, 1985).

While these voices in the correspondence column of the *British Journal of Psychiatry* were fluent and robust, and other contributions to the journal also offered different perspectives (Papeschi, 1985; Rizzoli, 1987), the ship had sailed. The paper by Jones and Poletti undoubtedly contributed significantly to the lack of engagement with the Italian experience among psychiatrists in Great Britain and Ireland. Jones and Poletti wrote again about this topic elsewhere (Jones and Poletti, 1986a) and responded to their critics in the *British Journal of Psychiatry*, but they continued to insist that the apparent solutions in Trieste were not transferrable to Britain (Jones and Poletti, 1986b).

Five years later, George B. Palermo in Wisconsin (who practiced as a psychiatrist in Rome from 1969 to 1987) argued, in the *Journal of the Royal Society of Medicine*, that while aspects of the Italian experience were indeed particular to Italy, other countries might still learn important lessons from it (Palermo, 1991). In response, Jones re-emphasized that law is not sufficient to cure patients and that the Italian situation remained an upsetting muddle (Jones et al., 1991).

The net effect of this protracted exchange was that Irish readers of the *British Journal of Psychiatry* did not see a clearly positive account of Basaglain reforms either as they occurred or in their immediate aftermath. And because Basaglia's own works were not widely available in English, and Irish psychiatry was never prone to radical intellectual shifts in the first place, Basaglia remained essentially invisible in Ireland. A 2018 search for 'Basagalia' in the archives of Ireland's two leading daily newspapers, the *Irish Independent* and the *Irish Times*, revealed no mention of Basaglia in the former and only one in the latter—a short note announcing a public lecture about Basaglia and his democratic model of psychiatry given by Professor Nancy Scheper–Hughes at the University of Limerick in 2012 (Thompson, 2012). Pat Bracken, consultant psychiatrist and clinical director of West Cork Mental Health Services, was also speaking at the event.

It was, in fact, Scheper–Hughes who provided Irish psychiatry with one of its few exposures to Basaglian thought, with her book *Saints, Scholars and Schizophrenics: Mental Illness in Rural Ireland* (Scheper–Hughes, 1979 [2001]). In the book, an anthropological exploration of life in a remote Irish village, Scheper–Hughes refers to Basaglia's paper 'Silence in the dialogue with the psychotic' which he presented at the Sixth Congress of Psychotherapy in London in 1964 (Basaglia, 1964), and, later, to the volume of Basaglia's writings that she co-edited with Anne M. Lovell in 1987, *Psychiatry Inside Out: Selected Writings of Franco Basaglia*. Scheper–Hughes and Lovell had also written about the Italian psychiatric experience the previous year, in *Social Science and Medicine*, in a paper entitled 'Breaking the circuit of social control: lessons in public psychiatry from Italy and Franco Basaglia' (Scheper–Hughes and Lovell, 1986).

On publication, Scheper–Hughes' *Saints, Scholars and Schizophrenics* had a mixed reception in Ireland, with David Nowlan providing a positive review in the *Irish Times* (1979) and journalist Michael Viney, who had a strong pre-existing interest in mental health (Viney, 1971), taking his bicycle to visit the village in Dingle where Scheper–Hughes had performed her anthropological observations (Viney, 1980). Viney described local anger and hurt following the publication of Scheper–Hughes' book, to which the author duly responded, noting, inter alia, that this was not unexpected (Scheper–Hughes, 1981). However, not all anthropologists saw rural Ireland as being in decline (Kane, 1981), and the dialogue prompted by Scheper–Hughes' book continued for some time in the *Irish Times* during the 1980s (Viney, 1983; Pye, 1983; Bradshaw, 1983).

Perhaps most interestingly, however, the 1990s showed that the allegedly high rate of mental illness in Ireland which underpinned much of this discussion was, in fact, a myth or misunderstanding (Kendler et al., 1993; Waddington et al., 1995; Holmquist, 1990; Kelly, 2017a). This, of course, did not detract from many of the observations in Scheper–Hughes' book, and nor did it diminish many of the points she made about mental illness and mental health systems in Ireland: while Ireland turned out to have an unremarkable rate of mental illness, it undeniably had an elevated rate of mental hospitalization, and this was not without significance (Kelly, 2016a). Indeed, Ireland's unremarkable rate of mental illness combined with its remarkable rate of mental hospitalization actually underscored the importance of Scheper–Hughes' references to Basaglia, both in *Saints, Scholars and Schizophrenics* and elsewhere (Scheper–Hughes, 1990), and suggested that while Basaglia did not visibly penetrate Ireland to any significant extent, maybe—paradoxically—Ireland had particular need of him?

Searching for Basaglia behind the scenes in Ireland

So, if Basaglia did not overtly influence public psychiatric discourse in Ireland or explicitly prompt the dismantling of Irish mental hospitals in the 1970s and 1980s, did he possibly have an effect behind the scenes? Leane and Sapouna are clear that *social* demand for a more democratic psychiatry did not underpin mental health reform in Ireland (Leane and Sapouna, 1998; Sapouna 2006), but was there a *covert* demand for a more democratic psychiatry underpinning these changes?

Dermot Walsh—psychiatrist, policy-maker, and Inspector of Mental Hospitals (1987–2003) (Kelly, 2017b)—was one of the key actors in the reforms that saw the number of inpatients in Irish psychiatric hospitals decrease from 19,801 in 1963 to

3,658 in 2003 (a decrease of some 82% over four decades) (Kelly, 2007). Indeed, today, Ireland's rate of involuntary care is less than 50% of that in England, indicating the emergence of a remarkably non-custodial mental health system in Ireland (Gilhooley and Kelly, 2018). Walsh, one of Irish psychiatry's most perspicacious voices, was very familiar with psychiatric developments in continental Europe from the 1960s onwards, but he noted that, in Ireland, much of the impetus for change emanated not from any formal or professional grouping of psychiatrists seeking a more democratic psychiatry but, rather, from the government's Department of Health:

> The Irish division of the Royal College of Psychiatrists has been a singularly inactive body and it has had little impact on pointing the future direction of psychiatry in this country. Instead the initiative in all these fields has been taken by the Department of Health. This has led to a devaluation of professional input from psychiatrists in the future direction of our psychiatric services, in their planning, organisation and administration.
>
> **(Walsh, 1992, p. 12)**

There were also, however, important international influences, most notably in the area of human rights. The early 1990s saw the emergence of the first comprehensive statement of the rights of the mentally ill—the United Nations' *Principles for the Protection of Persons with Mental Illness and the Improvement of Mental Health Care* (UN, 1991). In parallel with this, the European Convention on Human Rights from the Council of Europe was especially influential in Ireland (Kelly, 2016a). This ethos was reflected in the work of certain other Irish psychiatrists in addition to Walsh, including Robert McCarthy in Cork (Anonymous, 2014) and, perhaps most notably, Ivor Browne in Dublin.

Browne was a psychiatrist, medical director, professor of psychiatry, and key figure in the phased closure of St. Brendan's Hospital in Grangegorman, Ireland's best-known mental hospital. He was also familiar with Basaglia's work. In his 2008 book, *Music and Madness*, Browne noted both the success of Basaglia's reforms in Trieste and the inadequacy of community alternatives elsewhere in Italy, resulting in the emergence of the *abandonati* (Browne, 2008). Browne also referred to Basaglia in a paper he presented on the occasion of the twenty-fifth anniversary of the Mental Health Association of Ireland, a patient advocacy group which held its inaugural meeting on 24 February 1967 (Browne, 2013). Browne himself saw patient numbers at St. Brendan's decline significantly from 1,627 in 1962 to 942 in 1980, was publicly well known for this work, and remains a crucial, if controversial, figure in the history of psychiatry in Ireland (Crumlish, 2013). Today, looking back, Browne acknowledges that 'Basaglia was a considerable influence on me. I took him very seriously':

> In 1963 when I was working in St Loman's [psychiatric hospital, Dublin], I started the first psychiatric clinic in Ballyfermot [a Dublin suburb] and that started me

> on addressing social problems and community development. As soon as I set the clinic going I met all these horrendous social problems ... I was interested in Basaglia. I've always had a very strong interest in Italy. I spent a lot of time in Italy and visited Trieste to see the services he set up there. I was asked to join a group in the [European Union] to look at and report on the situation in Greek psychiatric hospitals in the 1980s. As part of that we visited Italy several times including Trieste. That is how I became so familiar with Basaglia and his work.
>
> **(Browne, private interview, 2018)**

According to Browne, the key difference between Italy and Ireland lay in the relationship between psychiatry and politics in the two jurisdictions:

> Basaglia's contribution in Italy was very socialist, left-wing and political. This did not carry over to Ireland. There wasn't that same relationship between psychiatry and politics, especially left-wing politics, in Ireland that you had in Trieste. Psychiatrists in Ireland are not generally very politically connected whereas Basaglia's socialism was as important as the psychiatry. For Basaglia, psychiatry was almost a lesser part of his left-wing political activity. When he was in his heyday, they would hold a parade getting patients to bring a boat to the sea and things like that. It was a left-wing community movement as well as psychiatry. I don't think there was that kind of psychiatric connection in Ireland at all.
>
> **(Browne, private interview, 2018)**

More recently, Dr. Pat Bracken, the psychiatrist and clinical director who spoke alongside Scheper–Hughes at the University of Limerick in 2012 (Thompson, 2012), has written extensively and convincingly on the subjects of trauma (Bracken, 2002), moving beyond the current paradigm in psychiatry (along with Browne and others) (Bracken et al., 2012), critical psychiatry (Thomas and Bracken, 2004), and 'post-psychiatry' (Bracken and Thomas, 2005). Bracken, like Browne, acknowledges the influence of Basaglia's work:

> Basaglia was not around when I graduated as a doctor in 1982. He died in 1980. But his ideas and actions inspired a whole bunch of people who I had the privilege to work with. These were people who challenged the *status quo* and who argued that we needed to create alternatives to hospitalisation for people with mental health difficulties. They were people who valued critical thought and who demanded more imaginative ways of thinking about and responding to such difficulties. They were not afraid to say that psychiatry, its ideas and its interventions, could be damaging and toxic for patients and families. We should never forget this.
>
> **(Bracken, private interview, 2018)**

Conclusions

Basaglia's life and work have proven as controversial as they are fascinating. The publication in 2015 of John Foot's book, *The Man Who Closed the Asylums: Franco Basaglia and the Revolution in Mental Health Care*, usefully reignited the debate about Basaglia and the enduring impact of his philosophy on psychiatry and beyond (Jones, 2015; Wise, 2015; Jay, 2016]. In Ireland, radical psychiatry did not gain a significant foothold in the 1900s, largely due to the imperviousness of the mental hospitals to any form of outside influence, be it the Roman Catholic Church, psychoanalysis, or even Basaglia and his democratic psychiatry. The difficulty of finding Basaglia's writings translated into English, and the limited, generally negative coverage of his work in English-language psychiatric journals available in Ireland, were additional obstacles to the propagation of Basaglian philosophy in Ireland.

Change, when it finally arrived to the Irish mental health system, was largely attributable to governmental initiatives and international human rights standards emanating from the UN and the Council of Europe, rather than from radicalized psychiatrists (Kelly, 2016a). But while there was no significant public *social* demand for a more democratic psychiatry in Ireland (Leane and Sapouna, 1998; Sapouna, 2006), and Basaglia was essentially invisible, it is now clear that Basaglia has influenced the thoughts of certain influential Irish psychiatrists, behind the scenes, over past decades.

Therefore, while public and general professional awareness of Basaglia was low, the revolutionary and historic episode he triggered in Italy might nonetheless have exerted some indirect influence on the eventual reform of the Irish mental health system. After all, challenging the status quo and engaging in critical thought are both very Basagalian activities, and are both essential components of any such change. As Bracken wisely advises: 'We should never forget this' (private communication, 2018).

Acknowledgements

I am very grateful to Professor Ivor Browne and Dr. Pat Bracken for their assistance. Material from the *Irish Journal of Psychiatry* is reproduced by kind permission of the late Dr. Dermot Walsh, to whom this chapter is dedicated.

References

Anonymous (2014). Obituary: Dr Robert A. McCarthy. *Irish Medical Journal* 107:62.

Basaglia, F. (1964). *Silence in the Dialogue with the Psychotic*. London: Sixth Congress of Psychotherapy.

Bourne, H. (1985). Misunderstanding the Italian experience. *British Journal of Psychiatry* 147:452.

Bracken, P. (2002). *Trauma: Culture, Meaning and Philosophy.* London and Philadelphia, PA: Whurr Publishers.
Bracken, P. and Thomas, P. (2005). *Postpsychiatry: Mental Health in a Postmodern World.* Oxford: Oxford University Press.
Bracken, P., et al. (2012). Psychiatry beyond the current paradigm. *British Journal of Psychiatry* 201:430–4.
Bradshaw, J.S. (1983). The yank in the corner. *Irish Times* 15 August 1983.
Brennan, D. (2014). *Irish Insanity, 1800–2000.* Abingdon, Oxfordshire: Routledge.
Browne, I. (2008). *Music and Madness*. Cork: Atrium/Cork University Press.
Browne, I. (2013). *The Writings of Ivor Browne—Steps Along the Road: The Evolution of a Slow Learner.* Cork: Atrium/Cork University Press.
Commission of Inquiry on Mental Illness (1966). *Report of the Commission of Inquiry on Mental Illness*. Dublin: The Stationery Office.
Crumlish, N. (2013). Browne's vision both inspires and infuriates. *Sunday Business Post* 4 August 2013.
De Girolamo, G. (1985). Misunderstanding the Italian experience. *British Journal of Psychiatry* 147:451–2.
Fitzgerald, M. (2003). Psychoanalytic psychotherapy in Ireland. In: M. Fitzgerald (ed.), *Irish Families under Stress (Volume 7)*. Dublin: South Western Area Health Board, pp. 115–19.
Foot, J. (2015). *The Man Who Closed the Asylums: Franco Basaglia and the Revolution in Mental Health Care*. London and New York: Verso.
Holmquist, K. (1990). Studies show lower rate of schizophrenia. *Irish Times* 19 October 1990.
Gilhooley, J. and Kelly, B.D. (2018). Return of the asylum. *British Journal of Psychiatry* 212:69–70.
Jay, M. (2016). 'I'm not signing'. *London Review of Books* 8 September 2016.
Jones, K. and Poletti, A. (1985). Understanding the Italian experience. *British Journal of Psychiatry* 146:341–7.
Jones, K. and Poletti, A. (1986a). The Italian experience in mental health care. *Hospital and Community Psychiatry* 37:795–802.
Jones, K. and Poletti, A. (1986b). The 'Italian experience' reconsidered. *British Journal of Psychiatry* 148:144–50.
Jones, K., Wilkinson, G., and Craig, T.K.J. (1991). The 1978 Italian mental health law: a personal evaluation: a review. *British Journal of Psychiatry* 159:556–61.
Jones, T. (2015). The Man Who Closed the Asylums: Franco Basaglia and the Revolution in Mental Health Care. *Guardian* 22 August 2015.
Kane, E. (1981). Reply to 'Ballybran'. *Irish Times* 13 April 1981.
Kelly, B.D. (2007). Penrose's Law in Ireland: an ecological analysis of psychiatric inpatients and prisoners. *Irish Medical Journal* 100:373–4.
Kelly, B.D. (2012). *The Irish Journal of Psychological Medicine* and the College of Psychiatry of Ireland. *Irish Journal of Psychological Medicine* 29:3–6.
Kelly, B.D. (2016a). *Hearing Voices: The History of Psychiatry in Ireland.* Dublin: Irish Academic Press.
Kelly, B.D. (2016b). *The Irish Journal of Psychological Medicine*: expanding horizons, moving on. *Irish Journal of Psychological Medicine* 33:1–2.
Kelly, B.D. (2017a). Ego, id, and Ireland. *Lancet Psychiatry* 4:281–2.
Kelly, B.D. (2017b). Dr Dermot Walsh, 1931–2017. *Irish Journal of Psychological Medicine* 34:217–20.
Kendler, K.S., McGuire, M., Gruenberg, A.M., O'Hare, A., Spellman, M., and Walsh, D. (1993). The Roscommon Family Study: I. *Archives of General Psychiatry* 50:527–40.

Leane, M. and Sapouna, L. (1998). Deinstitutionalisation in the Republic of Ireland: a case for re-definition? In: J. Campbell and R. Manktelow (eds), *Mental Health Social Work in Ireland*. Aldershot, UK: Ashgate, pp. 101–20.

Lunatic Asylums, Ireland, Commission (1858). *Report of the Commissioners of Inquiry into the State of the Lunatic Asylums and Other Institutions for the Custody and Treatment of the Insane in Ireland: (Part 1)*. Dublin: Thom and Sons, for Her Majesty's Stationery Office.

McQuaid, J.C. (1963). Introduction. In: E.F. O'Doherty and S.D. McGrath (eds), *The Priest and Mental Health*. New York: Alba House, pp. ix–xi.

Nowlan, D. (1979). Death by suppression. *Irish Times* 4 August 1979.

Palermo, G.B. (1991). The 1978 Italian mental health law—a personal evaluation. *Journal of the Royal Society of Medicine* 84:99–102.

Papeschi, R. (1985). The denial of the institution. *British Journal of Psychiatry* 146:247–54.

Pye, P. (1983). The yank in the corner. *Irish Times* 15 August 1983.

Ramon, S. (1985). Understanding the Italian experience. *British Journal of Psychiatry* 147:208–9.

Rizzoli, A.A. (1987). Italian psychiatry. *British Journal of Psychiatry* 151:276.

Sapouna, L. (2006). Tracing evidence of institutionalisation in the process of de-institutionalisation—the Irish case. In: L. Sapouna and P Herrmann (eds), *Knowledge in Mental Health*. New York: Nova Science Publishers, pp. 85–99.

Scheper-Hughes, N. (1979 [reissued 2001]). *Saints, Scholars and Schizophrenics: Mental Illness in Rural Ireland*. Berkeley, CA: University of California Press.

Scheper-Hughes, N. (1981). Reply to 'Ballybran'. *Irish Times* 21 February 1981.

Scheper-Hughes, N. (1990). Three propositions for a critically applied medical anthropology. *Social Science and Medicine* 30:189–97.

Scheper-Hughes, N. and Lovell, A.M. (1986). Breaking the circuit of social control: lessons in public psychiatry from Italy and Franco Basaglia. *Social Science and Medicine* 23:159–78.

Scheper-Hughes, N. and Lovell, A.M. (eds) (1987). *Psychiatry Inside Out: Selected Writings of Franco Basaglia*. New York: Columbia University Press.

Select Committee on the Lunatic Poor in Ireland (1817). *Report from the Select Committee on the Lunatic Poor in Ireland*. London: House of Commons.

Select Committee of the House of Lords (1843). *Report from the Select Committee of the House of Lords Appointed to Consider the State of the Lunatic Poor in Ireland*. London: House of Commons.

Tansella, M. (1985). Misunderstanding the Italian experience. *British Journal of Psychiatry* 147:450–1.

Thomas, P. and Bracken, P. (2004). Critical psychiatry in practice. *Advances in Psychiatric Treatment* 10:361–70.

Thompson, S. (2012). Health board. *Irish Times* 4 December 2012.

United Nations (1991). *Principles for the Protection of Persons with Mental Illness and the Improvement of Mental Health Care*. New York: UN, Secretariat Centre for Human Rights.

Viney, M. (1971). Mental illness: an inquiry. *Irish Times*.

Viney, M. (1980). Geared for a gale. *Irish Times* 24 September 1980.

Viney, M. (1983). The yank in the corner. *Irish Times* 6 August 1983.

Waddington, J.L., Youssef, H.A., and Kinsella, A. (1995). The prevalence of schizophrenia in Ireland. *Archives of General Psychiatry* 52:509.

Walsh, D. (1992). Brief historical review. *Irish Journal of Psychiatry* 13:3–20.

Walsh, D. (2006). Mental illness in Ireland and its management. In: D. McCluskey (ed.), *Health Policy and Practice in Ireland*. Dublin: University College Dublin Press, pp. 29–43.

Wise, S. (2015). Taking over the asylums. *Financial Times* 15–16 August 2015.

13
Asylum
A magazine for democratic psychiatry in England

Helen Spandler

Introduction

Most accounts of Franco Basaglia and Psichiatria Democratica[1] tend to focus on the closure of the asylums. Whilst this was clearly important, it would be a mistake to see the movement's impact solely in terms of legal and administrative changes in 'managing the mentally ill'. The movement provided inspiration and motivation to a new generation of mental health workers and activists keen to initiate social change—beyond dismantling the asylum system. Whilst Psichiatria Democratica may have had little influence on mainstream British psychiatry, a significant number of mental health professionals, workers, and activists in England took an active interest in the movement, and especially in Trieste, where the movement had its most profound impact. Arguably, Trieste played a significant role in radical mental health movements in England, both symbolically and physically (Harrington, 2008; Crossley, 1999). Most notably, it directly inspired *Asylum: the magazine for democratic psychiatry* which was established in 1986. (For the rest of this chapter I will just refer to it as *Asylum*.)

This chapter uses my research into the first 30 years of *Asylum* to explore how it functioned—and, I argue, still functions—as a concrete legacy of Psichiatria Democratica. Although I was not involved in setting up the magazine, I have been part of its editorial collective for over 20 years and am currently its managing editor. This gives me a unique vantage point through which to analyse these developments. I will use the contents of the magazine to explore the movement's influence on the UK mental health field.[2] Mirroring Psichiatria Democratica itself, where the movement was much stronger in Northern Italy, much of this influence occurred in the north of England, where I highlight some specific developments. I will suggest that *Asylum* continues the struggle for democratic psychiatry, adapted for contemporary times.

[1] Psichiatria Democratica was the name of the organization set up to pursue the aims of the movement, but I use it here as shorthand for the movement as a whole.

[2] Rather than listing each article in the reference list, I will refer to the author in the main text, and reference the issue of *Asylum* in which the article appeared.

I have reservations about reinforcing the status of an individual male psychiatrist, Franco Basaglia, as so central to the movement, especially since he died before most of the major changes and impact occurred.[3] However, given the focus of this book, and the importance of Basaglia's writing to the movement, I will reference his work to make this case.

The creation of *Asylum* magazine

Despite Psichiatria Democratica's apparent lack of influence on mainstream British psychiatry, some psychiatrists and mental health professionals did take an active interest in the movement. For example, Alec Jenner was 'one of the first psychiatrists in the UK to take a serious interest in the [Italian] movement' (*Asylum*, 1993, 7(2):29). Based in Sheffield in the north of England, Jenner was not known as a radical or an anti-psychiatrist. He had been a research biochemist, was involved in many trials of psychiatric drugs, and, controversially, helped introduce benzodiazipines into psychiatry. Yet he was intrigued by the radical psychiatrists and open-minded enough to think they might have something to offer. As such, he became acquainted with R.D. Laing and other psychiatric radicals. He also took a keen interest in the international politics of psychiatry. For example, he initiated professional protests against the use of psychiatry in oppressing political dissidents in Russia (*Asylum*, 2007, 16(1):9). He visited Trieste a number of times and was impressed by what he saw and heard. He was initially reassured that Psichiatria Democratica 'did not deny the reality of mental disorder, or the effectiveness of anti-psychotic drugs' (*Asylum*, 2013, 20(1):9). However, he wanted to 'put medical hegemony under scrutiny' and 'pose questions about the appropriate borders of medicine, to learn from others and shake up ourselves from any complacency' (*Asylum*, 2007, 16(1):2). In particular, he wanted to raise awareness in the UK about the movement.

It is important to note that there was very little of Basaglia's writing available in English until 1987, when Nancy Scheper–Hughes and Anne Lovell's inspired selection of his work was published as *Psychiatry Inside Out*. Moreover, Basaglia died in 1980, before interest in the movement took off in the UK. Although he left behind a powerful legacy, misinformation and misunderstanding about the movement grew. Therefore, Jenner, and Shula Ramon[4] (a social work academic based in London), organized a visit to the UK of four Italian mental health professionals from Trieste who were active members of Psichiatria Democratica. At various events in England, during March and April 1984, they spoke about the movement and led discussions about it in Manchester, Sheffield, and London.

[3] See my critical appreciation of John Foot's *The Man Who Closed the Asylums* (Spandler, 2016).

[4] Ramon was another key individual who helped introduce the Italian developments to a UK audience. She advocated for similar changes in UK mental health services and often defended the movement (e.g. Ramon, 1989).

Lyn Bigwood,[5] a psychiatric nurse and active trade unionist in York, heard about the Italians' visit and contacted Jenner. After talking with her, Jenner persuaded a couple of the Italian visitors to stay on to speak at a conference she was organizing in Wakefield. The event was for 'rank and file' health and social service workers to discuss the implications of closing the mental hospitals and of emerging community care policies. The conference ended up being 'dominated by reports and discussions of the Italian experience of just such a policy' (*Asylum*, 1986, 1(1):2). At the end of these discussions, a decision was made to set up a magazine to introduce and promote the idea of democratic psychiatry to a British audience. The three co-founders:—Jenner, Bigwood, and her partner, Phil Virden[6]—established *Asylum* to continue discussions and debate the possibilities of democratic mental healthcare in the UK. The Department of Psychiatry at the University of Sheffield had made a slight profit from the visit which Jenner was able to use to start publishing the magazine. It was produced with the help of a small group of Yorkshire-based mental health workers, ex-patients and other interested parties. Appropriately, given its connections to Psichiatria Democratica, the magazine was printed by a local ex-patients' cooperative for a number of years.

Jenner worked with, and mentored, another psychiatrist, Tim Kendall, who also took an active interest in the Italian situation (see Kendall, 1996). Kendall was acutely aware of the 'particularly negative' views of Trieste expressed by the British psychiatric establishment and decided to visit and see the situation for himself (see Kendall, 1996). He recalled that he 'slept, ate, breathed' Trieste for three weeks in 1985. The psychiatric establishment in the UK often argued that the Italian developments only *appeared* impressive because the situation in Italy prior to the changes was so appalling, and much worse than the situation in the UK. However, Kendall's experience of British psychiatry at the time suggested that it was not much better. He was working in an acute psychiatric ward in a general hospital, and on a long-stay ward in the old mental hospital in Sheffield. He observed the terrible conditions of patients, including their physical abuse and neglect. In comparison, he felt the reforms inspired by Psichiatria Democratica had had a positive impact on Italian mental healthcare.

That same year, 1985, the *British Journal of Psychiatry* had included a number of what Kendall called 'misinformed, outspokenly critical and at times frankly scornful' accounts of what it called the 'Italian experience' (Kendall, 1996). Rectifying this situation was undoubtedly one of Kendall's motivations for being involved in *Asylum* magazine. The title 'Asylum' was suggested by Barbara Jenner, Alec's wife.[7] It was

[5] From 1983, Bigwood had been trying to expose two Yorkshire-based psychiatrists who were systematically sexually abusing female patients. It took 20 years for these allegations to result in a formal investigation, the Kerr–Haslam Inquiry, which vindicated her claims, but Bigwood had been bullied, demoted, and subsequently sacked over her allegations (*Asylum*, 2006, 15(1)).

[6] Phil Virden was a former Sociology lecturer at York University who was illegally sacked during the Thatcher era.

[7] Barbara Jenner was a frequently supportive presence at editorial meetings, which were usually held at her and Alec's farmhouse outside Sheffield. Like Franca Ongaro, she is probably another unsung hero in this story.

seen as an ironic nod to the name of the journal which preceded the *British Journal of Psychiatry*.[8] At first glance, the title may seem at odds with the Italian movement's focus on *dismantling* the asylum system. However, the name was an attempt to reclaim asylum's original Greek origins as a place of sanctuary and refuge, a space that cannot be violated. Moreover, the magazine was intended to be as much a sanctuary for unpopular, controversial, and disturbing *ideas*, as for disturbed and disturbing *people*. Jenner and Kendall were both involved in the early years of the magazine. Jenner's involvement lasted for many years, until ill health forced him to retire, whilst Kendall went on to take up various senior-level positions with the National Institute of Clinical Excellence (NICE) and the Department of Health (NHS England). Although their paths diverged, both Jenner and Kendall kept up contact with their Italian counterparts. Therefore, it is possible that the movement did influence some aspects of psychiatry, albeit less directly and explicitly.

The magazine's indebtedness to Psichiatria Democratica is clearly signalled by its subtitle, 'a magazine for democratic psychiatry', and later (in 1993), '*the* magazine for democratic psychiatry'. This was also clear in its mission, recalled by Jenner in 2002:

> Our aim was . . . to struggle towards achieving what we thought was the best of the system in Trieste in the late eighties. There the great Asylum San Giovanni was now a complex of apartments for ex patients, with art studios for everyone, space for theatres and cinema performances and a *perpetual discussion of what more could be done to humanise mental health services* [emphasis added].
>
> **(http://asylummagazine.org/home/history-of-asylum-magazine/)**

The central idea was to create a forum for open, ongoing debate and discussion about what democratic mental health services might look like, especially if they were organized and controlled by the people most affected, especially workers 'on the ground' and service users, and not just hospital managers and doctors. The first issue of the magazine was published in Spring 1986 and its editorial explained its roots in Psichiatria Democratica, for which it expressed explicit admiration (Figure 13.1).

This first issue included numerous articles about the politics of mental health, including articles by Jenner about Franco Basaglia and the Italian mental health reforms. It also included an article by Givoanna Battaglia, a psychiatric nurse in Trieste, who gave an illuminating description of the complex process involved in nurses being relocated from the hospitals into the community, and the ideological shifts and learning involved.

Later, *Asylum* included features about mental health services in other countries that had been influenced by Psichiatria Democratica. For example, it included an article about Sicilian villages where 'the whole population accepts "madness" and the

[8] It was initially called the *Asylum Journal* (1853–1855); then, the *Asylum Journal of Mental Science* (1855–1857), the *Journal of Mental Science* (1858–1962), and the *British Journal of Psychiatry* (1963–present).

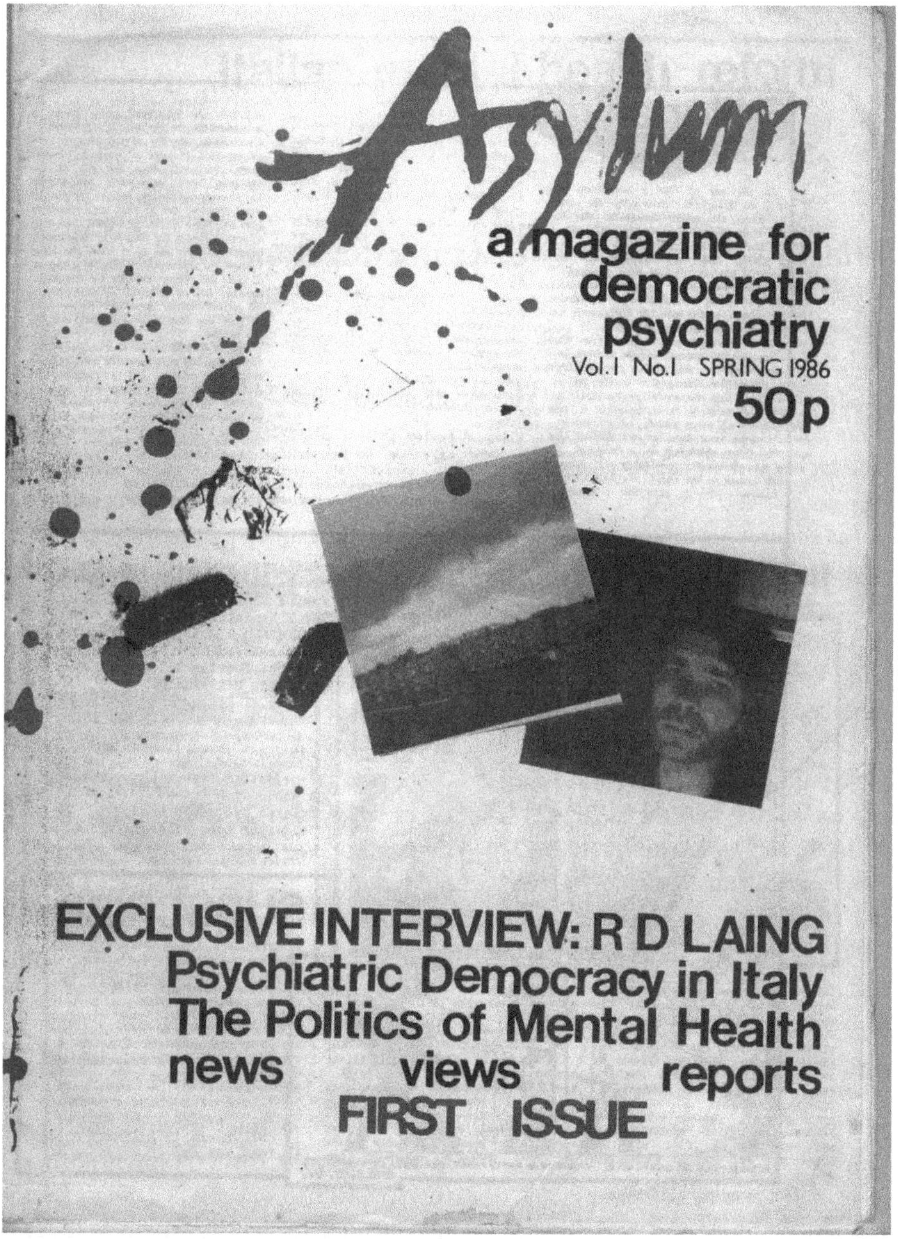

Figure 13.1 *Asylum* magazine is launched in Spring 1986.

people manage to live together' (*Asylum*, 1990, 4(1):10). It also included an article about Liege Belgium, which had close links with Trieste (*Asylum*, 1991, 5(1):6–8). More recently, it included an article about a Brazilian mental health programme in Santos which was inspired by the Basaglian experience of a left-wing government striving for radical change in mental health services beyond an individual clinical approach (*Asylum*, 2002, 13(3):21–23).

The next section focuses on developments in England, where Trieste seemed to offer both a philosophical system and an alternative model of practice than what was being developed in the UK.

Trieste as inspiration for service developments in England

The closure of the old asylums was not a new policy in the UK. Psychiatric hospitals had been discharging long-stay patients from the 1960s onwards. However, there were concerns about this policy being accelerated in the 1980s under a cost-cutting and highly individualistic Conservative Government. Given the devastation that this Government was inflicting on industrial working-class communities, there were concerns about what their policies would do to mental healthcare. Many mental health workers and activists in the north of England had actively supported the long and courageous, but ultimately defeated, miners' strike of 1984–1985. Indeed, many had families directly involved in the strike. They were anxious that patients might be liberated from the old mental hospitals but end up being isolated, stigmatized, and unsupported in the community. Government policy of closing the old asylums might have seemed similar to the situation in Italy. However, mental healthcare under Thatcherism would be very different from the collective provision and workers cooperatives that were the hallmark of services in Trieste.

In this context, activists looked to Trieste to see how community care could be implemented differently (i.e. if they were underpinned by a socialist ideology of collectivism, social responsibility, and cooperation). Trieste was seen as more politically progressive than Laing's more individualized approach which had been popular amongst radicals in the 1960s and 1970s. Laing's approach had been criticized for its conservative undercurrents by the socialist scholar Peter Sedgwick in his influential book *Psychopolitics* (Sedgwick, 1982). Many mental health workers who had been radicalized in the 1960s and 1970s were looking for genuine workable alternatives to the mental health system. In Trieste, they found a system 'they could connect with, one which articulated their concerns in a coherent form' (Crossley, 1999, p. 814).

Jenner's article in the first issue of *Asylum* bemoaned the absence of any 'clearly formulated principles and policies' in the UK for creating 'realistic new ideas or understanding and caring for emotionally distressed people' (*Asylum*, 1986, 1(1):3). He claimed that the 'medical model' in the UK had 'merely been reproduced outside of the hospitals with people "maintained" on long-term drug therapy, the occasional visit from a community nurse and a ten minute out-patient appointment' (*Asylum*, 1986, 1(1):3). Many aspects of Trieste appealed to workers and activists who shared his concerns. In particular, they were inspired by the creativity, optimism, and sense of community in Trieste. After all, these very qualities were being attacked in the Thatcher years in the UK. Jenner visited Trieste in August 1985 and recalled how:

> We were impressed by the political outlook and inclusive services in Trieste and the inspiration of the Basaglias. Amongst other things there we saw the importance of offering to everyone the cultural riches of the arts, entertainment, sport, and freedom of expression. They wanted society in general to be made aware of the mental health services and the human needs involved. Perhaps more importantly they produced an atmosphere of optimism, and celebration, a conviction too that [by] working together much can be achieved and richly enjoyed. Everyone could also be shown that we are all part of the problems in our own society.
>
> **(*Asylum*, 2007, 16(1):2)**

Activists were impressed by practices like the assemblies in Trieste where, at least in theory, everybody involved in the services had a right to speak their mind. These various forums for debate were key to the collectivization of responsibility, accountability, and anti-institutional practice. These practices had been adapted from therapeutic community ideas and practices in the UK. Jenner was attracted to the idea of making the society therapeutic, rather than isolating and excluding patients from society and creating psychoanalytically informed mini 'therapeutic community' institutions. Jenner recalled wanting to imitate the development of Italian democratic psychiatry in the UK (*Asylum*, 2013, 20(1):9). He even tried to convince the University of Sheffield's Department of Psychiatry (where he was based) to run a service, modelled on Trieste, in the more deprived areas in Sheffield:

> because I was very influenced by the Italian idea that ... a psychiatric service should be part of the community ... It shouldn't allow people to ignore what was perhaps causing a lot of the problems which was social and interaction with other people. And the only way to do that was to implant it in a real community.
>
> **(*Asylum*, 2007, 16(1):2)**

Whilst this proposal did not materialize, Jenner, Kendall, and colleagues attempted to democratize local services, and they believed in the movement's emphasis on the 'right of the patient to be part of the debate about their own treatment' (*Asylum*, 2013, 20(1):9). It is worth noting that whilst service user involvement is more accepted in the UK now, even if it is still underdeveloped, it was very much in its infancy in the early 1980s. As Kendall later recalled: 'during its early years, *Asylum* magazine was viewed by the psychiatric profession as scandalous. The idea of spending much time listening to patients—let alone listening to their views on mental disorder or psychiatry—was anathema' (*Asylum*, 2016, 23(2):3)

Asylum drew in others who were inspired by Trieste—most notably, a group of mental health workers and activists across the Pennines, in Manchester, who were also trying to democratize local mental health services. For example, members of the *Asylum* editorial collective included workers from a new resettlement team in Harpurhey, North Manchester, set up to 'resettle' patients from Springfield Psychiatric Hospital in 1987. Like Gorizia, when Basaglia first arrived and where he initiated the movement (Foot, 2015), Springfield Hospital desperately needed change. Its physical conditions were described as appalling, and its practices were considered controlling and oppressive (Harrington, 2009). The resettlement team was made up of a small number of nurses and support workers who were redeployed from Springfield Hospital. One of the resettlement workers was Mark Greenwood—a psychiatric nurse, and an active member of the *Asylum* collective. He explained that the first activity the new team undertook was a week-long overland trip to Trieste by minibus. He recalled that they did not want to be just simply a 'small micro-project' but, rather, part of a much bigger global movement for social change:

> We were very excited by that, you know, we were very sort of fired up by that... [We] proposed, I'm not quite sure where it came from, but we came up with the idea that the new team, which was sort of ten, eleven of us, would spend the first week of our working together, it amazes me to think that we had the resources to do this, but we went to Trieste ... and we organised a very, very memorable trip overland in a mini-bus all the way to Trieste ... One of their co-operatives ran a hotel and we were put up on people's floors and stuff, and we met other people who were there.
>
> **(Harrington, 2008, p. 245)**

According to Greenwood, this visit had a profound impact on the group and became a major influence on how they would go on to frame their practice:

> We were kind of blown away with what we saw. [It was] very much, I suppose, how people would go to kibbutz in the '70s and '80s and be inspired by what they saw ... It kind of honed up ... it was deeply influential because it gave us lots and lots of ideas ... The predominant influence [was] the ideology that you transferred resources from a hospital base into a community ... rather than you just simply settled onto a community and drained the community's resources. That was a very ... crucial part of our thinking.
>
> **(Harrington, 2008, p. 245)**

In other words, they wanted to harness the resources that had gone into the psychiatric hospital and ensure that they directly benefitted the communities where patients would be resettled.

In addition, echoing Trieste, some of the workers were involved in writing practical proposals, such as the idea of fully integrated community mental health teams, offering a 24-hour, open-access service which would eventually replace all hospital-based acute facilities (Harrington, 2008). However, not everyone in the team shared their values and, according to Harrington (2008), this led to a fundamental tension. On the one hand, the 'radicals' saw the resettlement team as just one element in a much broader 'Trieste-like' project to break the power of the hospitals and transfer resources into community. On the other hand, the 'conventionals' still framed the service in terms of traditional professional values and saw the resettlement team as constituting a discrete service for a particular group of clients, connected only tangentially to broader social movements (Harrington, 2008). This division mimicked the splits that were also apparent in the Italian situation. It also suggests that although the movement's impact was significant, it was certainly not widespread and it did not go unchallenged.

Radical mental health workers and academics organized a number of subsequent trips to Trieste over the next few years. For example, *Asylum* included an advert for an 'opportunity to take part in an organised visit to Trieste to see at first hand the work of the mental health service' which would take place in May 1993 (*Asylum*, 1992/1993, 7(1):7). This visit was organized by the third-sector campaigning organization, the Manchester Alliance for Community Care, some of whose members were involved in *Asylum*.

It may be that Psichiatria Democratica's influence was strongest in the north of England. For example, *Asylum* magazine has always been produced by a collective primarily based in Sheffield and Greater Manchester. In addition, the resettlement team was not only in Manchester, but in the more socially and economically deprived north of the city, rather than in the more prosperous and seemingly fertile environments in the south. This is important not only because radical developments are often portrayed as London-centric, but also for what it means about the conditions for this kind of innovation. Harrington has suggested that Springfield Hospital's position as a marginalized and neglected institution may have created the conditions for this kind of innovation (Harrington, 2009). Rather like the situation in Gorizia when Basaglia first arrived there, Springfield Hospital's relatively marginalized, peripheral, and neglected position—away from regulation and influence from more mainstream psychiatric developments—may have allowed activists more freedom and opportunity to innovate (Harrington, 2009). It is beyond the scope of this chapter to fully understand Trieste's impact or influence on services. However, it is important not to overstate the influence of Trieste on these developments. Other influences were also important. For example, socialist feminist public health officers were an important influence on radical developments in North Manchester at the time.[9]

Whether Psichiatria Democratica had any lasting impact on service development in the UK is difficult to discern. However, it certainly had a significant impact on the consciousness and confidence of a group of mental health activists eager to create

9 See Harrington (2009) for a fuller account of the Harpurhey resettlement team.

social change. The 'pilgrimages' to Trieste did not just inspire *Asylum* magazine or specific service developments: the connections made with, and within, Trieste played an important part in galvanizing international networks of activists (Crossley, 1999).

A broader network of mental health activists

The international lure of Trieste is well-documented (see Donnelly, 1992). Crossley (1999) has suggested that Trieste functioned as a 'working utopia' for mental health activists in the 1980s and 1990s in the UK (as Kingsley Hall had earlier).[10] Working utopias embody concrete mini-realizations of the desires of a social movement. They are important to social movements because they boost the 'imaginative force' of activists. This allows them to envisage the possibility of alternatives, providing them with added impetus to continue with their struggle for social change (Crossley, 1999, p 814). For example, after his visit in 1985, Jenner commented that Trieste was 'the most obvious remnant of the turbulent 1960s' (*Asylum*, 1986, 1(1):4). It thus helped to keep alive some of the radical hopes of that generation.

Trieste became a meeting ground for key intellectuals with an interest in democratic psychiatry. Jenner recalls how it felt like 'everybody went to Trieste'. He met key figures there who played a part in the emerging international intellectual anti-psychiatry scene. For example, he met Félix Guattari (co-author of *Anti Oedipus*); Robert Castell (author of *The Psychiatric Society*); and David Cooper, the South African/British (anti)-psychiatrist and author of *Psychiatry and Anti Psychiatry* (Jenner, in Crossley, 1999, p. 822). Spaces like Trieste were not only important as concrete 'working utopias' which fed activist's imagination. They also functioned as places for debate and discussion, which in turn created and sustained social networks of activists—and this helped 'make things happen'.

Arguably, Trieste played a role in the development of the international Hearing Voices movement. The Dutch psychiatrist Marius Romme, and Sandra Escher, talked about their research on hearing voices at the World Health Organization (WHO) conference which was hosted by Trieste in 1988. Key activists who attended the event from the UK took up these ideas and helped translate them into action. They invited Romme and Escher to come to the UK to talk about their research and discuss emerging new approaches to hearing voices. Their subsequent visit to the UK was supported and sponsored by Jenner and led to the development of the Hearing Voices Network in the UK. Whilst the ideas underpinning an alternative approach to hearing voices were already forming, this connection helped ignite the movement. This is not to say that Trieste is responsible, or can take credit, for the international Hearing Voices movement. Credit for this must go to voice hearers themselves and their allies. However, it is an important part of the overall history of the movement.

[10] Kingsley Hall was the therapeutic community in east London associated with R.D. Laing and the Philadelphia Association in the 1960s and 1970s.

Critical engagement with Trieste

Mental health activists in the UK have been criticized for over-romanticizing the situation in Italy, especially in Trieste (Jones and Poletti, 1985). Indeed, Crossley noted that his interviews with key mental health activists revealed 'frequent and often eulogistic' references to Trieste (Crossley, 1999, p. 811). However, whilst Trieste was clearly an inspiration to activists, it was not without criticism. For example, the first issue of *Asylum* also included a long and exclusive interview with R.D. Laing, by Lyn Bigwood, where he explicitly criticized Basaglia and the Italian movement (*Asylum*, 1986, 1(1):13–21). Laing was cautious that the magazine did not publish a 'put down on the Italian thing' especially as he was 'friends with some of them'. However, his objections were serious and noteworthy.

Laing thought Basgalia was a 'decent doctor', but he found him distinctly naive in matters of serious mental ill health. He took particular exception to the fact that Basaglia had taken charge of a mental hospital with little knowledge of psychiatry or the 'depths of human misery'. Laing noted that Basaglia had 'never been in a mental hospital in his life'. In addition, Laing thought the movement's alliance with the Communist Party was disastrous, not least because of Russia's chequered history of using psychiatry to oppress political dissidents (which Alec Jenner had highlighted). Laing criticized Basaglia for imposing a particular political ideology on patients with little understanding about their situation. As such, he accused Basgalia of adopting a rather 'sentimental' kind of Marxism which culminated in a lack of care and concern for patients. He gave the often-cited example of the long-stay 'catatonic schizophrenic' patient who was discharged from hospital to live with his mother who could not cope and was accused of his murder after he died in her house due to neglect. Laing suggests he was 'not just let out of the door, but kicked out of the door'. He is unequivocally scathing about this situation: 'That's no solution ... that is not psychiatric revolution. That is no progress. I disassociate myself from the Italian experiment in that sense, totally' (*Asylum*, 1986, 1(1):15).

It was not only Laing who expressed criticisms of the movement. Ian Parker, who would later become another member of the *Asylum* collective, was amongst another group of about 10 people to visit Trieste in May 1988, 10 years after Law 180 had been passed. This visit was planned in order to speak to people involved in the community mental health centres and, by this time, San Giovanni was functioning as one of the community centres, which included a café and a workers' cooperative. Parker was generally impressed by the visit and appreciated the barriers faced by the movement in making radical changes. However, he also recalled dimensions of the Trieste experience that some visitors found problematic. For example, the lack of attention to questions of culture, gender, and curiously, given the influence of Marxism in Basaglia's thinking, social class. Parker recalls observing that even in the so-called democratic spaces, the male psychiatrists, especially those with a charismatic presence, did most of the talking. Moreover, he got the impression that it was rather naively assumed that just putting patients back to work would solve their problem of integration into 'the community' which, in turn, was never really defined or interrogated.[11]

In addition, Jenner was also cautiously critical. For example, he suggested that 'perhaps it was the great mistake of Basaglia's and the Italian movement for Democratic Psychiatry, the original leaders of the movements, that they said it was cheaper as well as better' (*Asylum*, 2002, 13(3):23). As we shall see later, many of these concerns were echoed by psychiatric survivors.

Notwithstanding these important criticisms, however, the magazine continued to take inspiration from the movement. For example, a later editorial (*Asylum*, 1991, 5(1):9) refers to 'the unique national reform of psychiatric care in Italy' as 'the vanguard of state provision with a human face'. The editorial concluded that 'there is much to be learnt from Italy's example'. Later, it included articles defending the Italian reforms. For example, Mark Greenwood argued that it was 'important not to confuse the financial crisis of state funding for mental health services, with the perception that community care is failing in Italy as a result of the impracticality of law 180. The two issues should be kept separate if a clear analysis is to emerge about what is going on' (*Asylum*, 1993, 7(3):28).

Beyond mental health service reforms

Another consistent theme in Psichiatria Democratica, and one that animated Basgalia's work, was the importance of changing society's relationship with madness. In other words, not just focusing on reforming mental health services, but radically changing society in order to accommodate madness and to find new ways for the mad to be in society. This theme was emphasized more strongly when Terence McLaughlin, an activist in the Manchester hearing voices network, took over editing the magazine at the turn of the millennium (2000–2006). He was undoubtedly very familiar with Basaglia's work, and clearly appreciated the magazine's heritage. Most notably, McLaughlin embodied Basaglia's radical spirit, especially his dialectical revolutionary zeal. For example, he wrote in one of his editorials:

> Inspired initially by the movement Psichiatria Democratica and, we argue, still has a historical mission ... We clearly still believe, along with Basaglia, that as much as the power to repression and conformity looms, as divisions are explored, the possibilities for political change are deepened.
>
> **(*Asylum*, 2001, 12(2):3)**

In 2002 (13:2), *Asylum* included a special feature about 'the struggle for democratic psychiatry 25 years on' (see Figure 13.2). At this time, UK mental health activists

[11] Parker, personal communication with the author, 2018.

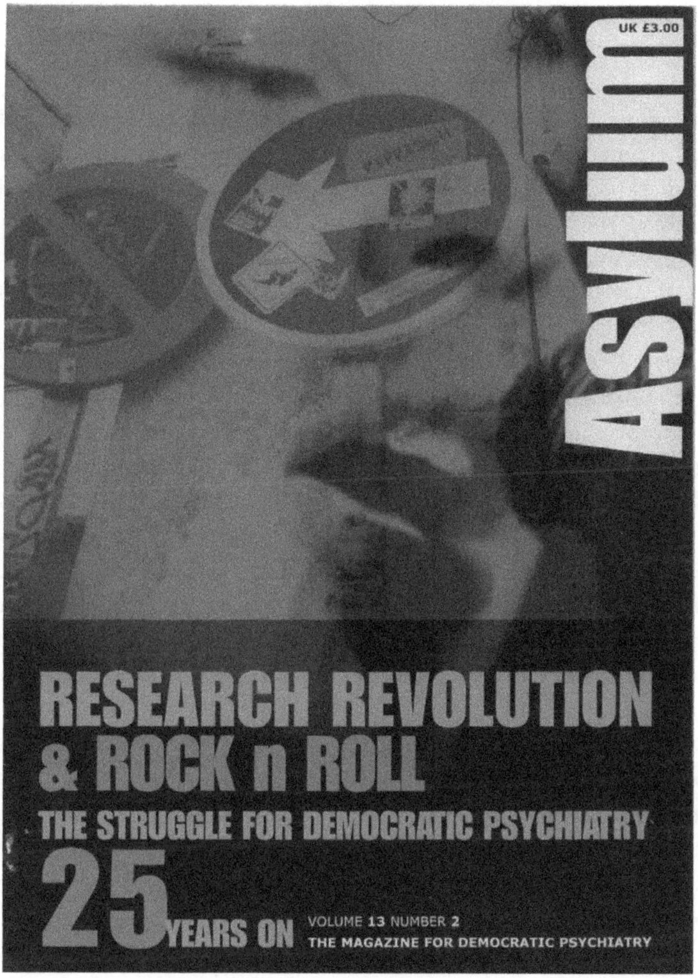

Figure 13.2 *Asylum: the struggle for democratic psychiatry 25 years on.*

were campaigning against proposed changes to mental health law and, specifically, the introduction of Community Treatment Orders. In his editorial, 'The Trieste Experiment revisited', McLaughlin expressed his hope that demonstrations and activism 'will be reminiscent of the spontaneous assemblies of the Trieste Experiment which unlike " 'care plans" always got to the heart of the matter—to find a community alternative to exclusion' (*Asylum*, 2002, 13(2):3). In particular, he highlighted the importance of Basaglia's wider vision of social change, and his fear that developments would ossify into mere legal reforms:

> While Trieste remains a beacon for community mental health services internationally, the asylum closing policies of Thatcher and Reagan during the same period

> combined to give both 'community' and 'care' a bad name. However, the virtual extension of the walls of the asylum into the community—the recuperation of coercion and exclusion by other means—came as no surprise to the democratic psychiatry movement led by Franco Basaglia. The law was not the endgame (in fact the law was a compromise). The real struggle was ideological, against the class nature of exclusion and for the decriminalisation and depsychiatization of irrationality and distress. The Trieste Experiment taught how the sane only hold a temporary truce against madness.
>
> (*Asylum*, 2002, 13(2):3)

A few years later, *Asylum* included a special feature about Soteria House, a pioneering minimal medication therapeutic community in the USA for people experiencing first episode psychosis (*Asylum*, 2006, 15(2)). A number of activists were campaigning for a Soteria House in the UK. McLaughlin took a typical and explicitly 'Basaglian' position on this. Basaglia had argued that therapeutic communities were important in increasing our understanding of how mental patients are scapegoats for a society riddled with contradictions. However, he was clear that the ultimate aim was to deprive society of any places created to internalize its contradictions (Basaglia, 1987). In other words, therapeutic communities should be merely 'transitional' projects, not ends in themselves. McLaughlin's editorial, entitled 'Critical Soteria', argued:

> The focus should be less about creating (Soteria) 'houses' and more about housing—more about changing social contradictions and relationships ... maybe it is about building Soteria Communities—the struggle for equality and democratic rights ... Hopefully, this is not seen as a too simplistic expression of the Italian democrats position.
>
> (*Asylum*, 2006, 15(2):5)

Asylum and 'democratic psychiatry'

When *Asylum* was relaunched in 2010 (see Figure 13.3), after a few years hiatus following McLaughlin's untimely death, the re-formed editorial collective decided to keep its subtitle, 'democratic psychiatry', despite it coming under some criticism. For example, when the US radical psychiatrist Thomas Szasz was asked to offer his support for the magazine's relaunch. he said: 'I regret that I cannot support the idea of a "democratic psychiatry". For me, the issue is coercion versus non-coercion ... Democratic psychiatry is a term associated with Basaglia's Italian version of locking up mental patients' (*Asylum*, 2013, 20(1):3). Szasz was arguably the most 'anti-psychiatry' of all the radical psychiatrists and was opposed to any form of state mental health provision. Given his negative experience of growing up in communist Hungary, he was suspicious of any state intervention in individuals' lives. He believed that distressed people

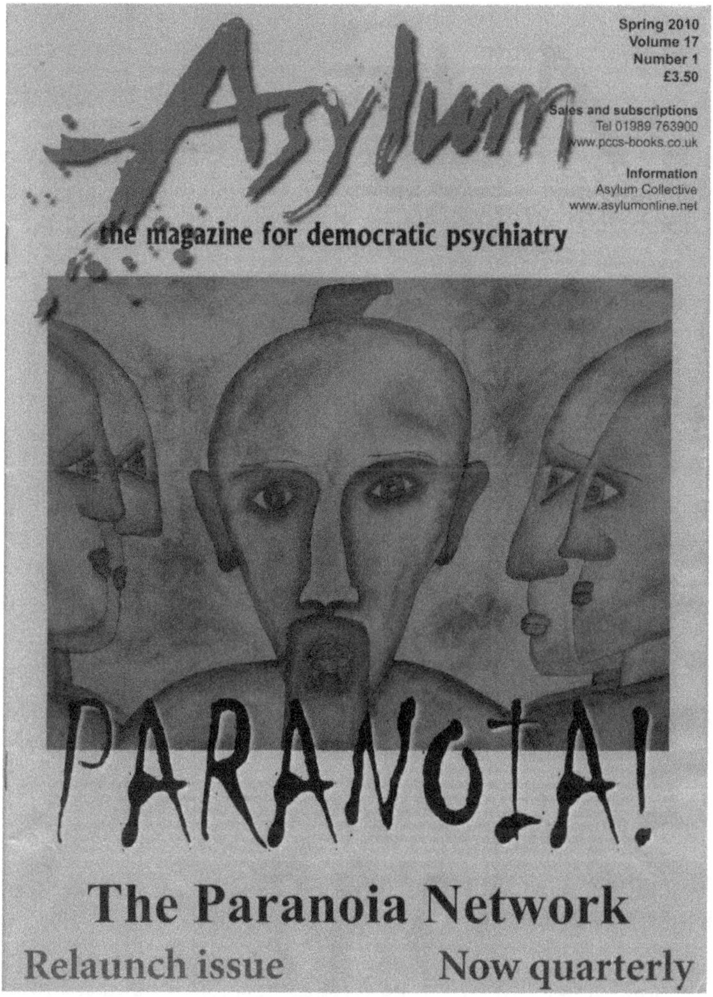

Figure 13.3 *Asylum* relaunch issue (2010).

should, if they wish, enter into an entirely voluntary contractual agreement with private mental health providers.[12]

Phil Virden, one of the magazine's founders, returned to the collective to act as its executive editor. He defended the magazine's continued use of 'democratic psychiatry' as follows:

> 'Psychiatry' = the management of mental disorder; 'Democracy' = government by the people; 'Democratic psychiatry' = managing mental disorder by way of the democratic

[12] Despite, or perhaps because of Szasz's critique, *Asylum* devoted a whole issue to discussing his work when he died (*Asylum*, 2013, 20(1)).

decisions of everyone involved. Obviously, this raises many questions. Hence ASYLUM magazine = a forum for debate.

(*Asylum*, 2013, 22(2):28)

Szasz's criticisms, however, were echoed by some psychiatric survivors. They thought the notion of 'democratic psychiatry' was an oxymoron due to psychiatry's complicity in coercion, detention, and forced treatment. For example, when *Asylum* asked for other readers' views on the issue, two psychiatric survivors responded:

When I first spotted Asylum on a bookstand at one conference—its subtitle was a reason for me to leave it where it was. It was only much later, after I was given a couple of issues and actually read them that I started liking the content very much. I know Democratic Psychiatry as an Italian political movement, with some significant achievements. Beyond that—the phrase itself has no meaning to me. It sounds like democratic slavery, democratic patriarchy or democratic apartheid. I think that theories and practices that are fundamentally wrong are best abandoned because no attributes will make them better.

(Jasna Russo, 2013)[13]

The idea of a 'democratic psychiatry' has always perplexed me. I have heard it championed by Italian psychiatrists though never by Italian survivors. They are far more reserved about the democratic psychiatry movement and its legacy.

(Debra Shulkes, 2013)[14]

Trieste, *Asylum*, and the psychiatric survivor movement

As previously suggested, whilst Trieste certainly inspired a number of radically inclined mental health professionals in the UK, it was much less of an inspiration to the psychiatric survivor movement. Some survivor activists did find parts of Basaglia's writings helpful to their cause. For example, Frank Bangay, a key activist in early patient organizations like Protection of the Rights of Mental Patients in Treatment (PROMPT) and the Campaign against Psychiatric Oppression (CAPO), recalled some of Basaglia's writings being of interest. He recalls being impressed by Basaglia's assertion that 'psychiatrists acted like criminals in peacetime, like the Nazis were criminals in war time'.[15]

In addition, notable survivor activists from the UK visited Trieste. For example, Louise Pembroke, who was a key activist in many notable survivor organizations in

[13] http://asylummagazine.org/2013/06/asylum-quiz-this-is-no-ordinary-quiz/
[14] http://asylummagazine.org/2013/06/asylum-quiz-this-is-no-ordinary-quiz/
[15] Personal communication with the author, 2018.

the 1980s and 1990s in the UK,[16] was an invited speaker at a WHO conference entitled 'The Question of Psychiatry' held in Trieste in 1988.[17] However, whilst survivor activists were impressed with some of the reforms, and especially the informality of services in Trieste, they had some important criticisms. For example, some expressed concern about the seeming (over)use of medication. At the WHO conference, some activists organized a separate space to discuss survivor perspectives and decided to deface drug-company sponsored posters which were displayed at the event as an objection to drug-company involvement in proceedings. Like other critics, they were also sceptical of the central role played by male psychiatrists in the movement and the continuing reverence shown to Basaglia.

At least in theory, Basaglia had welcomed patient rebellion and criticism because it helped highlight and open up key contradictions that needed attention (Foot, 2015). Moreover, the movement did support internal initiatives like a patients' magazine and some of its publications included patients' perspectives. For example, large sections of the movement's key text, *The Negated Institution*, was written by patients (although edited by psychiatrists). However, the extent of service-user involvement in Psichiatria Democratica is hard to assess. The movement did not appear to support, or benefit from, an autonomous patients' movement, unlike in the UK and other parts of Europe and in North America. An independent movement of service users or psychiatric survivors was not apparent in Italy, even in areas where Psichiatria Democratica was strong.

Some Italian service users did visit the UK to talk about developments in Trieste (e.g. at an event held at Camden's branch of MIND). However, they saw Psichiatria Democratica as primarily a movement of mental health professionals such as psychiatrists, psychologists, and psychiatric nurses, not service users. This did not endear them to UK service user activists who were demanding active involvement in mental health services and were setting up their own organizations. Not surprisingly, they took their primary inspiration from prominent patient activists and psychiatric survivor-led initiatives and movements. For example, networks and links forged around prominent patient activists like Judi Chamberlain[18] in the USA and the Dutch Patients' Councils were more long-lasting and influential.

Understanding the extent of engagement with the broader survivor movement, or the reasons for the lack of engagement, is beyond the scope of this chapter. Suffice to say that Psichiatria Democratica *was* led by mental health workers and that theirs was a different, if related, struggle to the psychiatric survivors' demand for patient-controlled services. Addressing the synergies *and* tensions between these two important struggles was—and still is—high on *Asylum*'s agenda.

[16] Such as Survivors Speak Out and the Self-Harm Network.

[17] Also present were Alec Jenner (*Asylum*), Paul Baker (Manchester MIND), and Mary Boyle (author of *Schizophrenia: a Scientific Delusion?*).

[18] Judi Chamberlain wrote the book *On Our Own: Patient-Controlled Alternatives to the Mental Health System* (Chamberlain, 1978). This had a very significant impact on the emerging patients' movement.

As the years progressed, *Asylum* kept its roots firmly within the broader philosophy of democratic psychiatry. However, it became as much influenced by the emerging survivor and Mad movements. For instance, many survivor-led activist groups such as Survivors Speak Out and CAPO in the 1980s, and many others over subsequent years (e.g. the emerging Self-Harm, Hearing Voices, and Mad Pride networks), used the magazine to express their views. Whilst explicit references to Psichiatria Democratica became less apparent, there are still examples which have a distinctly 'Basaglian' flavour. For example, the editorial in the special issue put together by Mad activists from Toronto included the following:

> There is no institution, big or small that can protect us from the violence and discrimination that we experience in this world. No government, no justice system, no asylum . . . I would rather live my whole life plotting to bring down the asylum than another moment propping it up.
>
> (*Asylum*, 2013, 20(4):3)

Rather than Trieste inspiring the Mad movement, however, it is more accurate to say that Psichiatria Democratica's vehement opposition to the segregation, discrimination, and oppression of the asylum system was shared by the emerging Mad movement. In addition, *Asylum*'s initial founding vision, inspired by Psichiatria Democratica—to create a forum for debate between workers and service users—only materialized in a piecemeal form. For example, in the early years, Kendall and Jenner noted that 'sadly, professionals seem unenthusiastic about this debate and rarely send articles' (Kendall and Jenner, 1989, p. 571). Despite attempts to encourage trade unions and statutory mental health organizations to support and subscribe to the magazine, it has always had a relatively small circulation and limited reach.

Precisely because of this, the broader, and unfinished, project of democratic psychiatry remains central to *Asylum*. As a longstanding member of the *Asylum* editorial collective, and its current editor, I have followed and been influenced by Psichiatria Democratica and Basaglia's work.[19] Therefore, I conclude this chapter by explaining how I think *Asylum* continues the struggle for democratic psychiatry today, adapted to contemporary concerns.

The struggle continues

In its thirtieth anniversary issue, *Asylum* included a cautiously positive appraisal of *Trieste: Before and After* by Daniel Magalhães Goulart (*Asylum*, 2016, 23(3):20–1) (see

[19] For example, I used Basaglia's critique of anti-psychiatric 'alternatives' that do not address their internal and external contradictions in my research about radical therapeutic communities in the UK (Spandler, 2006, 2009).

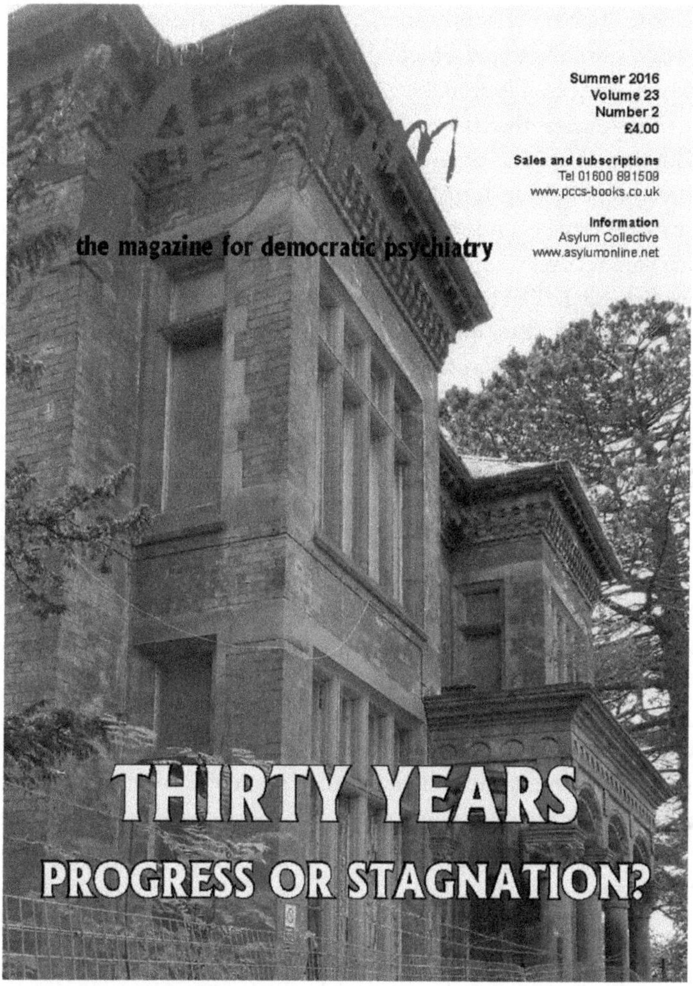

Figure 13.4 *Asylum* magazine 30 years on.

Figure 13.4). Goulart, a Brazilian mental health activist and researcher, visited Trieste 30 years after his English predecessors in *Asylum* had done so. He was similarly impressed by the open, informal, and dialogical approach to mental healthcare of the Italians, and critical of the central role of psychiatrists and the assumed necessity of medication. He perceptively concluded:

> As with any social and political movement, what is most important is not its history but . . . what is yet to be achieved. If this story [Trieste] is still a source of inspiration, it is precisely due to the contradictions that is has been able to expose. Which inevitably still persist today.
>
> (*Asylum*, **2016, 23(2):21)**

The current situation certainly poses unique new challenges, tensions, and contradictions. For a start, the English mental health system has not only moved away from asylum-based services, it is arguably moving away from community care-based services, too. This suggests that Basaglia's concern about creating new forms of institutionalization is perhaps less of an imminent danger, at least in mental health, as there is little investment in long-term therapeutic community-type services or long-term community care services and support structures. This situation, alongside the current policy focus on 'recovery' and 'social inclusion' through paid employment, could be seen as meeting the Italian movement's desire for wider social change 'beyond service reforms'. However, the situation is unlikely to be characterized as 'Basaglian', given the individualized, marketized, and cost-cutting focus of its neo-liberal context, and the increased use of compulsion and coercion.

In this context, current tensions have emerged around the rise of new, alternative 'recovery' models, frameworks, and policies. Many have argued that what began as a survivor-led 'recovery movement' has resulted in practices which are equally as oppressive as the ones they sought to replace. For example, the UK survivor organization Recovery in the Bin have suggested that 'recovery' is increasingly imposed on service users and used as an excuse not to provide people with financial or social support, and fails to address wider societal conditions, inequalities, and exclusions (*Asylum*, 2016, 22(3):21–2). Basaglia's warning is apposite here:

> [Ideas] become fixed in pre-established patterns even though, having acquired their birthright through a repudiation of a particular reality, they should, as a safeguard against their becoming an element of oppression themselves, be constantly reverting to reality to reinvigorate the *spirit of renewal* that originally informed them.
>
> **(Basaglia, 1985, p. 42)**

Basaglia argued that progressive mental healthcare innovations can only happen through continual crises and self-criticism. This, he maintained, is necessary to prevent the premature 'resolution' of ongoing contradictions and tensions by a seductive new idea, model, or project. He was especially worried that these efforts would become crystallized into new oppressive structures which ignore their own inevitable contradictions. Instead of ignoring or denying these contradictions, he argued that we should try to understand and confront them.

Asylum can be seen as an attempt to keep this 'spirit of renewal' alive by providing a space for ongoing and new contradictions to be aired and discussed. Rather than championing a new idea, service, or policy, it tries to maintain a space where alternatives can be discussed and critiqued. Crucially, this spirit demands critical attention to tensions *within* the project of democratic psychiatry itself.[20] for example, Psichiatria

[20] See for example, http://asylummagazine.org/2018/05/so-what-is-democratic-psychiatry-by-validconsent/

Democratica's lack of engagement with the depth and diversity of the psychiatric survivor movement. This is why *Asylum* foregrounds psychiatric survivor and Mad perspectives. Rather than surrendering itself to any illusions of a 'democratic psychiatry', or creating a permanent substitute for psychiatry, *Asylum* tries to widen, strengthen, and deepen the space for democratic dialogue. This means trying to remain open to criticism itself. Whether it achieves any of this is a moot point. However, I believe keeping this spirit alive is Psichiatria Democratica's enduring legacy. Paradoxically, this must include scrutinizing the demand for 'democratic psychiatry' itself.

Funding and Acknowledgements

The research for this chapter was funded by a Wellcome Trust Research Bursary Award (no. 208269/Z/17/Z). The author would also like to thank: Frank Bangay; Paul Baker; Peter Barham; Peter Campbell; Anne Plumb; and the editors of this volume.

References

Basaglia, F. (1985). What is psychiatry? *International Journal of Mental Health* 14(1–2):42–51.

Basaglia, F. (1987). The institution negated. In: N. Scheper–Hughes and A.M. Lovell (eds), *Psychiatry Inside Out: Selected Writings of Franco Basaglia*. New York, Guildford: Columbia University Press.

Chamberlain, J. (1978). *On Our Own: Patient Controlled Alternatives to the Mental Health System*. New York: Haworth Press.

Crossley, N. (1999). Working utopias and social movements: an investigation using case study materials from radical mental health movements in Britain. *Sociology* 33(4):809–30.

Donnelly, M. (1992). *The Politics of Mental Health in Italy*. London: Routledge.

Foot, J. (2015). *The Man Who Closed the Asylums: Franco Basaglia and the Revolution in Mental Health Care*. London: Verso.

Harrington, V. (2008). 'Voices Beyond the Asylum: A Post-War History of Mental Health Services in Manchester and Salford', PhD thesis, University of Manchester.

Harrington, V. (2009). Innovation in a backwater: the Harpurhey Resettlement Team and the mental health services of North Manchester, 1982–1987. *Health & Place* 15(3):664–71.

Kendall, T. (1996). 'Trieste: The Current Situation': Plenary address to the Third International Conference on 'Psychosis: Integrating the Inner and Outer Worlds', University of Essex, Colchester, England, September 1996. http://www.triestesalutementale.it/english/doc/triestekendall.pdf

Kendall, T.J.H. and Jenner, F.A. (1989). 'Asylum': a new magazine. *Psychiatric Bulletin* 13:571–2.

Ramon, S. (1989). The impact of the Italian psychiatric reforms on North American and British professionals. *International Journal of Social Psychiatry* 35(1):120–7.

Sedgwick, P. (1982). *Psychopolitics*. London: Pluto Press.

Spandler, H. (2006). *Asylum to Action: Paddington Day Hospital, Therapeutic Communities and Beyond*. London, Philadelphia: Jessica Kingsley Publishers.

Spandler, H. (2009). Spaces of psychiatric contention: a case study of a therapeutic community. *Health & Place* 15(3):841–7.

Spandler, H. (2016). Book review. *The Man Who Closed the Asylums: Franco Basaglia and the Revolution in Mental Health Care* by John Foot. *Critical and Radical Social Work* 4(2):438–41.

14
'Visions of another world'
Franco Basaglia and German reform

Chantal Marazia, Heiner Fangerau, Thomas Becker, and Felicitas Söhner

Introduction

The celebration of the silver jubilee of the *Psychiatrie-Enquete*, in 2000, was an official event in Germany (Aktion Psychisch Kranke, 2001). It commemorated the publication of the 'report on the state of psychiatry in the Federal Republic of Germany', which had been prepared for the German parliament by an ad hoc commission of experts between 1971 and 1975 (Deutscher Bundestag, 1975). The report painted a devastating picture of German psychiatry, detailing the inhumane living conditions most asylum patients had to endure. It mandated immediate measures and actually resulted in practical reform on various levels of German psychiatry and psychiatric care (see Kersting, 2003). In the inaugural speech of the *Enquete* jubilee, then Minister of Health, Andrea Fischer, celebrated this 'awakening of psychiatry' (Fisher, 2001), placing a special emphasis on its political import, as well as on its connection with the Italian mastermind Basaglia. She argued that:

> There were radical ideas at the origin of the psychiatric reform ... The complete destruction and dissolution of the 'madhouse' was demanded. 'Freedom heals', the patients wrote on the walls of the former madhouse that Basaglia closed in Trieste in the late 1960s (sic!). This awakening was radical and it had to be radical, because only with visions of another world such strong a structure could be broken.
>
> **(Fisher, 2001, p. 10)**

This assessment of Basaglia's early impact on German psychiatric reform resonates with much of the academic literature on the subject, although with hardly the same emphasis (but see Somma, 2006). However ubiquitous, references to the Italian contribution and its timing remain very vague, generally alluding to an indefinite 1968. Basaglia is usually acknowledged as having a key role in the 'socialisation of psychiatry' (Kersting, 2003; Klein, 2015; Beyer, 2016) and the 'unsettling of the defenders of the out-dated care system' (Häfner, 2003, p. 126). Recent articles pleading for a 'theoretical reanimation' of German social psychiatry recognize in Basaglia—next to Michel Foucault and Erving Goffman—the 'scientific foundation and the legitimation' (Salize, 2012) or the 'fundamental theoretical matrix' of early socio-psychiatric reform in Germany (Thoma, 2012). Psychiatrist Asmus Finzen, one of its protagonists, was even more specific as he argued that by 1973—by the time of the *Enquete*—*L'istituzione negata* [*The Institution Denied*] (Basaglia, 1968) 'had become the leading text of the social-psychiatric movement in Germany' (Finzen, 1998, p. 42).

And yet, in the 1,800 pages of the *Enquete*, the name of Basaglia does not appear once, while references to other experiences, such as those of England, Sweden, Denmark, Canada, and the USA, pepper the report (Bauer and Becker, 2001). Basaglia's absence could be easily explained by the fact that his most tangible and renowned achievement, which projected him onto the international stage—Italian Law 180—was only passed in 1978, three years after the publication of the *Enquete*. It may, however, be more complex than that. Unlike in some other European countries, Basaglia's writings were soon available in the German language, arguably enough to be at least acknowledged by the report. Suhrkamp was the second European editor to propose a translation of *L'istituzione negata*[1], appearing as *Die negierte Institution* in 1971 (Basaglia, 1971). *Die abweichende Mehrheit* [*The Deviant Majority*] appeared in 1972 (Basaglia and Basaglia Ongaro, 1972), one year after its original publication. *Was ist die Psychiatrie?* [*What is Psychiatry?*] reached the German market in 1974 (Basaglia, 1974). Basaglia sold well. The first reprint of *Die negierte Institution* was issued in 1973, the second in 1978 (the year of the Italian Law), and the fifth in 1980 (the year of Basaglia's death). It was therefore unlikely to be just a matter of timing. The *Enquete* simply overlooked Basaglia. Yet, this indifference was reciprocated.

Communists and Nazis

When Basaglia visited Brazil in 1979, whilst on a lecture tour (Basaglia, 2005), he was hailed as the leader of an ongoing revolution. Law 180 had been passed one year before, making Italy a model of psychiatric reform worldwide. Consistent with his role as 'padre nobile', Basaglia understated his own accomplishment by repeatedly framing it in a global context of change, and one not limited to psychiatry. In Rio de Janeiro, for instance (26 June 1979), he commented on the experience in Gorizia almost 20 years before: 'Nothing extraordinary', he minimized, 'nothing exceptional, this [humanisation of the asylum] was already happening in England and France' (Basaglia, 2005). Not a single word was spoken about Germany and its reform programme—not even for the sake of contrast, as he did with the French 'secteur' and English community psychiatry. Basaglia's silence was surely not due to ignorance—he knew German psychiatry extremely well. It may be an eloquent omission rather than an oversight, and deserves a closer consideration.

1 The first having been the French editor Seuil, in 1970.

At this time, both Germany and Italy had been hit by a bloody wave of left-wing terrorism (by the Rote Armee Fraktion (RAF) and the Brigate Rosse (BR), respectively), and their relationship was particularly tense. The mutual perception was mostly dismissive, showing the resilience of established stereotypes. On the Italian side, the German way of dealing with terrorism (and dissent in general) was perceived through the lens of a tired cliché of cold Teutonic efficiency, inevitably associated with the Nazi regime. In turn, Italy was depicted in regional and national German media as the country of chaos, violence, and communism. 'PCI [Partito Comunista Italiano] and BR from the same family album: kindred spirits with the same origin' was the headline in the *Saarbrücker Zeitung*, while the *Rheinische Post* proclaimed that 'Everyone who invokes Lenin and Marx stems from the same vipers' nest!' (quoted in Riegler, 2016). The implicit allegation was, if not of direct complicity with the terrorists, then of a 'climate of unquestioned freedom of opinion that allows fumes of class hatred and threats to blow over the country' (Riegler, 2016). In the 1970s, Italy was not only a popular holiday destination for German families, it became a veritable 'revolutionary dreamland' for young West German militants (Riegler, 2016, p. 23)—something conservatives feared.

In the second half of the 1960s, Basaglia had contributed to a political magazine, unequivocally titled *Che fare (Bollettino di critica e azione di avanguardia)* [*What is to be done (Bulletin of critics and avant-garde action)*], later to become the theoretical paper of the Partito Comunista (Marxista–Leninista) Italiano. It was not hard to identify him as a proselyte-seeking agitprop. The reception of Basaglia in West Germany (and vice versa) must be read against this background of typecasts and distrust—culminating in the 1977 *annus horribilis* in West German–Italian relations. Basaglia's invitation: 'Venite a vedere Trieste!' ['Come see Trieste'] (see Basaglia, 1979, p. 212) resounded in Germany at the same time as the *Bunte Illustrierte* warned its readers, on 31 March 1977, 'Do not travel to Italy', a message reinforced by the front cover of the leading magazine *Der Spiegel* on 25 July 1977, which showed a serving of spaghetti topped with a gun (Figure 14.1).

At stake, of course, was more than just diplomatic relations. In the very first phase of his career, Basaglia had deeply drawn on German-language psychiatric culture, or at least a part of it. He belonged to a not insignificant, but marginal, cohort of young Italian psychiatrists that included Bruno Callieri, Eugenio Borgna, and the slightly older Danilo Cargnello. These were inspired by the phenomenological thoughts of (the Swiss) Ludwig Binswanger and Karl Jaspers. The former's *Daseinsanalyse*—existential analysis in its English rendering—provided the methodological and interpretative framework for Basaglia's early scientific publications, throughout the 1950s (see Colucci and Di Vittorio, 2001). At the time, he worked as an assistant at the psychiatric clinic of the University of Padua, a position he kept until 1961 when, aware that he could hardly hope for an academic career, he applied for the directorship of the public asylum in Gorizia. Here, almost overnight, he woke up from his own 'dogmatic

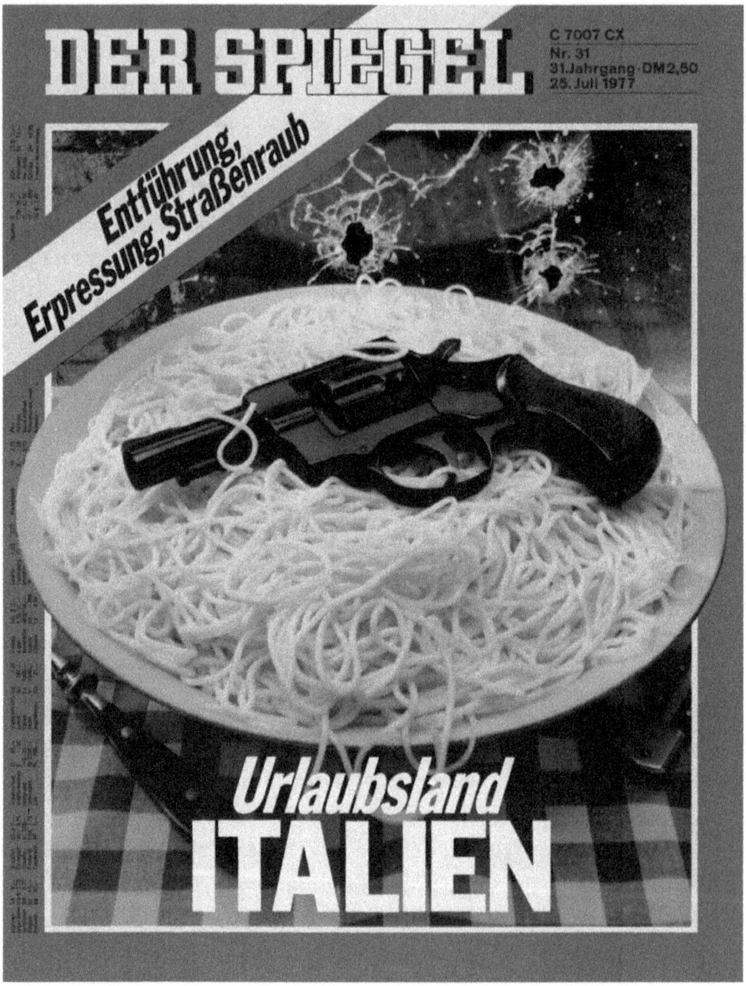

Figure 14.1 Magazine cover of *Der Spiegel* (25 July 1977) reading 'Holiday destination Italy. Abduction, blackmail, assault'.

Reproduced from *Der Spiegel* (1977).

slumber' and threw out Binswanger and the whole of anthropological psychiatry. As he wrote in 1974, in a long and analytical curriculum vitae:

> Contact with the violent, destructive and segregating reality of the psychiatric institution [demonstrated that] there are no terms to define the modalities of existence of [the] patient destroyed by [these] institutes. Phenomenology, as a method of investigation and understanding of the diseased reality [*realtà*

> *malata*], is a privileged instrument for privileged patients and falls when in contact with this reality ... It is the same distance between conceptual elaborations and this violent reality, that undermines the validity of the classical definition of illness.
>
> **(Basaglia, 2017, p. 28)**

There is, here, a not so veiled reference to Binswanger, who had directed the private Sanatorium Bellevue in Kreuzlingen: 'that institution on Lake Constance where pampered lunatics from wealthy households are gently and expensively treated and the staff are as tender as midwives', as Joseph Roth lyrically put it in his 1932 novel *Radetzkymarsch* (see Marazia, 2005). This was, basically, the same socioeconomic profile of the patients that Basaglia himself had 'daseinsanalysed' at the University clinic in Padua: mostly young bourgeois ladies and students (cf. Basaglia, 2017, pp. 47–259). Nothing could be more remote from the population of the public psychiatric hospitals that he and colleagues had to deal with later:

> The fact that the internees of our mental hospitals all belong to a single class—the proletariat and the underclass—testifies to the existence of a double psychiatry, which applies different scientific definitions and practical sanctions, depending on the social and economic conditions of the patient.
>
> **(Basaglia, 2017, p. 26)**

Existential–anthropological psychiatry simply was not translatable into the asylum. Even worse, 'a phenomenological analysis of the-being-in-restraint or of the-being-together-in-segregation' ['analisi fenomenologiche dell'essere-nella-contenzione o dell'essere-con-nella-segregazione'], he wrote, aping the anthropo-phenomenological jargon, would be 'an insult to reality' (Basaglia, 2017, p. 28).

Basaglia's newfound disdain for the German anthropo-phenomenological tradition was rather harmless in comparison with his merciless condemnation of that other pillar of German phenomenological psychiatry, Karl Jaspers. Although Jaspers had abandoned psychiatry for philosophy shortly after the First World War, he was still regarded as an authority in the field, and—despite having moved to Switzerland—as a moral guide for the country. [2] It was therefore no small thing that in a 1967 essay, bearing the eloquent title 'The final solution' ['La soluzione finale'] (Basaglia, 1967), Basaglia overtly accused Jaspers of fascism.

The occasion had been provided by an excerpt of Jaspers' forthcoming book published by *Der Spiegel* (Jaspers, 1967), in which the philosopher had declared—'without any hesitation and modesty' (Basaglia, 1967, p. 443) that Russians and

[2] His 1913 handbook *General Psychopathology* (Jaspers, 1913), then in its seventh edition, was still a reference manual among German psychiatrists.

Americans should ally and threaten Maoist China with atomic weapons. How could, asked Basaglia,

> a man who had refused to identify with Nazi Germany, propose the deletion of 700 million people in a single act of exclusion as a solution to a state of world tension? Are his words any different from those that, more than thirty years ago, decreed the death of 6 million Jews?
>
> **(Basaglia, 1967, p. 444)**

After quoting Julius Streicher, a prominent member of the Nazi party prosecuted in Nuremberg for crimes against humanity, and Joseph Göbbels, he concluded that Jaspers' distinction between 'the understandable and the incomprehensible in mental illness could not but run aground on a racist and classist terrain' (Basaglia, 1967). The target here was not merely a questionable geopolitical stance. His point was about a 'science that, born revolutionary, had ended up endorsing the game of power'. It was about epistemology, ethics, and politics. Basaglia mused that:

> The meaning of Jaspers' statement ... [appeared] consistent with the premises: the father of what had been the new anti-positivist psychiatry (which had nonetheless accepted the determinism of the incomprehensible) revealed, at the end of his career, his racism, even if at the time of the Hitler conflict he had taken sides with the excluded.
>
> **(Basaglia, 1967, p. 443)**

In this article, Basaglia was adamant that, to his eyes, Jaspers' latest statements on international politics 'had the power to unmask the bad faith evidently underpinning his philosophical approach' (Basaglia, 1967).

In short, to Basaglia, the old positivist German psychiatry—deemed, inter alia, responsible for Italy's backwardness (Basaglia, 1968)—was not the only foe, as often suggested. Also, the preposterous attempts at overcoming it (like anthropological psychiatry), or the outright dangerous ones (such as Jaspersian psychopathology), deserved condemnation. While in Italy, the anthropo-phenomenological school was at the margins of official discourse, in Germany it was becoming more and more influential (Janzarik, 1974), especially among young, progressive psychiatrists. Many of them would later turn to social psychiatry and/or have an active role in the reform (see Söhner et al., 2017; Thoma, 2019). It was precisely against them that Basaglia directed his most severe criticism.

In the *Die negierte Institution*, Basaglia called the enemy by its name:

> German-speaking countries ... bound to the rigid Teutonic ideology, are still trying to solve the problem of psychiatric asylums by ever more perfect

> structures, in which the custodial attitude continues to dominate. Suffice it to mention the example of Gutersloh, Herman (sic) Simon's hospital, now headed by Winkler, where there is only the technical perfection of Simon's ergotherapeutic ideology.
>
> **(Basaglia, 1971, p. 136)**

His chastisement continued:

> The same social psychiatry, now in vogue . . . does not express any awareness of the failure of asylum psychiatry (with consequent awareness of the patient's objectification at the institutional and scientific level), but is rather the fruit of a need for intellectual updating that can only lead to the building of social psychiatric institutions, such as the one that will arise—the new Brasilia of German psychiatry—in Mainz (sic!), under Haefner's leadership.[3]
>
> **(Basaglia, 1971, p. 136)**

A critique of Hermann Simon could not have been more untimely. The German translation of *L'istituzione negata* appeared, as said, in 1971. That very same year, the German Psychiatric Society (Deutsche Gesellschaft für Psychiatrie und Nervenheilkunde, DGPN) instituted an award to honour the memory of that very man. The prize, rewarding 'outstanding scientific achievements in the field of social psychiatry', was assigned by an independent board of trustees. Five of its seven members where part of the Psychiatrie-Enquete-Kommission: Walter Theodor Winkler, Hanns Hippius, the social worker Helmtraud Schmidt–Gante, its president Caspar Kulenkampff, and the vice-president Heinz Häfner.[4]. Moreover, the institute Basaglia hints at in this passage is, in all likelihood, the Zentralinstitut für Seelische Gesundheit, inaugurated in Mannheim (and not Mainz, Magonza) in 1975 under the directorship of Häfner himself. The misspelling of Häfner's name was reproduced in the Suhrkamp edition of *L'istituzione negata* but, to the cognoscenti, the reference was unequivocal.

The German reaction

This critique of social psychiatry was surely not out of the blue. Basaglia had first presented his radical programme for 'the distruction (sic) of the mental hospital as a place of institutionalisation' at the first international congress of social psychiatry, held in London in 1964. According to a later account (Giannichedda, 2005), his

[3] Here, the comparison with Brasilia is unequivocally dismissive, and not positive or even deferential as sometimes stated (e.g. see Payk, 2004, where it is erroneously associated with Hannover).

[4] See Kersting, 2018, p. 220. In 2009, the prize was destituted, following recognition of Simon's involvement with the Nazi regime.

presentation had been a disaster, with a lot of rumblings of dissent in the audience. At one point, judging that the problem might lie in Basaglia's uncertain pronunciation, an English colleague had taken over the reading of the paper. This only proved that the problem was not that the audience failed to understand, but that they did. According to Giannichedda, the disquiet was a reaction by the British, seeing themselves side-lined on their 'own turf'. It is however safe to assume—given the international nature of the congress—that the response was more composite than that. Basaglia's radical stance must have left a long-lasting impression on the many German attendees, too.

The psychiatrist Erich Wulff, one of Basaglia's few German fellow travellers,[5] recalled how coldly Basaglia and his collaborators had been received in Germany a few years later, at the time of the *Enquete* (Wulff, 1980). Except for an article about 'the courageous doctors of Gorizia' appearing in the weekly *Die Zeit* (on 24 September 1971), *Die negierte Institution* did indeed not receive much attention in the German press. Despite Wulff's own effort to introduce Basaglia to carefully selected audiences—such as the group gathered around the magazine *Das Argument*, the so-called Mannheim Circle [Mannheimer Kreis], and the German Society for Social Psychiatry [Deutsche Gesellschaft für Soziale Psychiatrie, DGSP], founded in 1970 (Wulff, 1980)—the overall reaction had been 'a mixture of disregard and silent distrust' (Wulff, 1980, p. 250).

Wulff had met Basaglia in 1970, during a visiting professorship in France. At that time, Wulff was an editor of *Das Argument*, a Marxist independent magazine and essentially an organ of the student movement inspired by critical theory. It was against the grain of this current of thought that *Die negierte Institution* was first reviewed in the journal (Abholz and Gleiss, 1972). Unsurprisingly, it did not stand the test. Although there are some allusions in *L'Istitutzione Negata* to Herbert Marcuse's *One-Dimensional-Man* (Marcuse, 1964), this is clearly not the first intellectual reference of the book (see Mollica, 1985). Two years later, *Das Argument* conceded a second opinion, also covering further contributions by Basaglia and collaborators (Autorenkollektiv, 1973) in a wider analysis of the international anti-psychiatric scene. The verdict of the *Argument* was still critical, but subtler, and—at least according to Agostino Pirella, co-author of *L'istituzione negata*—not entirely wrong: 'From what I can gather', Pirella wrote to Basaglia, 'it seems to me that they also say things that are right, but that you (and us) are taken for Marcusian utopianists— (!)' (Pirella to Basaglia, 7 April 1973, Archivio Basaglia, hereon AB). The Italian 'meta-psychiatry' (as the authors specified, denoting a fine-grained reading of the reviewed texts) was, here, painstakingly compared to the position of R.D. Laing and David Cooper, and to that of the German Socialist Patients' Collective (SPK or, from 1973 onwards, Patientenfront).

The SPK had been founded in 1970 by the psychiatrist Wolfgang Huber, his wife, two other doctors, and 40 patients of the Heidelberg Psychiatric University Clinic. The tolerance, initially granted by the University, was soon reversed, as the collective's

[5] Wulff is the only German author acknowledged in the edited volume *Crimini di pace* (Basaglia and Ongaro Basaglia, 1975).

radicalism grew more and more evident. Their motto was 'Turn illness into a weapon!' (SPK, 1972). In April 1971, a SPK patient had committed suicide. That June, following the shooting of a policeman near Heidelberg, flats and houses of SPK members were searched in the hunt for suspected RAF terrorists.[6] Huber and other members of the SPK were arrested for participation in a criminal association, manufacture of explosive materials, and forgery of documents. In a first dramatic trial in November 1972, Huber, his wife, and a third member were sentenced to prison. A second trial was held in 1973.

Although they pursued opposing goals (e.g. see Brückner and Wulff, 1973), the association between Italian 'meta-psychiatry' and the SPK outlined by the *Argument* was not far-fetched. Basaglia was in close contact with the group, at least from 1972 onwards. His reference person was Werner Schork, a former patient turned SPK leader thanks to his erudition and dialectic skills (Pross, 2016). In mid May 1972, some members of the former SPK travelled to Trieste, in order to visit the mental hospital and disseminate informative material about their group and the trial. According to Basaglia, the initiative had provided the local neo-fascists with the occasion for 'a frontal attack on the hospital and to all those who work there' (Basaglia to Schork, unsent letter, 15 July 1972, AB). The visit may well have provoked the neo-fascists in town. The fact that a patient had killed his parents in June must have done the rest (see Foot, 2015).

At the time, Schork had his own legal troubles: The day after the shooting of the policeman in June 1971, weapons were found in his apartment, and he was arrested with the allegation of being an inside man of the RAF. Waiting for the first trial, he pleaded for explicit support from the Italian group. More specifically, he asked for an official declaration of solidarity to be transmitted from a local radio in order to attract attention (Schork to Basaglia, undated letter, AB). The four-page typescript on the SPK, kept in Basaglia's archive, was arguably written for this occasion (unpublished typescript, file 11.5, AB). On the other hand, the hypothesis cannot be excluded that the text was intended for publication, perhaps as a foreword to the Italian edition of SPK's manifesto. In an unsent letter to Schork, Basaglia mentions the plan of submitting the SPK pamphlet (SPK, 1972) to an 'editor and friend' (Basaglia to Schork, unsent letter, 15 July 1972, AB), probably alluding to the progressive publisher Feltrinelli. The project was never realized, although, two years later, Feltrinelli was still showing sustained interest for it (letter from Brega to Basaglia, 23 November 1974, AB). Whatever its destination, the document is a clear and dense declaration of support to the group and, at the same time, a pitiless attack on German psychiatry, past and present.

According to Basaglia, the SPK affair had historical roots and meaning. German psychiatry had indeed played a key role in the emergence of psychiatry in Europe, but its 'practical verification' had clarified 'its true meaning'. The same man that German psychiatrists had 'minutely investigated, codified, diagnosed in his symptoms and

[6] More than a dozen SPK members later actually joined the RAF.

syndromes and so well incorporated in medical science, was eliminated and killed to safeguard and protect the race and production' during the Second World War. Neither phenomenology, nor Anglo-Saxon pragmatism had been able to redeem the German scientific spirit in any way. On the contrary, they 'had continued to refine and modernize the techniques and thinking of the old masters'. However 'confused' and 'limited', Basaglia diagnosed, the 'technical' action of the SPK critically targeted this very science as an expression of the ruling class's values (Basaglia, unpublished typescript, file 11.5, AB).

For Basaglia, the SPK had become a target of repression primarily because of the subversive potential of its 'technical action' to unmask those 'new' psychiatric experiences which 'by simple transformation of the formal aspect, kept true to the rigid scaffolding on which Germanic psychiatric culture is based'. By interrupting 'the soliloquy of its prophets', the SPK had shown that the king was naked. Their sanction, therefore, had an explicitly political character, its purpose being the elimination of a small number of 'technicians' who had initiated 'the—unfortunately—only practical transformation in German psychiatry'. At first, only hindered by the university establishment, 'the young people of the SPK found their precise role in German psychiatry when the police qualified their action by blocking it' This meant that 'the true face of German psychiatry is that of the police who protect and defend it, as they are guarding the established norm, whose limits the police are delegated to maintain'. Thus, the SPK had already accomplished its task, concluded Basaglia—a task going far beyond the results obtained on its specific terrain: 'the crisis of a science that needs the courts and the police to survive, is that of a justice incapable of protecting itself' (Basaglia, unpublished typescript, file 11.5, AB).

Despite their own troubles with the courts—or perhaps because of them—Basaglia and his collaborators did not abandon the members of the SPK. On the eve of the trial, a delegation from Trieste attended a 'teach-in' with 1,000 participants, organized in Heidelberg by the Informationszentrum Rote Volksuniversität [Information Centre Red People's University], the successor organization to the SPK. According to the eyewitness Mario Reali, their declaration of solidarity brought the house down at the words 'All Italy is behind you' (see Pross, 2016, p. 180, n. 638). The endorsement, which could not have been more explicit, must have added to the German perception of Basaglia's radical potential (see Glatzel, 1974; Hartmann, 1974). This was a prejudice he was well aware of, and tried to dispel. In a speech in Berlin, in 1980, Basaglia sought to explicitly mark the distance between his own experience and the parable of terrorism. His fight, he conceded, had first grown underground, 'so to speak illegally'. He was quick to specify, however, that his concept of 'illegal fight' did not overlap with that of the terrorists (Dörner and Basaglia, 1981, p. 208).

Basaglia's solidarity with the SPK in 1972—concurrent with the first translations of his texts—was not the best position for gaining approval from the members of the Mannheimer Kreis (MK), and the Society for Social Psychiatry that had grown out of it. The DGSP had been founded in open opposition to the DGPN (see Bauer, 2003). Unlike its 100-year-old counterpart, the DGSP was not restricted to doctors, but included psychologists and sociologists working in psychiatric clinics or closely related institutions. This pluralism, together with an emphasis on the social dimensions of disease, conferred an aura of progressivism on the Society. Both the MK and the DGSP, however, had converged in their early condemnation of the SPK, in order to protect the 'fragile little plant of social psychiatry' from the 'overflowing surge of enthusiasm for anti-psychiatry' (Finzen, 1998, p. 41). Finzen retrospectively admitted the tendency, among social psychiatrists, 'to underestimate [the] social-psychiatric content [of *L'istituzione negata*] in favour of the anti-psychiatric rhetoric posturing and to simply deny Basaglia's clear distancing from anti-psychiatric theory' (Finzen, 1998, p. 42). It is worth noticing that the term 'anti-psychiatric', adopted in the Italian original (as synonymous with 'anti-specialized'), was expunged—it is not clear whether by Basaglia's will or on the translator's initiative—from the German translation. Nevertheless, Basaglia was put into this overcrowded cauldron (i.e. Glatzel, 1974; Hartmann, 1974).

This explains why, in the early 1970s, in social-psychiatric circles, Basaglia and his associates were, in one way or another, *personae non gratae*. As previously stated, Wulff (founding member of both the MS and the Society for Social Psychiatry) vainly attempted to forge bonds of collaboration between these new, progressive associations and the pressure group 'Psichiatria Democratica' that gathered around Basaglia. In 1973, he eventually managed to invite, with the consent of the advisory board, Basaglia and Gian Franco Minguzzi (first secretary of 'Psichiatria Democratica') to the annual meeting of the DGSP in Heidelberg. The event, however, turned into a farce: the Italians were literally and metaphorically *left* aside ['links liegen gelassen'] during the whole meeting, and Minguzzi was allowed a 20-minute talk only at 1.00 a.m. (Wulff, 1980, p. 251). Wulff gives two reasons for this ostracism, or 'fear of contact' ['Berührungsangst'] as he calls it: first, the veil of ignorance regarding the actual developments in Italy; second, the 'Enquete-euphoria' reigning in the DGSP and the consequent 'concern of many involved board members of jeopardizing their work in the Enquete by contact with partners perceived as too radical' (Wulff, 1980). Considering that that very year German psychiatry had twice been under the spotlight (the second SPK trial and the deadline for the interim *Enquete* report), this argument sounds particularly convincing.

Law 180 removed both these barriers in one fell swoop. Was the law, then, the watershed?

After Law 180

Basaglia's achievement was promptly acknowledged north of the Alps, even beyond psychiatric circles (see De Girolamo, 1989). In November 1978, *Der Spiegel* sympathetically reported on the Italian experience (pp. 196–207): in the Bel Paese, 'schizophrenia could be dealt with just like a cough' ['Schizophrenie austragen wie Schnupfen'], a measure 'unthinkable in Germany' . For the magazine, the passing of Italian Law 180 provided the occasion for an assessment of the four-year-long *Enquete*: 'The Italians seem to have succeeded in what social psychiatrists have been announcing for years', teased the article. Indeed, the suggested German reform was found defective in all its four pillars: community orientation; patient-centred care; coordination of all service institutions and providers; and equal treatment and opportunities for the mentally and physically ill. On top of that, it had not even been discussed by the Bundestag.[7]

Visibility brought consensus to Basaglia, even among initial sceptics. The 1979 special issue of *Das Argument* (AS30) scrutinized the practical outcomes of Italian reform, asking (positively) if this could provide a valuable 'alternative to German social psychiatry' (Zencker and Zencker, 1979). Meanwhile, the 'Enquete-euphoria' had cooled down, even among some social psychiatrists, who feared the inquiry would prove a dead letter, 'gathering dust in shelves and drawers of the offices' (Finzen and Schädle-Deininger, 1979, I). Suddenly, the embargo on critical psychiatry was lifted, starting from the Lower Saxony Section of the DGSP. Under the leadership of Hans Werner Jenz, the Wahrendorf Clinic in Ilten had been one of the headquarters of the *Enquete*. It was therefore no little thing that at the 1978 conference in Ilten, the leadership of Psichiatria Democratica of Arezzo was received with full honours. Not only were caregivers present, political authorities had also been invited (Wulff, 1980, p. 251). German interest in the Italian psychiatric system grew exponentially. Texts were translated, invitations multiplied, mutual visits intensified, and conferences organized. In October 1979, for instance, 700 caregivers from the two countries gathered for three days in Munich, to discuss their respective experiences (Berger, 1980). Sil(vana) Schmid's 120-page report about Psichiatria Democratica, bearing the militant title *Freiheit heilt* [*Freedom heals*] (Schmid, 1977), went through 21 editions within four years.

The endorsement was not universal, however. Not everybody converted. The first number of *ZI Dokumentation*, the in-house magazine of Häfner's Zentralinstitut für Seelische Gesundheit (the 'Brasilia' of German psychiatry), was a special issue on Italian reform (Zentralinstitut für Seelische Gesundheit Mannheim, 1980/81, p. 118). Apparently, no copy of the report is left (Hans Salize, personal communication), but it is safe to assume that it was extremely critical throughout. The *Deutsche Ärzteblatt* [*German Medical Journal*], organ of the Bundesärztekammer [AK, Medical Chamber], had come to the same conclusions, but with a print run of more than 100,000 copies. In 1979, a delegation of the AK visited Trieste at the initiative of Erwin Odenbach, head of science and training at the Chamber. The report was anything but supportive (Burkart, 1979).

According to Thomas Simons, the Italian experience had elicited a 'decidedly ambivalent echo' in the Federal Republic (Simons, 1980, p. 9): 'The undivided enthusiasm of the ones stood against an often sharp and equally fundamental rejection of

[7] This happened only in 1979.

the others. A remarkably polarised climate, ideal for a fight' (Simons, 1980, p. 10). The point here is not to make a census of those who were with Basaglia and those who were against him, nor of those who were for and against Law 180.[8] The opposing fronts, as it were, are not so easily defined, as Basaglia's last appearance in Germany illustrates.

In May 1980, Basaglia featured at the first Gesundheitstag (Dörner and Basaglia, 1981)—a counter-event to the official Bundesärztetag organized by the Bundesärztekammer, hosted of course by the Freie Universität, Berlin. The *Ärzteblatt* had dismissed the initiative as an act of 'extra-parliamentary opposition' (Ausserparlamentarische Opposition, APO—the allusion being to the evanescence of the 1968 movement). The *Ärzteblatt* had constantly warned its readers against the anti-psychiatric drift (i.e. Glatzel, 1974; Hartmann, 1974) in general, and against 'Basaglia's revolutionary delusion' in particular. It would be simplistic, however, to split the camp of German psychiatry between those who attended the Ärztetag (the dominant establishment) and those who went to listen to Basaglia and his friend Klaus Dörner (the ineffective 'opposition').

Dörner had cared to distance himself from the Italian way. He never called for the closure of the asylums, not even during the 1980 rally organized under this very motto (see *Sozialpsychiatrische Informationen* special issue, 1980). A year before, he had given the reason for the missed call: 'We consider a drastic closure of all major psychiatric hospitals by law ... to be sensible only if humane accommodation and care alternatives are simultaneously implemented in the community' (Dörner et al., 1979, pp. 143–4). What is remarkable here is not so much Dörner's procrastination,[9] as his recourse to the same argument deployed by Basaglia's opponents: the inhumane consequences of the Law.

Railing against a new anti-psychiatric *Der Spiegel* article published shortly before the Gesundheitstag (December 1980, pp. 98–124), the director of the Düsseldorf University Psychiatric Clinic, Kurt Heinrich, compared Basaglia to Till Eulenspiegel, a popular trickster character of German mediaeval literature (Heinrich, 1980, p. 1013). Heinrich made explicit reference to the bitter episode when Eulenspiegel promised the city council to empty the hospital from all the annoying, money-consuming patients. Although the wag succeeded with a lazy trick (threatening to burn the last patient in the hospital), they were all back after three days. This story, Heinrich added, was not at all funny, just as Basaglia's psychiatric revolution was not at all humanitarian. This criticism became a sort of mantra for Basaglia's opponents, as articles and letters on Italian patients pleading for rehospitalization were regularly highlighted in the *Ärzteblatt* (van der Beeck, 1980). According to Wulff, one leading German social psychiatrist even went so far as drawing an explicit association between Basaglia's programme and euthanasia (Wulff, 1980). The inhumanity argument proved powerful, at

[8] On the risk of crystallizing the fronts as 'Basaglians' and 'not Basaglians', see for instance Fiorani (2010). His considerations are applicable to the historiography of German psychiatry as well.

[9] As Erich Wulff recalled some years later, Dörner had pleaded for the destruction 'of a programme, a system, a posture'; that is, of 'the asylum inside us', and not for the asylum qua institution (Wulff, 1991).

least for the German media. In 1983, a long article in *Der Spiegel*, denouncing the dark fields into which the Law had plunged the 'matti' and their families, bore the title: 'Endless shame' (44/1983, p. 44). Tellingly, the pictures accompanying this infamous issue were exactly the same as those illustrating the first, supportive one.

Conclusions

What most irritated Heinrich in the first, sympathetic *Der Spiegel* article from 1978, was that Basaglia's devilment had been put on the same plane as German reform. Basaglia did not want any reform, i.e. an 'improvement of the situation, but an overturning of the whole society', Heinrich explained (Heinrich, 1980). If Basaglia could be perceived as a model [Vorbild], he concluded, it was because his radicalism had been misunderstood as reform.

This misunderstanding proved particularly hard to beat, and was the origin of new and powerful misinterpretations. Thus, in retrospect, Basaglia was turned into an icon of postmodern deinstitutionalized psychiatric reform, just as Philippe Pinel has been refashioned as the releasing icon of modern psychiatry (Weiner, 1994). A first trace of this metamorphosis is found in Basaglia's German obituaries. Here, the Italian psychiatrist is celebrated as an 'impulse', an 'idol', for the German reform movement (Finzen, 1980) and—quite ironically—as 'an institution, a model, a monument' (Abram, 1980, p. 217). This picture contrasts with the reactions Basaglia had evoked in large swathes of German psychiatry before and around 1980. Generally speaking, the impression is rather that Basaglia's radicalism represented, at least in the first phase (until Law 180), more a problem than a driving force for German reform. It took a new generation of psychiatrists, with a different take on German reform and its concrete perspectives, to lump Basaglia's stance together with the promises of the *Enquete*. It also required a reassessment of Basaglia's role and cultural currency (see Trivelli, 2016) to allow for statements like that of the Minister of Health on the occasion of the silver jubilee of the *Psychiatrie-Enquete*. To a significant extent, the retrospective smoothing of this contrast has been grounded on a narrow and overemphatic focus on the common intellectual roots of the two movements. As shown, Basaglia openly rejected any association with the German antropo-phenomenological tradition and the social psychiatric movement inspired by it.

All in all, the relation between German psychiatry and Basaglia was at least complicated, and marked by mutual prejudices: communism and terrorism on the one side, and (crypto)Nazism on the other.[10] Both sides accused each other of being inhumane in the practical consequences of their theories. In the light of the German reaction

[10] Just how powerful the left-extremist label was (in Germany) can be appreciated from an article in 2001 by Häfner: 'The political lever [for Law 180] was his wife (a far-left member of the Italian Parliament)'. Franca Ongaro Basagalia actually only became a member of the parliament in 1983, three years after her husband's death.

to Law 180, it is still an open question whether the German reform movement really needed Italy and Basaglia as radical counterparts in order to come to grips with its own reforms, and to 'frame' them as the better organized and better planned solution against the background of a 'social state' (cf. Schmid, 1980). As some of the attendants at the large Munich conference (already in 1979) put it, in a short overall assessment of the event, the difference between the reform of Psichiatria Democratica and the programme of the German 'Soziale Psychiatrie' was easy to define: while for the Italians, the therapeutic community was only the first (and necessary) step towards the abolition of the asylum, for the Germans it was already the final objective of the reform—'community psychiatry despite the asylum, not *instead* of it' (Lohmer et al. in Berger, 1980, p. 164).

Acknowledgements

The authors would like to express their thanks to Fabio De Sio and Heinz-Harald Abholz for their valuable suggestions. We also wish to acknowledge the liberality of the Fondazione Basaglia in granting access to the Basaglia Archive, and Leonardo Musci's generosity in helping with the archival sources.

References

Abholz, H.-H. and Gleiss, I. (1972). Zur Frage der Anpassung in der psychiatrischen Therapie—dargestellt am Beispiel des Buches 'Die negierte Institution'. *Das Argument* 71:79–87.

Abram, M. (1980). Franco Basaglia 1924–1980. In: T. Dersee and S. Dupke (eds), *Bankrott der Gesundheitsindustrie. Eine Kritik des bestehenden medizinischen Versorgungssystems.* Berlin: Verlagsgesellschaft Gesundheit, pp. 215–17.

Autorenkollektiv (1973). Psychiatrie und Politik. *Das Argument* 78:69–93.

Basaglia, F. (1967). La soluzione finale. Reprinted in: *Scritti 1953–1980*. Milano: Il Saggiatore, pp. 443–50.

Basaglia, F. (ed.) (1968). *L'istituzione negata. Rapporto da un ospedale psichiatrico*. Torino: Einaudi.

Basaglia, F. (ed.) (1971). *Die negierte Institution oder die Gemeinschaft der Ausgeschlossenen. Ein Experiment der psychiatrischen Klinik in Görz*. Frankfurt/Main: Suhrkamp.

Basaglia, F. (1974). *Was ist Psychiatrie?* Frankfurt/Main: Suhrkamp.

Basaglia, F. (1979). Conversazione con Venturini. In: E. Venturini (ed.), *Il Giardino dei gelsi*. Torino: Einaudi, pp. 211–12.

Basaglia, F. (2005). Conferenze Brasiliane. Milano: Raffaello Cortina Editore.

Basaglia, F. (2017). *Scritti 1953–1980*. Milano: Il Saggiatore.

Basaglia, F. and Ongaro Basaglia, F. (ed.) (1972). *Die abweichende Mehrheit: die Ideologie der totalen sozialen Kontrolle*. Frankfurt/Main: Suhrkamp.

Basaglia, F. and Ongaro Basaglia, F, (ed.) (1975). *Crimini di pace*. Torino: Einaudi.

Bauer, M. (2003). Reform als soziale Bewegung: Der 'Mannheimer Kreis' und die Gründung der 'Deutschen Gesellschaft für Soziale Psychiatrie'. In: F.-W. Kersting (ed.), *Psychiatriereform als Gesellschaftsreform*. Paderborn: Schöningh, pp. 155–63.

Bauer, M. and Becker, T. (2001). Die Psychiatrie-Enquete im europäischen Vergleich. In: Aktion Psychisch Kranke (ed.), *25 Jahre Psychiatrie-Enquete*. Köln: Psychiatrie Verlag, pp. 235–40.

Berger, P. (ed.) (1980). *Neue Psychiatrie: Erfahrungen aus Italien und Deutschland. Materialien zu einer Arbeitstagung 12–14 Oktober 1979 in München*. Bonn: Psychiatrie Verlag.

Beyer, C. (2016). 'Islands of reform': early transformation of the mental health service in Lower Saxony, Germany in the 1960s. In: D. Kritsotaki et al. (eds), *Deinstitutionalisation and After: Post-War Psychiatry in the Western World*. Basingstoke: Palgrave Macmillan, pp. 99–114.

Bopp, J. (1980). *Antipsychiatrie. Theorien, Therapien, Politik*. Frankfurt/Main: Syndikat.

Brückner, P. and Wulff, E. (1973). Anmerkungen zum sozialistischen Patienten-Kollektiv (SPK). *Kritische Justiz* 6(4):420–34.

Burkart, W. (1979). Franco Basaglia und die institutionalisierte Antipsychiatrie. Ein Besuch bei der 'Demokratischen Psychiatrie in Triest'. *Deutsches Ärzteblatt* 44:2872–6.

Colucci, M. and Di Vittorio, P. (2001). *Franco Basaglia*. Milano: Bruno Mondadori.

De Girolamo, G. (1989). Italian psychiatry and reform law: a review of the international literature. *International Journal of Social Psychiatry* 35(1):21–37.

Dörner, K. (1979). *Gemeindepsychiatrie*. Stuttgart: Kohlhammer.

Dörner, K. and Basaglia, F. (1981). Von der Irrenanstalt zur reformierten Großklinik–Fortschritt oder Getto neuen Stils? In: T. Dersee, S. Dupke (eds), *Bankrott der Gesundheitsindustrie. Eine Kritik des bestehenden medizinischen Versorgungssystems*. Berlin: Verlagsgesellschaft Gesundheit, pp. 205–14.

Deutscher Bundestag (1975). *Enquete-Bericht über die Lage der Psychiatrie in der Bundesrepublik—Zur politischen und psychotherapeutisch/psychosomatischen Versorgung in der Bevölkerung, 2 vols.*, Bundestagsdrucksache 7/4200 and 7/4201. Bonn: Bundestag.

Finzen, A. (1980). La liberta e terapeutica. Zum Tode von Franco Basaglia. *Psychiatrische Praxis* 7:207–9.

Finzen, A. (1998). *Das Pinelsche Pendel. Die Dimension des Sozialen im Zeitalter der biologischen Psychiatrie*. Bonn: Psychiatrie Verlag.

Finzen, A. and Schädle-Deininger, H. (1979). Einleitung. In: A. Finzen and H. Schädle-Deininger (eds), *'Unter elenden menschenunwürdigen Umständen': Die Psychiatrie-Enquête*. Wunstorf, Rehburg-Loccum, Bonn: Psychiatrie Verlag, pp. 1–2.

Fiorani, M. (2010). *Bibliografia di storia della psichiatria italiana 1991–2010*. Firenze: Firenze University Press.

Fischer, A. (2001). Rede von Bundesgesundheitsministerin Andrea Fischer zum Festakt und Kongress '25 Jahre Psychiatrie Enquete—Bilanz und Perspektiven der Psychiatrie-Reform' am 21. November 2000 in Bonn. *Psychosoziale Umschau* 16(1):10–11.

Foot, J. (2015). *The Man Who Closed the Asylums*. London, New York: Verso Books.

Giannichedda, M. G. (2005). L'utopia della realtà. Franco Basaglia e l'impresa della sua vita. In: F. Basaglia, *L'utopia della realtà*. Torino: Einaudi, pp. XLVIII–XLIX.

Glatzel, J. (1974). Psychiatrie und Antipsychiatrie—eine Wissenschaft kommt ins Gerede. *Deutsches Ärzteblatt* 19:1415–19.

Häfner, H. (2001). Hat Basaglia eine bessere Psychiatrie geschaffen? Zur Biographie der italienischen Psychoreform. *Der Nervenarzt* 72(7):485–6.

Häfner, H. (2003). Die Inquisition der psychisch Kranken geht ihrem Ende entgegen. Die Geschichte der Psychiatrie-Enquete und Psychiatriereform in Deutschland. In: F.-W. Kersting (ed.), *Psychiatriereform als Gesellschaftsreform*. Paderborn: Schöningh, pp. 113–40.

Hartmann, K. (1974). Antipsychiatrie, Antiautoritarismus—Antithesen. *Deutsches Ärzteblatt* 45:3255–61.

Heinrich, K. (1980). Die Psychisch Kranken tragen den Schaden. Anmerkungen zu einem 'Spiegel'-Artikel. *Deutsches Ärzteblatt* 16:1009–14.

Janzarik, W. (1974). *Themen und Tendenzen der deutschsprachigen Psychiatrie*. Berlin: Springer.
Jaspers, K. (1913). *Allgemeine Psychopathologie*. Berlin: Springer.
Jaspers, K. (1967). Bomben gegen Chinas Bombe? *Der Spiegel* 12:122–7.
Kersting, F.-W. (ed.) (2003). *Psychiatriereform als Gesellschaftsreform*. Paderborn: Schöningh.
Kersting, F.-W. (2005). Between the national socialist 'Euthanasia Programme' and reform: asylum psychiatry in West Germany 1940–1975. In: M. Gijswijt-Hofstra et al. (eds), *Psychiatric Cultures Compared: Psychiatry and Mental Health Care in the Twentieth Century*. Amsterdam: Amsterdam University Press, pp. 200–24.
Kersting, F.-W. (2018). Der Psychiater Hermann Simon im erinnerungskulturellen Kontext. In: M. Frese and M. Weidner (eds), *Verhandelte Erinnerungen. Der Umgang mit Ehrungen, Denkmälern und Gedenkorten nach 1945*. Paderborn: Schöningh, pp. 209–30.
Klein, A. (2015). Governing madness—transforming psychiatry. Disability history and the formation of cultural knowledge in West Germany in the 1970s and 1980s. *Moving the Social* 53:11–37.
Lohmer, M., et al. (1980). Was hat uns die Tagung gebracht? Einschätzung aus München. In: P. Berger (ed.), *Neue Psychiatrie: Erfahrungen aus Italien und Deutschland. Materialien zu einer Arbeitstagung Oktober 1979 in München*. Bonn: Psychiatrie Verlag, pp. 159–68.
Marazia, C. (2005). L'internamento dei grandi. Ludwig Binswanger e la clinica Bellevue di Kreuzlingen. *Medicina e Storia* 10:75–92.
Marcuse, H. (1964). *One-Dimensional Man: Studies in the Ideology of Advanced Industrial Society*. Boston: Beacon.
Mollica, R.F. 1985. The unfinished revolution in Italian psychiatry: an international perspective. *International Journal of Mental Health 14* (1/2): 22–41.
Payk, T.R. (2004). Antipsychiatrie—eine vorläufige Bilanz. *Fortschritte der Neurologie-Psychiatrie* 72:516–22.
Pross, C. (2016). *Wir wollten ins Verderben rennen. Die Geschichte des Sozialistischen Patientenkollektivs Heidelberg*. Köln: Psychiatrie Verlag.
Riegler, A. (2016). 'West Germany and Italy in the 1970s: mutual perceptions during a decade of crisis'. Thesis, University College London.
Sachverständigen-Kommission zur Erarbeitung der Enquete über die Lage der Psychiatrie in der BRD, Zwischenbericht (1973). Bundestagsdrucksache 7/1124. Bonn: Bundestag.
Salize, H.J. (2012). Sozialpsychiatrie—Wohin?. *Psychiatische Praxis* 39:199–201.
Schmid, S. (1977). *Freiheit heilt*. Berlin: Wagenbach.
Schmid, S. (1980). *Überlegungen zur Frage der Übertragbarkeit der italienischen Psychiatrie-Reform auf bundesdeutsche Verhältnisse*. In: *Wege zu einer neuen Psychiatrie, Protokolle einer Tagung*. HU-Schriften 9, München, pp. 22–4.
Simons, T. (1980). *Absage an die Anstalt*. Frankfurt/Main: Campus.
Söhner, F., et al. (2017). Die Rolle der anthropologischen Psychiatrie in der Vorbereitungszeit der Psychiatrie-Enquete und Psychiatriereform in der Bundesrepublik Deutschland. *Psychiatrische Praxis* 1(17):252–7.
Somma, A. (2006). Psichiatria e diritto: appunti sull'esperienza tedesca. In: V. Andreoli et al. (eds), *L'utopia dell'uguaglianza. Ricordo di Fabio Visintini*. Napoli: Edizioni Scientifiche Italiane, pp. 193–208.
Sozialistisches Patientenkollektiv (SPK) (1972). *Aus der Krankheit eine Waffe machen. Eine Agitationsschrift des Sozialistischen Patientenkollektivs an der Universität Heidelberg*. München: Trikont Verlag.
Thoma, S. (2012). Phänomenologisch-anthropologische Sozialpsychiatrie –Wegmarken für eine theoretische Wiederbelebung. *Psychiatrische Praxis* 39:407–9.

Thoma, S. (2019). ‚Der Mensch ist dazu gemacht, das Menschliche zu ergründen'. Zur konzeptuellen Bedeutung der phänomenologisch-anthropologischen Psychiatrie im Vorfeld der westdeutschen Psychiatriereform. *Medizinhistorisches Journal* 54: 209–240.
Trivelli, E. (2016). The Basaglian legacy in Italian psychiatry: remembering, myth-making and crystallising. In: D. Kritsotaki et al. (eds), *Deinstitutionalisation and After: Post-War Psychiatry in the Western World*. Basingstoke: Palgrave Macmillan, pp. 217–40.
van der Beeck, M. (1980). Hilflose Patienten. *Deutsches Ärzteblatt* 13:850.
Weiner, D. (1994). 'Le geste de Pinel': the history of a psychiatric myth. In: M.S. Micale and R. Porter (eds), *Discovering the History of Psychiatry*. New York: Oxford University Press, pp. 232–47.
Wulff, E. (1980). Nachwort. In: T. Simons (ed.), *Absage an die Anstalt*. Frankfurt/Main: Campus-Verlag, pp. 249–55.
Wulff, E. (1991). Einleitung: 20 Jahre Info. *Sozialpsychiatrische Informationen* 4.
Zenker, C. and Zencker, J. (1979). Demokratische Psychiatrie in Italien—alternative zur deutschen Psychiatrie. *Das Argument* AS 30:138–50.
Zentralinstitut für Seelische Gesundheit Mannheim (1980/1981). *Zweijahresbericht*.

15
Has the spirit of Basaglia affected Polish psychiatry?

Jacek Moskalewicz, Grażyna Herczyńska, and Katarzyna Prot-Klinger

Introduction

During the Second World War, over 20,000 patients in Polish psychiatric hospitals, as well as over 100 psychiatrists (about half their number) were killed following the Nazi extermination policy of *lebensunwerten Lebens* (Jaroszewski, 1993; Nasierowski, 2008; Ilnicki, 2012). This war-time trauma has affected Polish psychiatry over the decades since. The priority in Polish mental health policy has been to take care of the survivors and to offer them shelter and support.

Polish psychiatry after the War inherited several dozen huge hospitals with about 10,000 beds, dating back to the turn of the twentieth century, and with no more than 100 psychiatrists (Puzynski and Moskalewicz, 2001). Well into the 1950s, large hospitals dominated mental healthcare in Poland. Of 31 psychiatric inpatient units, 22 were psychiatric hospitals, which provided over 97% of all the beds. Over 90% of patients in residential institutions were treated in psychiatric hospitals (see Table 15.1). Three quarters of all beds were located in large hospitals, with between 500 and 2,000 beds in each. Only 5% were in hospitals with fewer than 100 beds. Over half of patients had a duration of hospitalization of over one year, and a fifth had spent more than five years in the hospital (Biuletyn statystyczny, 1963, pp. 21–5). Most of these were people without any family support or real home. These huge institutions were only able to satisfy very basic needs, including shelter and food. Often, one psychiatrist had responsibility for several hundred patients. The need for reform of the system grew over the 1950s, the 1960s, and 1970s, not only amongst psychiatrists, but also amongst social scientists and policy makers (Nasierowski, 2016).

A proposal for a mental health act to ameliorate the existing situation was launched in the late 1950s in the climate of the early political thaw. This debate was reinforced in the 1970s by a paper published in the academic journal *Państwo i Prawo* (Daszkiewicz et al., 1974), in which the authors (a psychiatrist and two lawyers) presented an outline of the new mental health law. Special meetings to discuss the draft of the law were held by the Polish Sociological Association in the early 1970s. In addition to sociologists, prominent criminologists and lawyers participated. The critical opinion of the

Table 15.1 Pace of reforms in mental healthcare in Poland 1955–2015

	1955	1975	1995	2015
Number of psychiatric hospitals	22	38	49	46
Number of beds in psychiatric hospitals	22,575	38,789	27,275	17,444
Percentage of beds in psychiatric hospitals	97.2	97.5	88.2	72.8
Number of beds per hospital	1,026	1,020	556	379
Number of patients in psychiatric hospitals[1]	53,097	107,876	159,043	154,622
Percentage of patients in psychiatric hospitals	91.0	99.1	84.2	63.9
Mean length of stay (in days) in psychiatric hospitals	150.7	89.7	52.4	31.1
Number of psychiatric wards in general hospitals	9	18	55	158
Number of psychiatric beds in general hospitals	654	990	3,642	6,527
Number of patients in psychiatric wards in general hospitals[1]	5,227	6,664	29,857	82,178
Mean length of stay (in days) in general hospitals	NA	44.1	35.6	28.1

Source for 1955: Biuletyn Statystyczny, 1963, pp. 21–25, Tables 7–8

Sources for 1975: Dziduszko et al., 1976, pp. 51, 86–93, Table 1.17, Table 13.29

Sources for 1995: Jaszczuk et al., 1996, pp. 74, 82, 134–135, Table 3.32, Table 3.35, Table 3.73

Sources for 2015: Data from Departament of Public Heath, Institute of Psychiatry and Neurology (DPH, IPiN)

[1] Since 1975—number of admissions

Section of the Sociology of Law of the Polish Sociological Association also hampered attempts to implement the law. On balance, the project had as many opponents as it did supporters and, therefore, could not be adopted for many years to come (Leszek Kubicki, a lawyer, personal communication).

The mental health act was eventually adopted as law in 1994. The long-lasting resistance to introducing the law was partially related to fears of how it might be used or abused (Pomorski, 1972; Szwedek, 1975; Daszkiewicz, 1975), particularly to violate the rights of patients, including political opponents who could be hospitalized involuntarily, as had happened in the Soviet Union. A director of a big psychiatric hospital near Warsaw, Zbigniew Jaroszewski, described those developments to his colleague, the prominent psychiatrist and phenomenologist Eugeniusz Minkowski, who had been living for decades in Paris:

> We hoped that this year the Parliament would adopt a psychiatric law (entitled 'on protection of mental health') which has been under preparation for 20 years. In a meanwhile, however . . . concerns were expressed among lawyers and sociologists, that the law may be used as a tool to detain in the psychiatric hospitals persons who were mentally healthy but inconvenient for someone. Even though such cases do not occur, the perception of the law in public opinion was bad and more time will be needed for its adoption . . . In fact, the law is probably least needed for psychiatrists.'
>
> **(Jaroszewski, 1971, p. 153)**

This quotation carries a number of important messages. First of all, that the Polish debate about how to reform psychiatric care did not come out of the blue but had been a longstanding process dating back to the 1950s. Secondly, that Polish psychiatrists were in direct contact with their colleagues in other European countries beyond the Iron Curtain. Thirdly, that the risk of abusing psychiatry for political purposes was understood, which confirmed direct contacts with Soviet psychiatry. Fourthly, that public opinion did matter, despite a one-party political system. And last but not least, that thereform was probably least desired by psychiatrists. Hence, the majority of psychiatrists were in favour of gradual reforms from inside the system rather than a top–down political process.

It is certainly the case that reforms had indeed been gradual. Over decades, large psychiatric hospitals had seemed to be the major treatment response to mental health problems, as shown in Table 15.1. Their number more than doubled between 1955 and 1995, to reach a peak of 49 hospitals in 1995. In the next two decades, until 2015, only three hospitals vanished from the system. The hospitals were renovated and modernized rather than closed down. However, the number of beds slowly diminished, from over a thousand per hospital in the 1970s to about 400 in 2015. Mean length of hospitalization has also come down from five months to about one month. In parallel, a network of psychiatric wards in general hospitals has been on the rise. Their number increased from nine in the 1950s to over 150 in 2015, with an increased momentum in last 20 years. Nevertheless, large hospitals still provide three quarters of Polish beds and serve two thirds of patients (Dziduszko et al., 1976, pp. 51, 86–93; Jaszczuk et al., 1996, pp. 74, 82, 134–5; DPH, IPiN, 2015).

In the following pages, we will try to consider to what extent Polish national debate and reforms were affected by Franco Basaglia's thoughts and reforms in Italy. To understand his potential influence (or lack of it) in a more systematic manner, elements of a theory of diffusion of innovations, developed by Everett M. Rogers (Rogers, 2003), will be applied. Rogers claims that diffusion of innovation is not a technical question but constitutes a gradual process of social construction, in which the meaning of innovation is worked out. He defines diffusion as the process that includes, in addition to innovation, communication channels, time span, and social system. For communication channels, he emphasizes informal ways and sources of information that may decrease the uncertainty of potential stakeholders associated with an innovation and support subjective evaluation of cost benefits of its adaptation. This is a multi-stage decision-making process covering the acquisition of knowledge and consideration of the potential benefits and disadvantages of adopting innovation. Therefore, in this chapter, particular attention is paid to communication channels, including interpersonal networks, as well as potential gains to be attained and interests to be preserved in reforming the system of mental healthcare in Poland.

Sources

To answer the question of how much Basaglia influenced Polish debate and reform, we made a search in the Polish scientific libraries. The Polish medical bibliography was reviewed for the years 1979–2017 using key words including 'Basaglia', 'Italy', 'Law 180', and mental health reforms. Then, resources of the library of the Institute of Psychiatry and Neurology, the leading national centre for psychiatry, were investigated. We also searched the library of the Department of Philosophy and Sociology of Warsaw University, where opposition against the new mental health law seemed to be most clearly articulated in the 1970s. In addition, a review of the journal *Polish Psychiatry* was made for the period 1970–1990. We systematically interviewed seven major actors of the Polish reform of those times (including one of the co-authors of this chapter) who had, since the 1990s, made efforts to disseminate experiences of the Italian reform and the 'Basaglia law'. In non-structured interviews, we asked about the time and circumstances surrounding when our respondents first heard about Basaglia, the perception of the Italian reforms among major stakeholders in Poland, and the extent to which Italian experiences affected reforms in Poland.

Finally, we used informal forms of communication—shorter and longer conversations with more than a dozen other people, who were active and likely to remember the time when the 'Basaglia' law was introduced and subsequent reforms were implemented. The majority of them had no clear recall of Basaglia being discussed, and reported that he did not influence the Polish reforms. However, few offered statements, interpretations, or impressions that helped us to better understand those times.

Basaglia's influence on Polish mental health reforms: communication channels and the diffusion of innovations

Libraries

In addition to searching for Basaglia's writings, we also sought other heralds of deinstitutionalization who could catalyse Polish psychiatric reforms. We found that the works of Erving Goffman (all in English) and, in particular, his *Asylums. Essays on the*

Social Situations of Mental Patients and Other Inmates, published in 1961, had been available in the library of the Warsaw University since 1966, along with a number of his other books. *Asylums* became a standard textbook in the sociological curriculum from the early 1970s, and may have contributed to the debate whose scope went far beyond psychiatry.

The first signs of Basaglia's thinking in Poland were identified in the library of the Institute of Psychiatry and Neurology. His book *Qu'est-ce que la psychiatrie?* (published in French in 1977) was available in the library in 1978. It can be assumed that the book was donated by the then director of the Institute, Stanisław Dąbrowski, who had personal and professional contacts with French psychiatry. Unfortunately, Dąbrowski and most of his contemporaries are no longer alive and we cannot make any direct assessment on the impact of the book in Poland. What we do know is that Dąbrowski was very influential as regards implementation of reforms of mental healthcare in Poland.

One of Dabrowski's reforms imitated the French approach of *sectorization*. Individual hospital wards were made responsible for relatively small catchment areas where outpatient community support could also be offered. Its initial name in Polish was *sektoryzacja*, and then *subrejonizacja* (subregionization). The reform led to a huge change in the psychiatric hospitals. Thousands of chronic patients who had been living in the hospitals for many years were suddenly able to identify relatives and support in their local communities. As a consequence, they could be discharged from the hospitals to the community, family home, or local social welfare institution (Wanda Langiewicz, an expert in organization of mental health care, personal communication).

Rumours

A psychiatrist working in the Institute of Psychiatry and Neurology during those times, reported to us how the reform was initiated there. It consisted of reviewing each individual patient, who could then be sent from the hospital back to the community. They closed one of the two hospital wards, and established a day ward and community team instead. The reform was followed by a rapid decline in the number of beds, shortening of hospitalization time, and better outcomes of treatment (Jarema, 2001, p. 72). The direction of the reform was not administratively imposed but actively promoted by the Institute team all over Poland. Nevertheless, the reform was not copied from the Italian experience. On the contrary, the interviewed doctor's first reaction to the mention of Basaglia's name was 'Basaglia? It was that Italian, who we attempted to imitate in Poland in the 1970s. But fortunately, it was given up.' Our respondent claimed that rumours were heard that Basaglia promoted an irresponsible reform that resulted in thousands of patients being thrown out of the hospital and forced to live in the streets without any support (Bożena Pietrzykowska, a psychiatrist, personal communication).

Second-hand sources

Franco Basaglia and his thoughts came to Poland through second-hand sources. The ideas of anti-psychiatry emerged in Poland from increasing contact of Polish psychiatry with colleagues in the USA and Western Europe after the political thaw of the late 1950s. Another respondent (a psychiatrist who graduated in the 1950s) reported that he had heard of Basaglia from Maxwell Jones in the late 1960s, when he spent a few months on a scholarship in the UK and had an opportunity to visit the first therapeutic communities (Andrzej Różycki, a psychiatrist, personal communication; Różycki, 1970). Maxwell Jones' opinion on the Italian movement was reported as less than enthusiastic. Basaglia seemed to be critical of the concept of the therapeutic community, which he considered to be a sophisticated way to isolate the patient from society. He insisted on more radical reforms.

Our respondent simply rejected the Italian experiences. He attempted to reform mental healthcare from the bottom up; from the individual hospitals where he was employed and performed managerial functions. In the largest psychiatric hospital in Poland at that time (Branice Hospital, with more than 2,000 patients) and in Drewnica Hospital near Warsaw, our respondent introduced very radical reforms for the times. These included the removal of iron bars, open mixed-gender wards, and elements of the therapeutic community, including addressing all members (both patients and staff) by their first name (Dobrowolska, 1976; Różycki, 1976; Jaroszewski and Herczyńska, 2003, pp. 81–102). This was real revolution in a Polish culture which respects hierarchy and, in particular, in the strongly hierarchical medical environment.

Direct first-hand accounts

The first ever direct report of 'Basaglia's law' and its outcomes was provided in 1988, to wider audiences interested in mental health reforms in Poland, by the Italian psychiatrist Antonio Balestrieri. Balestrieri published in the Polish bi-monthly journal *Psychiatria Polska.* His paper was in English and entitled 'Italian psychiatry in 1978'. Its Polish abstract was modest—indeed, it comprised only two and a half lines: 'The author presents major assumption of the Italian psychiatric law adopted in 1978 by the Italian Parliament and results of the psychiatric reform from a perspective of its ten year functioning' (Balestrieri, 1988, p. 469).

Balistrieri summarized the general principles of the Italian reform and its experiences, exactly 10 years after it was adopted, in a balanced but overall positive tone, challenging some of the myths about it. He confirmed that the Act of 1978 was considered as 'some kind of revolution carried out by a left wing cultural and political movement' but showed that the draft of the Law was 'brought before the Italian Parliament by a Christian Democratic politician and the law was passed with the support of all the major parties'. He also denied another myth—that all psychiatric hospitals were closed down overnight and thousands of patients emerged in the streets without any help. He stated that, to the contrary, 'mental hospitals are still active in Italy, since they must care for patients admitted before the law'. He stressed that 'the originality of the Italian situation lies in the attempt to introduce a new system at one point of time, instead of introducing reforms gradually'. He continued: 'Our actions can be considered as no more than another aspect of the Italian phantasy, but they can also be a fundamental experience for psychiatry everywhere in the world' (Balestrieri, 1988, pp. 472–3).

Antonio Balestrieri could not have submitted his paper to the Polish journal without encouragement from Polish colleagues, as the decision to accept and publish an article in English was quite exceptional. Mateo Balestrieri (a psychiatrist and son of Antonio) confirms that his father (who is 92 years old now) was invited to Poland for two weeks in the late 1980s by Stefan Leder. Leder was a prominent psychiatrist and psychotherapist who worked in the Institute of Psychiatry and Neurology. To date, we can find no other direct traces of Balestrieri's visit and publication in Poland, although we assume that he must have delivered a couple of lectures and had meetings with Polish professionals. Nor were we able to find any letters or comments to the editors of *Psychiatria Polska*, either critical or positive. The publication seems to have been simply ignored by mainstream psychiatry, including in academic circles.

A co-author of this paper (KPK), who completed her specialization in psychiatry in the early 1980s, never heard of Basaglia during her studies. This despite the fact that ideas of anti-psychiatry had been well known in Poland since the 1970s. She acquired first-hand knowledge and more details about Basaglia and his reforms from when she lived in Bologna for a year in the late 1980s. She attempted to promote his ideas during professional and scientific meetings after returning to work in Poland. However, her message was just ignored, as Basaglia's reforms were viewed as too radical. This resistance occurred against a background of the extremely rapid and radical transitions towards a market economy in Poland.

A wider debate on the Italian reforms was not initiated until 2007, after the publication (in Polish) of Vittorino Andreoli's book *I miei matti: Ricordi e storie di un medico della mente* (Andreoli, 2007). The author offered a very critical description of the Italian reforms and diminished Basaglia's contribution, calling him 'a dubious hero of psychiatry' whose 'ideas were not original, without any personal contribution'. Nevertheless, the author eventually admitted that the psychiatric hospital is a place where madness is born (Prot and Tibaldi, 2007). It seems that this book resonated with the expectations of the Polish audience and reinforced negative perceptions of Basaglia's reforms. In the same year, KPK made a plenary presentation at the Congress of the Polish Psychiatric Association on 'Italian reform—Basaglia law after 30 years'. Her presentation was received coldly, despite the presented facts showing that the reform reduced the number of involuntary admissions and was not followed by negative social consequences such as homelessness or increased suicide and homicide rates (Prot, 2007).

In 2010, a special discussion plenary session on the role of the psychiatric hospital was held during the Polish psychiatric congress 'Psychiatry after diploma'. Two papers were of particular relevance: 'Hospital as a basis for treatment' by Tomasz Szafrański, and 'Why a hospital is a barrier' by KPK. Szafrański quoted a list of 'false' assumptions published by Singh and Castle in *World Psychiatry* (2008), and claimed that demands to close down psychiatric hospitals are related to erroneous assumptions adopted in an 'idealistic and non-critical manner'. Further, he continued, criticisms of psychiatric hospitals are based on assumptions which he described as 'non-realistic, utopian, and ignoring medical facts and social reality'. According to Szafrański, psychiatric hospitals are needed as some disorders require hospitalization. He also claimed that there is a relationship between the quality and effectiveness of mental healthcare and the availability of hospital beds. He highlighted 'transinstitutionalization'—the phenomenon of shifting patients to other institutions of social control, starting with social welfare homes or prisons, and who eventually end 'under bridges, in railways stations or on the streets'. He believed that psychiatric hospitals could be reformed, and become modern, effective, profitable, and open. Additionally, he argued that some patients wish to be treated in a psychiatric hospital and 'depriving them of such an opportunity is a good instance of paternalism'. Szafrański's final argument was that psychiatric hospitals play a crucial role in small local economies, offering employment for hundreds of people, including medical personnel, administrative staff, and other workers (Szafrański, 2010).

In contrast, KPK stressed the stigma associated with psychiatric hospitals, and referred directly to Franco Basaglia and Italian Law 180, and the consequences of the reform inspired by his thoughts. As in her previous paper (2007), she underscored the fact that despite the closing down of 76 hospitals, the number of crimes committed by mentally ill persons and suicides did not increase in Italy. She showed that large hospitals in Poland consume the majority of funds, thereby limiting the financial resources of community care which is thus understaffed, weak, and unable to compete with the hospitals. Psychiatric hospitals, because of their great distance from patients' places of residence, constitute an obstacle for community care. She concluded that 'the hospital transforms a feature into an entity. Patients do not suffer from schizophrenia any longer, s/he becomes a schizophrenic.' Several hundred professionals from all over the country attended the session. Most of them supported Szafrański's position, but a significant minority were sympathetic to KPK's arguments that consider the psychiatric hospital as a barrier to proper mental healthcare (Prot, 2010).

Despite all these reservations, Franco Basaglia's presence in the Polish debate is on the rise involving translation of foreign publications (Altamura and Goodwin, 2011; Goanec, 2015). The leading psychiatric journal recently published an article (in Polish and English) entitled 'Deinstitutionalization in Italian Psychiatry—the course and consequences. Part I: the course of deinstitutionalization—the activity of Basaglia's group. Part II: the consequences of deinstitutionalization' (Mokrzycka-Markowska et al., 2015). The authors present the Italian reform from a historical perspective, against a background of anti-psychiatric movements, emerging community psychiatry and group therapy, and Basaglias's philosophical and ideological inspirations.

They offer objective, descriptive information about the pre-history of the reform and its implementation, and summarize its results. They seem to support critics of the reform, blaming its mainly administrative character. They claim that psychiatric hospitals were just replaced by psychiatric wards and outpatient clinics, where modes of treatment deviate from initial assumption and pharmacotherapy dominates. Nevertheless, they acknowledge that Basaglia's reform resulted in revolutionary changes in the social perception of mental illness and gave impetus to implement innovative methods of treatment, engaging non-medical sectors in the therapy, rehabilitation, and emancipation of people with mental disorders.

Discussion and conclusions

Travelling back in history to trace the potential impact of Basaglia's ideas and activities on Polish psychiatric reforms offers a unique opportunity to understand better the slow pace with which these reforms have progressed. Despite the first-hand reports that have been available since the 1970s, and in the following decades, opinions about Basaglia and Italian reform have continued to be based on initial rumours and second-hand sources. These spoke of an 'irresponsible' change that deprived thousands of patients of any care and left them alone 'in the streets and under the bridges'. These perceptions survived over three decades and can be identified in the present Polish debate on whether the hospital should remain as the most important bastion of psychiatric care.

Adoption of innovation does not depend solely on its technical content and expected benefits. There are also costs to be paid by reformers, both in terms of financial expenditure and non-monetary costs, including organizational engagement, power relationships, and other social costs. Major stakeholders in the Polish reforms held important managerial positions in large psychiatric hospitals, where they had enough power to implement the changes without external influence. They could improve the quality of care and the conditions in which this care is offered without much organizational burden. These reforms did not require power sharing or a weakening of their position within the system. The alternative of either introducing innovations within the system they control or destroying the foundations of their power may have led them to select the former.

In addition to these professional interests and considerations, closing down psychiatric hospitals located in the countryside could damage the local economy, depriving hundreds of people of employment. This would affect the prestige and influence of the hospital as a major employer, and thereby undermine the position of its managerial staff as a local elite.

Initiating a political process, as in Italy, may have produced additional risks in Poland, with its one-party political system that dominated until 1989. In that system, laws depended largely on arbitrary political decisions, thus increasing the sense of uncertainty among major stakeholders from the world of psychiatry. However, blaming the previous regime for delays in reforming the system would be a substantial oversimplification. As concluded by Pużyński and Moskalewicz in 2001, in the years of political and economic transformations, mental healthcare still suffered from major structural and functional shortcomings. These included uneven distribution of psychiatric facilities, concentration of beds in large psychiatric hospitals, and long distances between large hospitals and patients' places of residence (Pużyński and Moskalewicz, 2001; Pużyński et al., 2001).

In conclusion, it can be claimed that Basaglia's reforms were more of a negative reference point in Polish efforts to introduce change from the inside. Blaming Basaglia, as well as American psychiatry, for irresponsible reforms which affected thousands of patients gave moral legitimacy for slow, longstanding reforms without major costs for reform stakeholders. This experience from Poland confirms Rogers' theory of diffusion of innovations, where the stress is put on informal networks as important communication channels to adopt or reject an innovation. As shown in this chapter, major stakeholders also actively search for those communication channels, not excluding rumours and second-hand sources, that preserve their own interests or offer them optimal balance in cost–benefits evaluation.

References

Altamura, A.C. and Goodwin, G.M. (2011). W jaki sposób Ustawa 180 w ciągu 30 lat zmieniła psychiatrię: podejście w przeszłości, obecne trendy i niespełnione potrzeby. [Translation from the *British Journal of Psychiatry*] *Psychiatria po Dyplomie* 5:54–6.

Andreoli, V. (2007). *Moi wariaci* [*I miei matti: Ricordi e storie di un medico della mente*], M. Bielawski (trans.). Kraków: Wydawnictwo Homini.

Balestrieri, A. (1988). Italian psychiatry in 1978. *Psychiatr Pol* 6:469–73.

Biuletyn Statystyczny (1963). *Psychiatria 1956–1959*. Warszawa: Ministerstwo Zdrowia i Opieki Społecznej.

Daszkiewicz, W. (1975). Przymusowa hospitalizacja w zakładzie psychiatrycznym. *Państwo i Prawo* 3:122–6.

Daszkiewicz, W., Dabrowski, S., and Kubicki, L. (1974). Prawna regulacja ochrony zdrowia psychicznego. *Państwo i Prawo* 8–9:70–88.

Dobrowolska, M. (1976). *Analiza udanego eksperymentu socjotechnicznego*. Lecture at the International Symposium on Social Engineering, Warsaw. Archiwum Historii Psychiatrii Polskiej [Archive of History of Polish Psychiatry], Zakład Zdrowia Publicznego [Department of Public Health], Instytut Psychiatrii i Neurologii [Institute of Psychiatry and Neurology]. Folder: Andrzej Różycki.

Dziduszko, T., Bartoszewska, D., and Karewicz, Z. (ed.) (1976). *Zakłady psychiatrycznej oraz neurologicznej opieki zdrowotnej i społecznej. Rocznik Statystyczny 1975*. Warszawa: Instytut Psychoneurologiczny.

Goanec, M. (2015). Koniec szpitali psychiatrycznych, M. Madej (trans.). *Le Monde diplomatique. Polish edition*. 1(34):35.

Ilnicki, S. (2012). Straty wśród psychiatrów polskich podczas II wojny światowej. In: T. Nasierowski, G. Herczyńska, and D.M. Myszka (eds), *Zagłada chorych psychicznie. Pamięć i historia*. Warszawa: Eneteia, pp. 167–208.

Jaroszewski, Z. (1971). *Letter to E. Minkowski of 16 December. Drewnica.* Archiwum Historii Psychiatrii Polskiej [Archive of History of Polish Psychiatry], Zakład Zdrowia Publicznego [Department of Public Health], Instytut Psychiatrii i Neurologii [Institute of Psychiatry and Neurology]. Folder: Eugeniusz Minkowski 1885–1972, subfolder: Letters 1956-1973.

Jaroszewski, Z. (ed.) (1993). *Zagłada chorych psychicznie w Polsce 1939–1945.* Warszawa: Wydawnictwo Naukowe PWN.

Jaroszewski, Z. and Herczyńska, G. (2003). *100 lat Wojewódzkiego Szpitala dla Nerwowo i Psychicznie Chorych „Drewnica" w Ząbkach.* Ząbki: Szpital Drewnica.

Jaszczuk, H., Pietrzykowska, B., and Sobańska, M. (eds) (1996). *Zakłady psychiatrycznej oraz neurologicznej opieki zdrowotnej. Rocznik Statystyczny 1995.* Warszawa: Instytut Psychiatrii i Neurologii.

Jarema, M. (2001). III Klinika Psychiatryczna. In:Kulczycki, J. (ed.). *Instytut Psychiatrii i Neurologii 1951–2001.* Warszawa: Instytut Psychiatrii i Neurologii.

Morzycka-Markowska, M., Ewa Drozdowicz, E., and Nasierowski, T. (2015). Deinstitutionalization in Italian psychiatry; the course and consequence. *Psychiatr Pol* 49(2):391–412.

Nasierowski, T. (2008). *Zagłada osób z zaburzeniami psychicznymi w okupowanej Polsce. Początek ludobójstwa.* Warszawa: Wydawnictwo Neriton.

Nasierowski, T. (2016). Psychiatria. In: W. Noszczyk (ed.), *Dzieje medycyny w Polsce. Vol.3: 1944–1989.* Warszawa: PZWL, pp. 587–606.

Pomorski, S. (1972). Problematyka leczenia przymusowego na tle projektu ustawy o ochronie zdrowia psychicznego z 1970 r. *Państwo i Prawo* 3:45–59.

Prot, K. (2007). Reforma włoska—prawo Basaglii po 30 latach. *Psychiatr Pol* 41(Suppl. 3):122–3.

Prot, K. (2010). *Dlaczego szpital jest przeszkodą?* Lecture at Third Congress Akademia po Dyplomie, Warsaw. [Lecture Powerpoint Slide] Archiwum Historii Psychiatrii Polskiej [Archive of History of Polish Psychiatry], Zakład Zdrowia Publicznego [Department of Public Health], Instytut Psychiatrii i Neurologii [Institute of Psychiatry and Neurology].

Prot, K. and Tibaldi, G. (2007). *Vittorino Andreoli, Moi wariaci.* Book review. *Postępy Psychiatrii i Neurologii* 3:269–71.

Puzynski, S. and Moskalewicz, J. (2001). Evolution of the mental health care system in Poland. *Acta Psychiatr Scand* 104(Suppl. 410):69–73.

Puzynski, S., Langiewicz, W., and Pietrzykowska, B. (2001). Polska 2000: aktualne problemy psychiatrycznej opieki zdrowotnej. *Postępy Psychiatr Neurol* 10:95–107.

Rogers, E.M. (2003). *Diffusion of Innovations* (5th edn). London: Free Press.

Różycki, A. (1970). Realizacja zasad społeczności leczniczej na przykładzie wybranych ośrodków zagranicznych. *Psychiatr Pol* 3:333–41.

Różycki, A. (1976). *Udany eksperyment socjotechniczny we wprowadzaniu społeczności leczniczej.* Lecture at the International Symposium on Social Engineering, Warsaw. Archiwum Historii Psychiatrii Polskiej [Archive of History of Polish Psychiatry], Zakład Zdrowia Publicznego [Department of Public Health], Instytut Psychiatrii i Neurologii [Institute of Psychiatry and Neurology]. Folder: Andrzej Różycki.

Singh, B. and Castle, D. (2008). Why are psychiatric services getting better but looking worse. *World Psychiatry* 7(2):95–6.

Szafrański, T. (2010). *Szpital podstawą leczenia?* Lecture at the Third Congress Akademia po Dyplomie, Warsaw. Archiwum Historii Psychiatrii Polskiej [Archive of History of Polish Psychiatry], Zakład Zdrowia Publicznego [Department of Public Health], Instytut Psychiatrii i Neurologii [Institute of Psychiatry and Neurology].

Szwedek, E. (1975). Nowy środek zabezpieczający. *Państwo i Prawo* 2:115–17.

16
A spectre for some, a Mecca for others
The impact of Basaglia in the Netherlands

Gemma Blok

Introduction

> Italy, of course, was our role model. After all, it was a large and civilized European country. So if they could make it happen there, then surely, we were not talking nonsense? Besides, the Italian radical psychiatry movement was not made up of fools: some very prominent psychiatrists were part of it. These made us feel like we belonged to the avant-garde. We were absolutely sure that we were decades ahead of the troops.

This quote comes from an interview with a volunteer who, in the early 1980s, was working at the Runaway Shelter in the Dutch town of Utrecht. This Shelter had opened its doors in 1981 to people who had run away from psychiatric hospitals, escaping 'repression' and 'inhumane treatment'. In total, 11 such Shelters for psychiatric runaways were established in the Netherlands between 1980 and 1985 (Blok, 2004; Van de Wetering, 2007). For staff and volunteers working at the Shelters, Italy was the shining example, a country filled with innovative and brave people pioneering the future of psychiatry. The status of 'Italy' was very high. As another former volunteer from the Runaway Shelter in Utrecht remembered, at the time 'you only had to quote some South-Sicilian psychiatrist to make your point. And if you had actually been to Italy yourself, your star was definitely on the rise' (Van de Wetering, 2007).

In the Netherlands, the influence of Franco Basaglia and other psychiatrists that were part of the Italian anti-asylum movement was at its high point in the early 1980s. Whereas during the 1970s, the critical psychiatry of Ronald D. Laing and David Cooper had been all the rage, and progressive psychotherapeutic communities had been set up in several psychiatric hospitals based on their ideas, after 1980, the Dutch anti-psychiatry movement radicalized. Instead of Laing's Kingsley Hall or Cooper's therapeutic community Villa 21, the radical experiments in Italian 'democratic psychiatry' now became the leading example for those who longed for change in mental healthcare. The impact of challenging the 'medical model' from within had been too low. Many felt it was time to leave the asylum behind and try something new.

The impact of the Italian model was most obvious in Amsterdam. Critics of 'traditional' psychiatry, inspired by the events in Trieste in the late 1970s, were able to convince the newly arrived Amsterdam alderman for healthcare that the Dutch capital needed to adopt a radically different system of mental healthcare. After 1984, Santpoort, the large provincial psychiatric hospital for the Amsterdam region in the dunes of North Holland, was gradually dismantled. It was replaced with small-scale psychiatric clinics in the city that resembled the Italian *centri di igieni mentali* (CIM). The impact of Basaglia's democratic psychiatry manifested itself at national level as well when, in 1982, a successful appeal was made to the Dutch government to dismiss any further plans for the building of new psychiatric hospitals.

Towards an 'adult' form of treatment: the critical psychiatry movement in the Netherlands

As sociologist Nick Crossley and others have argued, 'anti-psychiatry' was one of the new social movements of the post-war period, partly overlapping ideologically with other social movements such as the youth counterculture movement of the 1960s, second-wave feminism, and the gay liberation movement (Crossley, 1998, 2006; Lewis, 2016). The most commonly used label for the movement, 'anti-psychiatry', is somewhat problematic. As historians have pointed out, not only does it refer to a very diverse myriad of ideas and practices, it was mostly a media term and one that many critics of psychiatry felt was not their own (Blok, 2004; Foot, 2015). In this chapter, therefore, the term 'critical psychiatry' or (when referring to Italian democratic psychiatry) 'anti-asylum movement' will be used as labels. Interestingly, the critical psychiatry movement was fuelled to a large extent by psychiatrists themselves; like the international superstar R.D. Laing (1927–1989) from England, his colleague and friend David Cooper (1931–1986), and Thomas Szasz (1920–2012) from the United States. Their ideas certainly were not identical, but they all shared the view that coercive psychiatry functioned as an instrument of social control. However, in the Netherlands, a strong client movement also existed, and criticism of psychiatry was very popular among psychologists and psychiatric nurses.

In the Netherlands, psychiatry came under attack at the beginning of the 1970s. Clients, family members, and their supporters made their voices heard, organized themselves, and published books and magazines; many journalists criticized the 'medical model' in mental healthcare; and last, but certainly not least, the Netherlands had its own 'anti-psychiatrist'—Jan Foudraine (1929–2016), who for a long time was the figurehead of the movement. This psychoanalytically trained psychiatrist was very critical of electroshock treatment and the dominance of psychotropic medication in psychiatry, and argued instead for a psychotherapeutic approach. He brought the ideas of Laing, Cooper, and Szasz to the Netherlands, stating that mental problems were not the result of a biological or neurological defect, but that they should be considered as 'problems in living'. In his bestseller *Wie is van hout ... Een gang door de psychiatrie* (1971), which sold about 200,000 copies within several years, Foudraine claimed that society actually made people ill. Parents, teachers, and clergymen—they all forced children to participate in a competitive and productive life style, based on self-restraint and massive repression of feelings and (sexual) urges. Listening to people and simply being kind to them would allow for them to liberate their 'true selves' (Blok, 1998).

In this climate of contesting psychiatry, Basaglia's works *La Maggioranza Deviante* and *Che Cos'è la Psichiatria?* were translated into Dutch in the mid 1970s. Remarkably, his major work *L'Istitutione Negata* (1968) was not translated into Dutch. However, its main argument was summarized in Dutch, in 1975, in the book *Antipsychiatrie. Een Overzicht* (*Antipsychiatry. An Overview*) written by Professor in Social Psychiatry, Kees Trimbos. Trimbos had been an active member of the Mental Hygiene Movement for most of his career and now, as he was approaching the age of retirement, he strongly sympathized with this new wave of 'anti-psychiatric' ideas. Trimbos called Basaglia one of the leading ideologists of 'anti-psychiatry', next to Laing, Szasz, Cooper, and others; and used the German translation of *L'Istitutione Negata* to present Basaglia's ideas and to write about his experiments in Gorizia.

However, in the Netherlands, the urge to reform psychiatry at the time was not yet aimed at dismantling psychiatric hospitals. Rather, it was directed at humanizing psychiatric treatment by protesting against the use of force and against the 'medical model' in psychiatry, symbolized by electroshock treatment, psychotropic medication, and the use of solitary confinement. Reform-minded workers tried to shape a new 'social model' of psychiatric treatment within the framework of existing institutions. In many psychiatric hospitals, reform-minded psychiatrists, psychologists, and nurses were given some leeway and were allowed to experiment in newly created 'therapeutic communities' or in specially designated wards. Instead of focusing on the individual, the focus of treatment shifted to incorporate the family as a pathogenic unit.

Workers tried to find ways to create a form of treatment that was non-coercive and empowering, instead of patronizing, repressive, and debilitating. This included (trying to) restrain from using medication, electroshocks, or solitary confinement, introducing family therapy and group therapy, and giving 'clients' or 'residents' more freedom as well as more responsibilities. Nurses got rid of their uniforms as the boundaries blurred between 'patients' and medical personnel. One sympathetic journalist wrote that it was time to get rid of the 'infantile' psychiatry of old, which was limited to 'soothing, adjusting and covering-up', using pills and a reassuring pat on the back; and to create instead a more 'adult' form of psychiatric treatment, which would strive for 'exposure, clarification, and discovery', using psychotherapy (Blok, 2004).

'To Basaglia!': enthusiasm about Italian democratic psychiatry

Towards the end of the 1970s, however, things started to change. First of all, psychotherapeutic enthusiasm within the psychiatric hospitals appeared to be reaching its limits. Results were disappointing and internal conflicts arose. Some experimental wards were overcrowded, as it had become the habit to admit not only the 'identified patients' but his or her family members as well. In this climate, the exciting developments in Italy started to attract a lot of attention, as people were looking for alternative ways to reform psychiatry. In Italy, they found one that they could connect with. Democratic psychiatry presented itself as the next radical step for mental healthcare reform. As Agostino Pirella put it, therapeutic communities, even the most radical ones, were never a true solution to the fundamental problem of traditional psychiatry, since in the end they still legitimized social exclusion. 'We have to abolish the mental hospital altogether, even if it has changed into a therapeutic community', he stated in an interview with a group of Dutch social science students (Van der Beek et al., 1980). In order to really change mental healthcare, one should work together with local populations.

Dutch interest in Italian events grew quicky after 1977 when, at a press conference, Basaglia famously announced the closure of San Giovanni, the city asylum of Trieste, of which he was the director at the time. Indeed, the hospital stopped admitting patients in 1980. The events in Trieste, writes Basaglia's biographer John Foot, 'led directly to a national law—the 180—the famous "Basaglia law"' that called for a closing down of all public asylums in Italy (Foot, 2015). In 1978, the story of Basaglia and Trieste entered the Netherlands through the Dutch translation of a book on Basaglia's experiment written by the Swiss journalist Sil Schmid: *Freiheit heilt. Bericht über die demokratische Psychiatrie in Italien* (in Dutch: *Vrijheid is de beste medicijn*). Schmid had witnessed the events in Trieste up close, interviewing and following Basaglia during and shortly after the press conference. Her book was reviewed in most leading Dutch newspapers and it was highly instrumental in attracting attention to the radical Italian variant of critical psychiatry.

The book inspired Hans Van der Wilk, for one. This former client of psychiatry, who had been admitted to psychiatric hospitals seven times when he was in his twenties, got his life back on track in his thirties and, in the late 1970s, became chairman of two influential Dutch client organizations—the Pandora Foundation and the Clients Union (Hunsche, 2008). Reading Sil Schmid's book turned him into an avid proponent of the anti-asylum movement in the Netherlands. He had always been very critical of the psychiatric hospital as a 'total institution', and in favour of dismantling them; in his words, 'there is no mental condition that justifies locking people up'. He described admission to a psychiatric hospital as an extremely traumatic event (Veldhoen, 1983). However, developments in Italy strengthened his belief that alternative forms of treatment were indeed a real possibility. 'Each time someone shouts at me: "what you want is quite impossible", I mention the Italian example', Van der Wilk told a journalist. 'It *is* possible' (Van der Meulen, 1979).

Moreover, Trieste became a place of pilgrimage for Dutch critics of psychiatry. As Foot and Crossley have already described, the Trieste experiment exerted a 'magnetic pull' and 'mobilized thousands of people', linking activists all over Italy and internationally (Crossley, 2006; Foot, 2015). Crossley typifies Trieste as a 'working utopia': a place that has a symbolic, almost utopian meaning for activists, since it lives in their imagination and motivates and inspires them to reform; but, it is a place that actually exists in reality as well, thus 'symbolizing the realistic nature of the movements aspirations' (Crossley, 1999). For Dutch members of the anti-psychiatry movement, Trieste certainly did function as a working utopia.

In September 1977, a Dutch delegation of about 25 people travelled to Trieste, on the occasion of the third conference of the International Network for Alternative Psychiatry, which was organized in this town. A group of Utrecht psychology students, client activists, and authors writing for the critical magazines *'t Narreschip* (*The Ship of Fools*) and the *Gekkenkrant* (*The Crazy's Paper*) visited the conference. Apparently, the conference was extremely popular; some members of the Dutch delegation had to stay the night in sleeping bags on the floor of an empty pavilion at San Giovanni, since all hotels in Trieste were fully booked. The terrain of San Giovanni slowly turned into a tent city and the place was crawling with visitors to the conference; according to one Dutch eyewitness, there were about 4000 of them (*'t Narreschip*, 1979).

Reports by Dutch visitors were mixed. Some, such as journalist Geert Mak, wrote about Trieste in glowing terms. Writing for the left-wing magazine *De Groene Amsterdammer*, he repeated key elements of what Foot calls 'the Trieste myth', such as the story about the horse Marco Cavallo. This story referred to a horse that used to cart away the hospital's dirty linen. Apparently, some of the older patients used to say he was the only one who managed to get out of the hospital. In the 1970s, Marco Cavallo became the ultimate symbol of the Trieste 'revolution', with artists creating a large, blue, papier mâché horse that was wheeled through town by patients, artists, and activists.

Others called the conference the 'Woodstock of antipsychiatry' and mocked the activists who were enjoying themselves with copious amounts of wine, sex, and endless discussions (Gekkenkrant, 1977). Others reported that the conference had been chaotic: radical students of the so-called autonomous movement had dominated it. Apparently, the students had been very loud and annoying, criticizing Basaglia and his colleagues for not being radical enough, for working within the system too much, and for focusing exclusively on just one group of socially excluded persons—the mad. For a while, a group of critical students even occupied the conference secretariat as a means of protesting against the fact that the conference was not free of charge; according to the students, this was exclusive. Language was a problem as well. Most lectures and tours were in Italian or French; some translators were present but many visitors ended up missing out on a lot of information. Still, as one Dutch visitor concluded, it had been a heart-warming experience to see so many people in one place who were all actively trying to reform psychiatry.

To a lesser extent, Dutch activists travelled to other places where democratic psychiatry had been put into practice. In 1976, three Dutch students in pedagogy and andragogy were deeply moved by a documentary film on the events in Parma: *Matti da Slegare* (translated into English as *Fit to be Untied*, and into Dutch as *Te gek om los te lopen*), which was made by a collective of movie directors. Sandro Petraglia was one of the collective, and went on to make the successful and well-known movie *La Meglio Giuventù* (2003). The documentary film *Matti da Slegare* was shown in Dutch art movie houses and appeared on Dutch television in the summer of 1976. Its focus was on Parma's psychiatric hospital, Colorno, where Mario Tommasini had been arguing for reform since 1965, when he had been appointed as the 'provincial assessor' of Colorno. Tomassino was appalled by the state the hospital was in, comparing it to Nazi concentration camps. He contacted Basaglia, and Gorizia and Parma began to work together. For a short while, in 1970 and 1971, Basaglia even became the director of Colorno (Foot, 2015).

The documentary film *Matti da Slegare* was based on extensive interviews with and life stories of (former) patients of Colorno. Many people who watched it were moved and inspired; 'Colorno has a crucial importance in the memory of the anti-asylum movement' (Foot, 2015). Among others, the French therapist and philosopher Félix Guattari praised the film. Basaglia and his colleagues made a point of working intensively with the general public, students, journalists, and artists, inviting them to participate in their movement. In Trieste, artists and their friends were given free run of the hospital grounds and the whole experiment was 'referred to as a laboratory' (Foot, 2015). As has been noted before, the Italian radical psychiatry movement was enhanced enormously by music and film and, as the Dutch example also proves, by the radical Italian film collective inspired by Basaglia (Portacolone et al., 2015).

Three Dutch students who watched *Matti da Slegare* were very impressed by the story of a woman who had been living in Colorno for 30 years, and was now living on her own, sharing an apartment with two friends. She did not use any medication, whereas during her decades in the hospital, pills had been a part of her everyday life. She had had to take them in order 'to make her a bit more gentle', she recalled in her own words (Van der Beek et al., 1980). The inspired students phoned one of the movie directors in Italy and inquired whether it was possible to come and work in Italy as volunteers. When he replied positively, they decided to give it a try and off they went, hitch-hiking to Italy. The students ended up working in Arezzo, among other places, and wrote a book about their experiences, *Democratische Psychiatrie. Niet de ziekte bestaat, wel het lijden* (*Democratic Psychiatry: there's no disease, there's only suffering*) (1980). The publication included an afterword by Agostino Pirella, who was invited to the Netherlands in 1980 to lecture at Utrecht University. The interest for this lecture was massive: about a thousand people signed up for it.

Another group of Dutch activists visited Arezzo as well, and even twice travelled to Naples to visit a 'socio-medical' centre for mental healthcare in Guigliano, a nearby village. Naples was probably even less well known than Perugia; the city was not on the forefront of psychiatric reform. However, it was interesting to Dutch visitors because of its Guigliano centre, which had been established in 1975 by a group of former co-workers of Basaglia in Trieste. The Dutch visitors had a great time in Guigliano, drinking wine with the workers and their friends, and being inspired by their working method. This method was very practical and focused on such things as creating jobs for unemployed clients or activities for teenagers with problems; also, the centre was running a very progressive, low-threshold morphine programme for opiate addicts (*'t Narreschip*, 1980, 1981).

The 'Italy hype' seems to have been at its peak by the late 1970s and early 1980s. In the summer of 1979, the events in Italian psychiatry were a news item on Dutch national television, and personal ads could be found in Dutch national newspapers of people who were going to Trieste and were looking for travelling companions: 'Naar Basaglia!' ('To Basaglia!'). Some Dutch psychiatrists and policy makers took the opportunity to go and see Basaglia at a conference in Ghent in 1979, in the neighbouring country of Belgium. Organized by the Belgium government and under the auspices of the World Health Organization, the conference was on alternatives to the psychiatric hospital. Basaglia was one of the speakers. The events in Italy were also closely followed by various groups of social scientists and Dutch university students (mostly psychologists). In 1980, Italian democratic psychiatry was one of the themes of a large Dutch conference on 'progressive developments in psychology' that attracted 1,400 visitors, who were mostly young, left-wing students and psychologists (Abma, 2001; Van der Kamp et al., 1989).

Most importantly, the Italian examples served as an inspiration for the establishment of Runaway Shelters for psychiatric 'refugees'. The first one was set up in the Dutch town of Haarlem in 1980. As one of the volunteers proudly stated, this was the first place in the Netherlands where the ideals of Italian democratic psychiatry were actually put into practice ('Wegloophuis', 1980). In 1979, the founders of the Haarlem Runaway Shelter invited two Italian psychiatrists to visit Amsterdam to lecture on democratic psychiatry and to offer advice on setting up a Shelter: Maria Grazia Cogliati and Giuseppe ('Peppe') Dell'Acqua from Barcola, a Trieste neighbourhood (*Gekkenkrant*, 1979). In the following years, 10 more Shelters were created all over the Netherlands. A number were located in squats and initiated by a mixture of people—politically engaged students, volunteers and professionals working in 'alternative' youth care, volunteers working for Release or other charity organizations offering free legal advice, and (former) psychiatric clients. Idealism was strong; the mental problems of clients ('residents') were characterized as 'healthy reactions to a sick system' and psychiatrists were considered to be 'scum bags' and 'sadists' (Van de Wetering, 2007). Workers in the Amsterdam Shelter described Italian democratic psychiatry as their 'philosophy of liberation' (*'t Narreschip*, 1982). Two Runaway Shelters were aimed in particular at women; feminism and anti-psychiatry strongly overlapped. 'Women often feel threatened in psychiatric hospitals' argued an employee of Hysterica, a Runaway Shelter for women in the Dutch town of Nijmegen. 'They easily become victims of sexual harassment in such an environment' (Wolfson, 1986).

Some Shelters disappeared quite quickly, however, because of dwindling subsidies, internal problems, or a lack of volunteers. Working with the runaways was not always easy; volunteers had to deal with aggression and suicide attempts, or unclean and psychotic clients. There were complaints that psychiatric hospitals attempted to get rid of their most troublesome and unwanted patients by sending them to the Shelters. Several Shelters, however, managed to remain in operation for decades. Gradually, the antagonistic attitude of the Shelters faded and a working relationship with traditional psychiatry developed. Nowadays, only the Shelter in Utrecht still exists. The working method there has become more pragmatic; however, workers are still proud if, in some cases, they manage to take care of people without having to use medication or force (Van de Wetering, 2007).

The most radical and direct impact of the ideas of Basaglia and his colleagues, however, could be seen in Amsterdam in the early 1980s, when activists sensed an opportunity to bring the Trieste experience to the Netherlands and to dismantle Santpoort—the largest psychiatric institution of the Netherlands, established in 1849 by the province of North Holland. Most Amsterdam citizens with mental health problems were sent to this hospital, which was situated about 45 kilometres from the Dutch capital, in a beautiful area near the sea. In the 1930s, the population of Santpoort had been at its peak with about 1,500 patients; by the early 1980s, this number had already fallen to some 1,200. Today, however, Santpoort is no longer in operation; it has indeed been dismantled completely.

The 'Amsterdam model'

Among the pilgrims who travelled to Italy were psychologist Mark Janssen and community doctor Egbert Van der Poel. Both would become very influential in changing the system of mental healthcare in Amsterdam and beyond, inspired by the Italian experience. Janssen—one of the founders of the first Runaway Shelter in Haarlem—visited an international conference on democratic psychiatry in Trieste in the early 1980s, in the hospital San Giovanni, which by then was 'almost empty' according to Janssen. He was very impressed with the whole experience of 'discussing psychiatric repression in those empty pavilions, those obsolete dormitories ... with "Freedom is therapeutic" written in big bold letters on the wall of the main building' (Blok, 1997).

Egbert Van der Poel worked at Stichting Interuniversitair Instituut voor Sociaal-Wetenschappelijk Onderzoek (SISWO), a social-scientific research institute that was partly financed by the Dutch government. In 1979, on behalf of SISWO, he embarked on a study trip to Italy to examine the ideas and practice of democratic psychiatry. In his report, he clearly showed his personal sympathies for the Basaglia project. 'Getting rid of so called mad persons by placing them in institutions that are isolated from society, is a common practice', he wrote (Van der Poel, 1980). Therefore, he thought, it was extremely interesting to see what would happen when those institutions were shut down.

First of all, Van der Poel visited a conference on the results of democratic psychiatry in Arezzo. He narrated how, in this city, Basaglia's friend and colleague, Pirella, had turned the local asylum into one of the centres of the movement against psychiatric hospitals, reducing the number of patients by more than 50% between 1971 and 1978 (Foot, 2015). In 1972, patients, nurses, and doctors had together demolished the walls of the Arezzo asylum, celebrating this as a liberating event. At the conference, Van der Poel met with and interviewed Basaglia as well. Also, he observed democratic psychiatry at work in Arezzo, as well as in Perugia, and interviewed health workers to learn about their experiences. On his return, he wrote several extensive articles educating the Dutch audience on the history and practice of democratic psychiatry in Gorizia, Trieste, and Arezzo. He was especially elaborate on the situation in Perugia, where he went on a field trip with his colleague, psychologist Joke Haafkens. Finally, he made a plea for using the Italian examples as an inspiration for the reform of mental healthcare in the Netherlands (Van der Poel, 1980; Van der Poel and Haafkens, 1980).

Van der Poel and Haafken's focus on Perugia is remarkable. Perugia never became as well known as Gorizia, Trieste, Arezzo, or Parma. According to John Foot: 'The Perugian movement was far less savvy about the use of the media than the Basaglians, and was less well connected intellectually and internationally' (Foot, 2015). Still, the movement was very successful in Perugia. ' n alliance of politicians, nurses, patients and psychiatrists managed not only to transform Perugia's huge asylum system, but also to set up alternatives to that system across the Umbrian region' (Foot, 2015). A network was created of decentralized mental health centres, or the CIM. Van der Poel and Haafkens were very interested in this kind of practical, concrete alternative to the psychiatric hospital, and interviewed the psychiatrist who was of crucial importance to the setting up of the CIM, Carlo Manuali. He told them at length about his philosophies and working method.

In 1981, Van der Poel was given the opportunity to bring the concept of the CIM to Amsterdam, when he was approached by an Amsterdam organization that was dead set against existing plans to build two new psychiatric hospitals in the Dutch capital. The Dutch government at the time was convinced that the large, 'old style' psychiatric hospitals that had been built in the nineteenth and early twentieth century, mostly in rural areas outside of town, were to be considered a thing of the past. They should be replaced by smaller-scale psychiatric hospitals in urban areas, each accommodating about 350 to 500 beds. These plans show that a reform-minded mentality was present at a national level as well.

In fact, in the Netherlands after the Second World War, a system of psychiatric care outside of the psychiatric hospitals had already grown into existence. It comprised child guidance clinics, clinics for adults with marital problems or 'questions concerning life and family', and social psychiatric services offering aftercare to patients who had been released from the psychiatric hospital. Some psychiatric hospitals set up halfway houses as well, where patients could slowly readjust to life outside of the asylum. All this was promoted, for a large part, by the efforts and ideals of the Dutch Mental Hygiene Movement (De Goei, 2001) and further stimulated by the psychopharmaceutical 'revolution' of the 1950s and 1960s, when new antipsychotic and antidepressive medications were introduced (Oosterhuis and Gijswijt, 2008).

Still, the progressive plans of the Dutch government were a thorn in the side for many members of the critical psychiatry movement. The governmental plans were nowhere near as radical as they felt necessary. 'When we heard about those building plans', Marc Janssen remembered, who played a leading role in the Amsterdam movement, 'we became furious. We wanted to demolish the asylums, and they were planning on building new ones!' (Blok, 1997). An Amsterdam-based neighbourhood organization asked Van der Poel to investigate how an alternative, community-oriented mental healthcare system could be set up. Van der Poel and his colleague Harrie Haaster wrote a glowing report based on the notion that persons with psychiatric problems should not be removed from their living situations. The starting point would be to ensure, as far as possible, that hospitalization was avoided. Mental healthcare should be community care as much as possible, in cooperation with families, friends, neighbours, general practitioners, and others.

Then, in 1982, a new council was installed in Amsterdam. The alderman for healthcare was Tineke van den Klinkenberg, a member of the Dutch Communist Party (CPN). According to Janssen, 'our heart rates accelerated when we heard this'. This is not surprising: in Italy, after all, communist politicians in some cities (for instance, Perugia) had been of great importance in supporting democratic psychiatry. In general, one of the big lessons of Basaglia and his colleagues was that in order to achieve anything political, support was crucial. So, it was very clear to the Amsterdam activists what needed to be done: Van den Klinkenberg should be convinced that building new hospitals was a bad idea and that Amsterdam should take control over its own mental healthcare policy, instead of having it dictated by provincial and national governments. Using the SISWO report written by Haaster and Van der Poel as a blueprint for the future, the Amsterdam anti-asylum movement started up a strong lobby for a radically new mental health policy in the Dutch capital.

The lobby was successful. In 1983, Van der Klinkenberg issued a report outlining the future of the local mental healthcare system. The report went a long way towards meeting the wishes of the reform-minded psychiatric activists. Van den Klinkenberg stressed that, in shaping her new policy, she had taken the recent criticism of psychiatry very seriously. In her report, she was not shy about showing her disgust with hospital care. The psychiatric hospital, she wrote, was the product of a society that excluded people instead of helping them. Hospital psychiatry did little to alleviate the suffering of psychiatric patients: on the contrary, it seemed to perpetuate it (Blok, 1997). She proposed to split up the city into five regions. In each region, a social psychiatric team would be primarily responsible for offering ambulatory psychiatric care. Next to this, a small-scale clinic of 20 to 40 beds, called the 'Social Psychiatric Service Centre' (SPDC), would be available to take care of the necessary short-term admissions in the region. The maximum duration of forced admission would be three months. Residential care facilities would be extended, and close cooperation between mental healthcare and general practitioners would be stimulated. Soon, this plan would become known as the 'Amsterdam model'.

Clearly, the Italian CIM that had been set up in Perugia and elsewhere were an inspiration for the concept of the SPDC in Amsterdam. However, the Netherlands, and Amsterdam itself, had a standing tradition of providing social psychiatric ambulatory care in the city, dating back to the 1920s. Working for the Amsterdam Municipal Health Services, psychiatrist Arie Querido (1901–1983) had established an elaborate system for emergency psychiatry and aftercare in the Dutch capital (Blok, 2014), with both psychiatrists and 'social psychiatric nurses' visiting patients at home. Still, the Amsterdam model promised to take this social psychiatric tradition an important step further. In 1984, the Amsterdam council unanimously accepted the report by Van der Klinkenberg.

Obviously, the Amsterdam anti-asylum activists were thrilled. They organized a conference on the upcoming changes in psychiatry in Amsterdam. As a grande finale to the conference, they staged a triumphant candle-lit walk to the location in town where Amsterdam was planning to build the first SPDC (Veldhoen, 1983). Another conference in the Netherlands, on democratic psychiatry, was organized for 1983. Clearly, many felt the moment was right to bring Italian ideas to Dutch mental healthcare.

The 'Amsterdam muddle'

However, turning the Amsterdam plans into practice was not as easy as the activists had imagined. In the years following the report by Van den Klinkenberg, there was a lot of squabbling about power and responsibility. Was Amsterdam, on its own, even able to determine where new psychiatric facilities would be built? According to Dutch law, the provincial and national governments should be involved in any plans for building new hospitals. Moreover, it was unclear at first who would run the SPDCs and be responsible for setting up and coordinating the new social psychiatric teams. At the time, the structure of Amsterdam mental healthcare was quite complex, with a number of different parties (e.g. policlinic centres for psychotherapy, the Municipal Health Service) involved.

The largest player in the field, Santpoort Psychiatric Hospital (Figure 16.1), protested in strong terms against the Amsterdam plans. In a formal reaction, directors of the hospital stated that, for many patients, the psychiatric hospital was a necessary and beneficial setting: their problems were severe to the extent that they needed long-term care in an institutional environment. For this group of people, the hospital was a safe haven. These people were better off in a quiet, rural, and green environment than in some urban apartment building. In fact, this was the ideal behind the psychiatric hospitals that had been set up in the nineteenth century: to remove psychiatric patients from the stressful hustle and bustle of the towns.

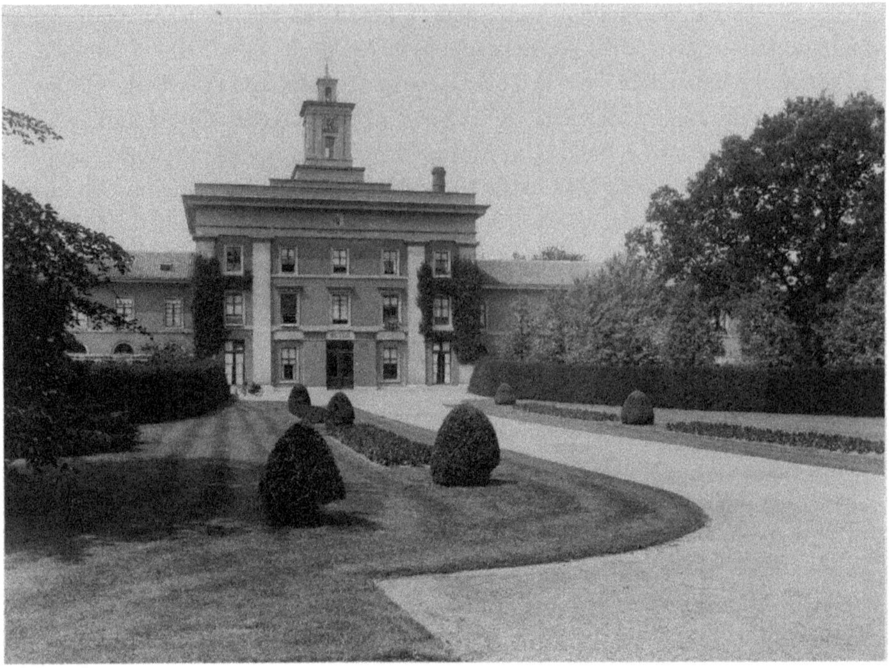

Figure 16.1 Santpoort Psychiatric Hospital.

However, at provincial level, there was strong support for the Amsterdam plans. In 1984, a Cooperation Agreement was signed between Amsterdam and the province of North Holland that they would cooperate in the years to come to bring about the changes outlined in the Van der Klinkenberg report. In the meantime, at national level, things were brewing as well. In 1982, two professors in Social Psychiatry (Kees Trimbos and his colleague Marius Romme), along with activists Hans van der Wilk (director of the Dutch Clients' Union) and Egbert van der Poel (SISWO) wrote a petition addressed to the Dutch Minister of State for Public Health and the Dutch parliament calling for a moratorium on the building of new psychiatric hospitals in the Netherlands. Psychiatric hospitals, in their view, were institutes from the past, based on old-fashioned ideas about how to deal with psychologically disturbed people; these hospitals were 'superfluous, useless, even harmful to the residents' (Romme et al., 1982). Many (former) clients of psychiatry had been protesting against 'hospitalization' for years; they should be listened to. Before building any more hospitals, a broad and fundamental discussion needed to be held on the future of mental healthcare (Romme et. al., 1982).

The petition was successful. In 1983, a majority in the Dutch Lower House voted in favour of a motion to freeze the plans for the building of new psychiatric hospitals, while a new report on the future of mental healthcare would be developed by the Secretary of State for Public Health. Furthermore, a public discussion did indeed follow the petition, as many articles were published in Dutch newspapers on the future of the psychiatric hospital. This created a favourable environment for the Amsterdam reforms.

In 1984, Secretary of State Van der Reijden presented his report outlining the future of mental healthcare. As he stated in the introduction, the report was written partly in reaction to the critical psychiatry movement. The Dutch mental health policy from now on would take into account the client's negative experiences with the 'closed nature' of psychiatric hospitals and their feelings of being 'excluded' from society (Van der Reijden, 1984). Deinstitutionalization was the guiding principle for the future. Psychiatric care should be provided in 'Multifunctional Units'—small-scale institutions in city areas, like the SPDCs in Amsterdam. Clients should no longer be removed from society and transported to hospitals situated 'in the woods or dunes', but stay within their own families as far as possible, with support from social psychiatric teams, or live in residential care facilities in urban areas. This trend of deinstitutionalization was confirmed in the next major government report on mental healthcare, *Onder Anderen* (1993).

Thus, the city of Amsterdam, the province of North Holland, and the Dutch government were thinking much along the same lines. The dismantling of Santpoort began in 1984, initially with the intention to keep facilities for about 500 chronic patients in operation at the Santpoort site, and thus effectively splitting the hospital into two parts. In 1986, however, a new member of the executive council of the province of North Holland stipulated that Santpoort would be dismantled completely. The main reason behind this move was that the province wanted to get rid of its administrative responsibility for Santpoort. Gradually, during the 1980s and 1990s, the hospital was closed. In 1991, the hospital board formally delegated their responsibilities for psychiatric treatment and care to two new SPDCs in Amsterdam (Schrameijer, 1991).

In Amsterdam, by 1993, about 750 places in residential care facilities had been created, and nine activity centres had been set up where clients could spend their days. By 1995, four new SPDCs were in operation (Blok, 1997).

Outside of Amsterdam, psychiatrists and other workers in the field of mental healthcare were interested in Italian democratic psychiatry as well. In the southern province of Limburg, Basaglia and Trieste inspired psychiatrist Detlev Petry to innovate the working method of the psychiatric hospital where he was employed, Vijverdal in the city of Maastricht. Petry had met Basaglia at the Ghent conference in 1979 and was very impressed; in his opinion, the English social psychiatrist Douglas Bennett and Basaglia were two psychiatrists who had done the most for improving the situation of chronic psychiatric patients (Petry, 1989). In 1987, he travelled to Trieste to see for himself how the new mental healthcare system was functioning. The most important difference with the Dutch working method, in his opinion, was that in Trieste, the emphasis was on 'the human being as a whole'. Clients were treated as individuals with a life story in a social context; in the Netherlands, the emphasis was on the history of their illness.

This different attitude inspired Petry to start working from a systems approach, involving family members in the treatment of clients and focusing on rehabilitation, later on adopting American concepts as well, such as case management and assertive community treatment. He stressed that psychiatrists and other professionals should behave as 'normal' as possible in their contacts with clients, and approach them not as objects of care but as equal partners in the 'triad' of care workers, clients, and family. From the late 1980s onwards, Petry organized conferences to put rehabilitation on the map in the Netherlands, inviting Douglas Bennett, Klaus Dörner, and others (Petry, 2011). In his own words, he wanted to see what 'Vijverdal Italian style' would look like, and started working towards creating a local Centro Mentale. In 1990, a Social Psychiatric Centre opened its doors in Maastricht; community care—or as the staff labelled it, 'customized transmural care'—was the guiding principle in the Centre. However, 30 beds were available for short-term clinical admissions. In the following years, many patients from Vijverdal were transferred to residential centres in the city of Maastricht (Klijn, 2007).

At national level, however, in the 1990s and early twenty-first century, the Dutch government pursued a cautious strategy of deinstitutionalization ('*vermaatschappelijking*') and residential care facilities were developed alongside mental hospitals (De Heer-Wunderink et al., 2008). In comparison to many other European countries, deinstitutionalization was a slow and gradual process in the Netherlands. The number of 'beds' in psychiatric clinics was about 21,000 in 1996 and 18,595 in 2008. When set against the rise in the Dutch general population, this is a substantial decline; but, in international comparison, a modest one. The reasons for this gradual deinstitutionalization are manifold. One was the fact that the emphasis on deinstitutionalization at national level faded into the background around 2000, when other developments demanded the attention of policy makers and workers in mental healthcare: the changing financial system for mental healthcare, with a growing neoliberal emphasis on privatization and more influence for healthcare insurance companies (Ministerie van Volksgezondheid, Welzijn en Sport, 2012). Secondly, in many towns, the old and new institutions for mental healthcare worked together abominably (Oosterhuis and Gijswijt-Hofstra, 2008).

Negative representations of mental illness and of deinstitutionalization did not help either. In Amsterdam in the 1990s, the number of homeless, psychologically troubled, and addicted persons on the streets was increasing. This was seen as the result of the 'failing' Amsterdam model, now mockingly referred to by critics as the 'Amsterdam muddle'. In 1993, when a psychotic neighbour killed a young girl in Amsterdam, worries about deinstitutionalization intensified. Amsterdam responded to these worries by setting up a system of hotlines. Worried citizens or housing associations could call these hotlines when mentally disturbed citizens caused nuisance or worry. In the meantime, for some policy makers, Italian developments served both as an inspiration *and* as a warning against too drastic deinstitutionalization. A big problem in Trieste, argued Jaap van Weeghel, after visiting this town in 1987, was the lack of suitable jobs for former hospital residents (van Weeghel, 1989). Creating ways of providing clients with a useful way of spending their days should be a focal point in deinstitutionalization, he argued. Others pointed out that in many Italian cities, homeless psychiatric patients were roaming the streets, left to their own devices. The Dutch Inspector for Mental Healthcare mentioned that in the Netherlands, 'Italian and American conditions' were increasing, referring to the growing number of homeless persons with psychiatric and addiction problems (Oosterhuis and Gijswijt-Hofstra, 2008).

Only quite recently did the Dutch government revive its earlier focus on deinstitutionalization. More drastic goals were formulated: in 2013, it was decided that the capacity of Dutch psychiatric hospitals should be reduced by a third by 2020, compared to 2008 (GGZ Nederland, 2014). Today, the number of teams for assertive community treatment is on the rise and the majority of patients are receiving ambulatory treatment.

Conclusion

All in all, the Italian experiments by Basaglia and his colleagues had a big impact in the Netherlands in the 1980s and 1990s, both in being an inspiration and a catalyst for reform. First of all, the fascinating events in Italy caused a revival of the critical psychiatry movement in the Netherlands. Visits to Trieste and other places stimulated renewed enthusiasm within this movement and resulted in new initiatives as well, such as the creation of Runaway Shelters. The experience of going to Italy was something new for activists: actually visiting the sites of 'anti-psychiatric' experiments and seeing what happened there with their own eyes, meeting like-minded people from other countries, strengthened the movement for reform immensely. Not only did democratic psychiatry provide activists with new ideals and practices, it also provided the critical psychiatry movement with a renewed vigour that may have been even stronger than during its first phase, when books and films had been the main instrument of transnational communication and inspiration. One Dutch activist wrote, after a visit to Trieste, about the enormous impact of actually being there: after having read Basaglia's 'muddle-headed and complicated books about the mad and capitalist society', his visit to Italy really turned him into a fan of Basaglia, stating that 'what this guy pulls off here in Trieste is formidable … Most of the madmen actually got out of the institution!' (Gekkenkrant, 1977).

In Amsterdam and Maastricht, the example of the CIM was an inspiration for the creation of a new system of mental healthcare and the setting up of social psychiatric centres. At national level, in governmental policy reports, small-scale 'Multifunctional Units' (much resembling the CIM) were presented as the future of psychiatry, although deinstitutionalization in practice was slow to happen.

The wave of enthusiasm for Italian democratic psychiatry had its indirect results as well. Several of those who visited Italy in the 1970s and 1980, and who sympathized with the ideas of Basaglia and his colleagues, went on to occupy posts where they were able to keep the ideals of Italian democratic psychiatry alive and on the Dutch agenda.

Rally Rijkschroeff, for instance, one of the students who travelled to Italy in 1976 after watching *Metta di Slegare*, went on to become a leading social scientist in the Netherlands and the director of the prestigious independent Verwey Jonker Institute, which advises the Dutch local and national government on social issues. He has published widely on rehabilitation and client participation in mental healthcare. Jaap van Weeghel, who visited Trieste in the late 1980s, is now professor in Rehabilitation and Social Participation of persons with severe mental problems. In the 1980s and 1990s, Mark Janssen, and various other members of the Amsterdam critical psychiatry movement, worked for the Trimbos Institute in Utrecht, a leading research organization focusing on mental healthcare and advising the Dutch government.

Still, it is important to realize that 'Italy' was not the only inspiration for reform: American, English, and German examples of deinstitutionalization and community care were also taken on board in the Netherlands. Moreover, the Dutch had been quite active in creating ambulatory mental healthcare since the interwar period, influenced by the ideals of the Mental Hygiene Movement. Psychiatrists, social workers, and nurses visited patients at home, and policlinic help was available in most cities as well. Furthermore, the circumstances in Dutch mental hospitals appear to have been far less dire than in Gorizia and elsewhere in Italy in the 1960s (Oosterhuis and Gijswijt, 2008). However, democratic psychiatry gave a more radical twist to this emerging trend towards creating community care in the Netherlands. Italy showed how community care should no longer be an 'extra' service, in addition to psychiatric hospital care; but conversely, psychiatric admissions into 24-hour care should be the 'extra' service, in addition to community care. Thus, for Dutch activists and policy makers, Italy in the early 1980s was instrumental in putting deinstitutionalization firmly on the map as the main goal of mental health policy in the Netherlands.

References

Abma, R. (2001). Afscheid van Psychologie en Maatschappij. *Academische Boekengids* 29 October:9–10.

Blok, G. (1997). Enkele reis op z'n retour. In: J. Vijselaar (ed.), *Gesticht in de duinen. De geschiedenis van de provinciale psychiatrische ziekenhuizen van Noord-Holland*. Hilversum: Verloren, pp. 238–68.

Blok, G. (1998). 'Messiah of the schizophrenics': Jan Foudraine and antipsychiatry in the Netherlands. In: M. Gijswijt-Hofstra and Roy Porter (eds), *Cultures of Psychiatry and Mental Health Care in Postwar Britain and the Netherlands*. Atlanta/Amsterdam: Rodopi, pp. 151–69.

Blok, G. (2004). *Baas in eigen brein. 'Antipsychiatrie' in Nederland, 1965–1985*. Amsterdam: Nieuwezijds.

Blok, G. (2014). *Achter de voordeur. Sociale psychiatrie vanuit de Amsterdamse GGD in de twintigste eeuw*. Amsterdam: Amsterdam University Press.

Crossley, N. (1998). R.D. Laing and the British antipsychiatry movement: a socio-historical analysis. *Social Science and Medicine* 47:877–89.

Crossley, N. (1999). Working utopias and social movements: an investigation using case-study materials from radical mental health movements in Britain. *Sociology* 33:809–30.

Crossley, N. (2006). *Contesting Psychiatry. Social Movements in Mental Health.* London: Routledge.

de Goei, L. (2001). *De psychohygiënisten. Psychiatrie, cultuurkritiek en de beweging voor geestelijke volksgezondheid in Nederland, 1924–1970.* Nijmegen: SUN.

De Heer-Wunderink, C., Caro-Nienhuis, A.D., Sytema, S., and Wiersma, D. (2008) Residential care: Dutch and Italian residents of residential care facilities compared. *Epidemiologia E Psichiatria Sociale* 17(2):162–5.

de Volkskrant (1980). Wegloophuis helpt patiënten. 29 April 1980.

Foot, J. (2015). *The Man Who Closed The Asylums. Franco Basaglia and The Revolution in Mental Health Care*. London/New York: Verso.

Gekkenkrant (1977). Vrouwen en vuistregels. November 1977:19.

Gekkenkrant (1979). Demokratische psychiatrie. August 1979:4–10.

GGZ Nederland (2014). *Sectorrapport ggz 2012. Feiten en cijfers over een sector in beweging.* Amersfoort.

Hunsche, P. (2008). *De strijdbare patiënt. Van Gekkenbeweging tot Cliëntenbewustzijn, portretten 1970–2000.* Amsterdam: Candide.

Klijn, A. (2007). *Vijverdal Maastricht. Biografie van een gebouw 1969–2007.* Hilversum: Verloren.

Lewis, A.J. (2016). 'We are certain of our own insanity': antipsychiatry and the gay liberation movement, 1968–1980. *Journal of the History of Sexuality* 25(1):83.

Ministerie van Volksgezondheid, Welzijn en Sport (2012). *Trendrapportage ambulantisering 2012.* Utrecht: Trimbos Institute.

't Narreschip (1979). April doet wat ie wil. April 1979.

't Narreschip (1980). Waarheen gaat de psychiatrie? November 1980.

't Narreschip (1981). Psychiatrie in onderontwikkeling. June 1981.

't Narreschip (1982). Wegloophuis-nummer 11. March 1982.

Oosterhuis, H. and Gijswijt-Hofstra, M. (2008). *Verward van geest en ander ongerief. Psychiatrie en geestelijke gezondheidszorg in Nederland (1870–2005).* Houten: Bohn Stafleu van Loghum.

Petry, D. (1989). Chroniciteit in Maastricht en Triëst. In: M. Van der Kamp, G. van der Laan, J. Wolf, and J. Zeelen (eds), *De patiënt als burger. Een bezoek aan de democratische psychiatrie in Triëst.* Utrecht: Stichting Welzijns Publikaties, pp. 81–91.

Petry, D. (2011). *Uitbehandeld, maar niet opgegeven.* Amsterdam: Sebes & van Gelderen.

Portacolone, E., Segal, S.P., Mezzina, R., Scheper-Hughes, N., and Okin, R.L. (2015). A tale of two cities. ehe Exploration of the Trieste public psychiatry model in San Fransisco. *Culture, Medicine and Psychiatry* 39:680–97.

Romme, M., Trimbos, K., van der Wilk, H., and van der Poel, E. (1982). *Adres van de initiatiefgroep 'Moratorium bouw psychiatrische ziekenhuizen'.* Available at: https://www.canonsociaalwerk.eu/nl/details_verwant.php?cps=3&canon_id=43&verwant=43

Schrameijer, F., ,Het Amsterdamse model; van droom naar daad en terug', *Maandblad Geestelijke volksgezondheid*, 46 (1991), 603–22.

Trimbos, K. (1975). *Antipsychiatrie. Een overzicht.* Deventer: Van Loghhum Slaterus.

Van der Beek, A., ter Laak, A., and Rijkschroeff, R. (1980). *Democratische psychiatrie. Niet de ziekte bestaat, wel het lijden*. Baarn: Ambo.

Van der Reijden, J. (1983–1984). *Nota Geestelijke Gezondheidszorg*. Tweede Kamer, vergaderjaar 1983–1984. 18463(1–2):4–5. Available at: www.statengeneraaldigitaal.nl

Van de Wetering, K.-M. (2007). *Te gek om vast te zitten. 25 jaar Wegloophuis Utrecht.* Utrecht: Hollandia Printing.

Van der Kamp, M., van der Laan, G., Wolf, J., and Zeelen, J. (1989). *De patiënt als burger. Een bezoek aan de democratische psychiatrie in Triëst*. Utrecht: Stichting Welzijns Publikaties.

Van der Meulen, M. (1979). Er bestaat geen psychische toestand die rechtvaardigt mensen op te sluiten. *Het Parool* 17 October 1979.
Van der Poel, E. (1980). Democratische psychiatrie in Italië. *Marge* 3:355–60.
Van der Poel, E. and Haafkens, J. (1980). Antwoord op de inrichtingspsychiatrie. *Psychologie en Maatschappij* 12:301–30.
Van Weeghel, J. (1989). San Giovanni en Sint Bavo. In: M. Van der Kamp, G. van der Laan, J. Wolf, and J. Zeelen (eds), *De patiënt als burger. Een bezoek aan de democratische psychiatrie in Triëst*. Utrecht: Stichting Welzijns Publikaties, pp. 47–62.
Veldhoen, L. (1983). Oproep tot wijzigingen in de psychiatrie. *NRC Handelsblad* 22 December 1983.
Wolfson, A. (1986). Wegloophuis biedt kans op zelfstandig leven. *de Volkskrant* 23 July 1986.

17
Basaglia in France

The marginality of exemplarity

Nicolas Henckes and Anne M. Lovell

Introduction

Many French mental health professionals and intellectuals have recognized Franco Basaglia, and the anti-asylum movement he developed, as a transformative cultural and social moment in Italian history and in the history of late twentieth-century psychiatry. Over 40 years' worth of articles in *Le Monde*, the most influential French daily, and other press, reveals a consistent presence. Sometimes articles concerned specific issues, such as Law 180 and its uneven consequences (Jaccard, 1984), and legal actions against Basaglia after a patient on leave committed a murder, known as 'the incident' (Basaglia and Basaglia Ongaro, 1987; Foot, 2015), and Basaglia's response (*Le Monde*, 1971). Other articles erroneously subsume Basaglia into anti-psychiatry, mentioning him indiscriminately alongside Laing, Cooper, Bonnafé, Guattari, Deligny, and others, as if they constituted a homogeneous social phenomenon (Escoffier-Lambiotte, 1971). Basaglia also appears in cultural reporting: he is present in Raymond Depardon's San Clemente celebrated asylum photographic series (Blanchard, 2017; Humblot, 1997), in film reviews (Guattari, 1976, Humblot and Devarrieux, 1976), and in theatre by people with disabilities (Marmande, 2005). Compared to Henri Ey, the most important figure of twentieth-century French psychiatry, Basaglia is ten times more present in the pages of *Le Monde* alone. Nevertheless, that daily newspaper, and others, paid little attention to Basaglia's direct influence on French psychiatric practices and debates.

In this chapter, we take up that challenge by focusing on the circulation of concepts and practices between France and Basaglia's anti-institutional work in Italy, their effects on French mental health policies and on scattered experimentation. We examine the extent to which Basaglia's ideas took ground in France through the efforts of a small network of psychiatric practitioners and intellectuals, within roughly three periods: 1960–1980, 1980–2000, and 2000 to the present. In conclusion, we ask what might explain the French paradox: the early receptivity to Basaglia's politically-oriented, community-based alternative to institutions, on the one hand; and a tenacious hospital-centric psychiatric system and increased use of constraints and high-security confinement, on the other hand.

The conditions of reception

The difficult dialogue between Basaglia and French psychiatry from 1970s on may be partly explained by the specific paths taken by psychiatric reform in both countries. In Italy, Basaglia, a political leftist and for years a phenomenological psychiatrist, emerged as a lone pioneer in the early 1960s. In a nation then far less economically and socially 'developed' than France, Basaglia spurned academia, gathered a core group of psychiatric reformers in Gorizia, created early political alliances with the Italian Communist Party, elected officials favourable to health reform, and finally built a broad following beyond psychiatry, in a society undergoing profound changes. By contrast, the French reform movement began much earlier, in the 1940s, and evolved over the next two decades.

France's first psychiatric reform experiments happened, famously, during the Second World War, in the asylums of Saint Alban in south-western France, and Charité-sur-Loire in France's centre, in response to war conditions (Fourquet & Murard, 1980; von Bueltzingsloewen, 2007). In particular, the psychiatrists Paul Balvet and François Tosquelles transformed the hospital environment at Saint Alban by introducing work and leisure activities for patients, while the hospital became a base for the Resistance (Ey et al., 1952). Young psychiatrists behind similar experiments included Georges Daumézon, Paul Sivadon, and Lucien Bonnafé; all moved into leadership roles in their profession after the War. Some belonged to the French Communist Party; others were closer to the Catholic or Protestant left. All shared an interest in new psychodynamic perspectives that since the interwar period had been transforming knowledge and treatment of psychopathology, influenced by psychoanalysis, phenomenology, and Marxism. In addition, all worked in public psychiatric hospitals.

By the late 1940s and early 1950s, these psychiatrists had articulated a doctrine and practice, *psychothérapie institutionnelle*, derived from their war experiences, as the basis of reform proposals they submitted to France's health authorities (Daumézon and Koechlin, 1952). These proposals included a new concept of the psychiatric hospital, translated into a reorganization of psychiatric work, nurses' training, and the architecture of the establishments. By the late 1950s, these reforms expanded to include experiments with prevention, post cure, and mental hygiene dispensaries (Henckes, 2007). The latter, soon redefined as mental health centres, became the first building blocks of community psychiatry, notably one practiced in a unique service and research model in Paris's Thirteenth Arrondissement, and later in Villeurbanne, near Lyon (Henckes, 2005).

During this post-war period, the Ministry of Health defined psychiatry as a priority, in reaction to decades of perceived neglect and underinvestment. In 1947, a permanent commission was created to advise the Minister of Health on psychiatric issues; by the end of the 1950s, this commission was working on a new scheme for mental health policy. The result was the '*secteur*' policy, launched in 1960 (Fourquet and Murard, 1980, Henckes, 2007)—an innovative reform aimed at transforming the psychiatric system by adding new institutions, including mental health centres and nursing homes, to the mental hospitals. The *secteurs* operated as both catchment areas and planning units, with about 70,000 inhabitants in each. Contrary to the Basaglian approach, *secteur* policy maintained psychiatric hospitals as central to the system. Hospital psychiatrists were to head up the psychiatric system and work in *secteur* facilities, with the help of a mental health team. In fact, from 1950 to 1970, the French state made its greatest impact ever in the renovation and construction of psychiatric hospitals: 30 new psychiatric facilities were constructed during this period, totalling 13,400 beds in 19 specialized and 11 general hospitals, with 7,290 new beds still under construction in 1972 (Laurenceau, 1972; Henckes, 2016). At its peak in 1967, the total number of psychiatric beds in the country reached 116,000.

The 1960 ministerial guidelines on mental health policy nevertheless left much room for interpretation, while providing few incentives to local authorities and professionals to really apply the reform. *Secteur* promoters within the psychiatric profession toiled to define 'good practices'. Ultimately, *secteur* psychiatry was a pragmatic movement using every available means to treat patients. While its promoters shared a humanistic vision of their mission, most adhered to a relatively traditional vision of psychiatry as a clinical medical discipline. In particular, following Henri Ey, they defended psychiatry as a specific way of creating knowledge about mental diseases. This explained their defensiveness, after 1968, towards what they saw as 'anti-psychiatry' (Ey, 1972). Thus, while the *secteur* provided a means for transforming the infrastructures of psychiatry, it was never meant to revolutionize its foundations.

From contesting psychiatry to developing alternatives

In this context, it is not difficult to understand a divergence between Basaglian and French psychiatry. In his first anti-institutional effort, at the Gorizia asylum, Basaglia and his colleagues sought inspiration from Maxwell Jones' therapeutic community in the United Kingdom, as well as from the French *secteur* policy and *psychothérapie institutionnelle*. Basaglia shared, with some of the latter's originators, a Marxist orientation and an experience of psychiatric institutions shaped by the Second World War. While never a member of the Resistance, which many French psychiatric reformers had been, Basaglia's anti-fascist activities led to his imprisonment towards the end of the War. That experience (as much, if not more, than his discovery of Erving Goffman's concept of total institutions) led him to compare, post hoc, the structure and dehumanization of asylums to those of concentration camps, much like French analogies two decades earlier.

Another (less-noted) footnote to both Basaglia and French reformers' analyses of the psychiatric institution concerns their reaction to the fate of chronic psychiatric patients who fled the asylums during the War. This led to the realization among these psychiatrists that categorization of psychopathology and the confinement of patients 'misread' and even suppressed the capacity of patients to act. In later years, Basaglia once remarked that patients who had escaped the bombing of the Ancona asylum were found 'not far from the asylum, living like anyone else. This led certain psychiatrists to think that the treatment of these patients, these inmates, could be conceived of differently. But it did not go any further' (Basaglia, cited in Pivetta, 2018, p. 24). In France, a formal study by Louis le Guillant of patients who fled the war-time asylum of Charité-sur Loire came to similar conclusions, but also influenced him and others to humanize the asylum and, in particular, to provide work opportunities (Le Guillant, 1947).

Although the Basaglian anti-asylum project diverged from the French reforms, Basaglia remained friends with Lucien Bonnafé until the end of his life, even participating in his retirement ceremony in Corbeil in 1977 (Basaglia, 1978). Ultimately, however, Basaglia drew more from Maxwell Jones's therapeutic community than the *secteur*. He also critiqued models like the American community mental health centres, which left hospital-centric psychiatry intact (Basaglia, 1987). More broadly, by the 1970s, Basaglia's democratic psychiatry had become part of a broader post-1968 and post-'Hot Autumn' (1969–1970) revolutionary movement. This mobilized many sectors of Italian society, from workers to feminists to the unemployed, for the democratization of everyday life itself and expansion of rights. Despite some parallels with achievements by French social movements (e.g. the legalization of abortion), the Basaglian movement's embeddedness within mobilizations for broader societal transformation, and Basaglia's collaboration with socialist and communist ministers and regional and local health officials, had no equivalent in France.

Basaglia's first articles in French appeared in the mid 1960s, in special issues on contemporary Italian psychiatry of two major psychiatric journals, *L'Evolution Psychiatrique* and *L'Information Psychiatrique*. The publications testified to the strength of the post-war relationship between French and Italian psychiatry and its many dimensions. The special issue of *L'Evolution Psychiatrique*, published in 1965, was introduced by Henri Ey, the journal's editor, as a 'tribute to Italian psychiatry' (Ey, 1965). It included contributions by leading Italian psychiatrists on current psychopathological perspectives. Basaglia's was a phenomenological reflection on the means through which a psychiatrist can reach the patient's subjectivity (Basaglia, 1965). The following year, the special issue of *L'Information psychiatrique*, the official journal of the Union of Psychiatric Hospitals Physicians ('Syndicat des Médecins des Hôpitaux Psychiatriques', which became the 'Syndicat des Psychiatres des Hôpitaux' in the late 1970s), published proceedings of a meeting organized in Varese on psychiatric reform in Italy. This time, Basaglia presented his work relating to Gorizia (Basaglia, 1966).

In early 1968, Basaglia addressed psychiatrists at Henri Rousselle Hospital (Paris). They reacted negatively to his representation of 'scandalous' asylum conditions and their transformation, accusing him of doing politics instead of psychiatry

(Castel, 1980, p. 15). The successful incursion of Basaglia's ideas into French psychiatry happened later that year, with the publication of the Gorizia team's analyses of their work in *L'Istituzione negata* (*'The Negated Institution'*) (published in France in 1970). In May 1968, Henri Vermorel (a psychiatrist, psychoanalyst, and practitioner of *psychothérapie institutionnelle*) organized the second French–Quebecois–Italian psychiatric conference in Courchevel, for *L'Information psychiatrique*. It is here that several young psychiatrists first heard Basaglia's radical critique of the institution (Carrino, 2018a).

One group particularly riveted by Basaglia's charismatic presentation at the conference were psychiatric residents (*internes*) at Le Vinatier Psychiatric Hospital in Lyon (Parizot, 2013). Their own mentors had already experimented with elements of therapeutic communities and *secteur* practices, including home visits, after visits to the USA (Sassolas, 2010; Amieux-Orsini, 2018). During the May 1968 events[1], information about the Italian experience circulated within a leftist union, the Syndicat des Psychiatres en Formation, recently founded by young psychiatrists (Roelandt, 2018). As the May events spilled into the streets of Lyon, the Vinatier *internes*, too, were radicalizing. Some rejected psychoanalysis and opposed the more conservative chiefs of staff. They invited Basaglia and other Marxist scholar-activists, like Serge Mallet and Lucien Goldman, to participate in dialogues with them. Marie-Claude Amieux and Luciano Carrino (himself Italian) left Le Vinatier to join Basaglia in Colorno (Parma) and then Trieste. Other Vinatier residents, including Marcel Sassolas, Claude Falconnet, Albert Jakubowicz, and Michel Gillet, became closely involved with Basaglian practices (Parizot, 2013).

Among these, Albert Jakubowicz's trajectory illustrates how Basaglian practices could influence even isolated areas (Amieux-Orsini, 2018; Jakubowicz, 2006; Carrino, 2018b). After his residency at Le Vinatier, Jakubowicz joined the health insurance regime for coal miners in Montceau-les-Mines. In reaction to the local, asylum-like atmosphere, he developed community alternatives and attempted to 'de-psychiatrize' psychiatric services by transferring them to general medicine. Jakubowicz analysed and treated miners' mental health problems as an effect of both coal-mine labour and conditions in the workers' town, which was organized hierarchically to facilitate mutual surveillance. His understanding reflected the spread of the Foucault-inspired notion of 'capillary' power and surveillance, or the ways in which power circulates in contemporary society and reaches all aspects of life and bodies, no matter how small (Foucault, 1991, p. 198). It also echoed analyses developed by Trieste's researchers and practitioners (Mauri et al., 1983). Jakubowicz visited Trieste annually, and often brought Carrino, by then a conduit between Italian psychiatry and France, to the Burgundy mining town.

[1] Between May and June 1968, France was shaken by its largest social movement in the twentieth century, consisting of massive student demonstrations and widely followed strikes in industry, services and government administrations. The Events were an important element in bringing De Gaulle's presidency to an end. They opened the way for a series of progressive social reforms in the early 1970s.

The diffusion of Basaglia's influence in the second half of the 1970s

Interest in Basaglia's work spread among other young psychiatrists in the early 1970s. Among the outcomes of the 1968 events were the separation of psychiatry and neurology into distinct specialties and the reform of psychiatric training (Bec, 1977; Pinell, 2005). The new psychiatric curriculum was closer to the human sciences. Moreover, the reform abolished the *concours* (competitive exam) which had controlled access to training programmes. As a result, within a few years, France witnessed an unprecedented increase in the number of practicing psychiatrists, from only 1,000 in 1970 to 4,000 by the mid 1970s and to more than 10,000 by the late 1980s (Ministère de la Solidarité, de la Santé et de la Protection Sociale, 1990). Most of these young psychiatrists were following in the footsteps of the post-war reformers, engaging *secteur* psychiatry and social psychiatry practices, more generally, albeit with a stronger commitment to psychoanalysis than the post-war generation. Some, inspired by leftist movements, sought inspiration in more radical or simply different ways of transforming psychiatry, including Lacanian psychoanalysis, British anti-psychiatry, and Basaglian ideas (Turkle, 1978).

From the 1970s on, French psychiatrists, sociologists, nurses, and students embarked on 'pilgrimages'—to Colorno (Parma), then Trieste (once Basaglia moved there), and to other cities of the 'Basaglian diaspora'. In turn, Basaglia often came to France, invited by young French colleagues. Psychiatrist Jean-Luc Roelandt thus recalls how, in the late 1970s, Basaglia agreed to visit Armentières Psychiatric Hospital near Lille, although he knew no one, after a simple phone call from Roelandt, then a young assistant psychiatrist. Basaglia stayed a week, organizing meetings with patients, professionals, and the wider community. Basaglia also influenced other leftist psychiatrists of the same generation, who were trained by the post-war reformers and their programmes (Roelandt, 2018). Among those young psychiatrists were Lucien Bonnafé's mentorees, Paul Brétécher, Claude Louzoun, and Jean-Pierre Martin. Still others included Guy Baillon, Stanislas 'Tom' Tomkiewicz, Bernard Doray, Anik Kouba, and Jean-Luc Metge; and the psychiatrist and film-maker Tony Lainé, who developed day hospitals, apartments, and other community-based facilities for children.

In 1977, the two-year-old international network Alternatives à la Psychiatrie ('Alternatives to psychiatry')—whose members included Italians, Félix Guattari, the Belgian Mony Elkaïm, and Robert Castel—held its congress in Trieste. Over 4,000 practitioners, intellectuals, and service users/survivors from 15 European countries witnessed the now largely empty psychiatric hospital. Elements of what Basaglians termed 'democratic psychiatry' were developing throughout Europe, from Dutch runaway houses to feminist critiques of psychiatry. The congress spurred young French in attendance to found a cultural organization, Le Cheval Bleu, named after the blue papier maché sculpture, Marco Cavallo, built by Trieste patient cooperatives and carried into the city of Trieste to raise awareness of the hospital's closure and reintegration of its former inpatients into urban everyday life.

Also attending the Trieste congress were psychiatrists, social workers, and others who, the following year, founded or joined the Association pour l'Etude et la Promotion des Structures Intermédiaires (ASEPSI) (Antoine, 2010). Le Cheval Bleu and ASEPSI often disagreed. However, along with the Centre d'Entraînement aux Méthodes de Pédagogie Active (CEMEA)—a much older progressive training and education organization for psychiatric nurses among other—they developed social and health-related community facilities. Prominent amongst these were social and therapeutic apartments and *lieux de vie,* micro-structures outside institutions aimed at 'put[ting] de-institutionalization into practice' (Antoine, cited by Sassolas, 2010). Drawing on Psichiatria Democratica, CEMEA also organized training for nurses, aimed at transforming their hierarchical relations with psychiatrists (Metge, 1980, p. 222). Articles by Basaglia and his collaborators appeared in mental health and rehabilitation journals like *Vie Sociale et Traitements (VST)* and *Fracture*, alongside general media and political journals like *La Nouvelle Critique*. Finally, Le Cheval Bleu lives on through the theatre company of the same name, made up of users from the sheltered workshop system (Centres d'Aide par le Travail).

Several characteristics of these innovations are worth recalling. First, they were run by mental health and social work professionals, alongside psychiatrists; a rare configuration in the mental health field but a frequent one in the field of disabilities. Second, though influenced by Basaglia, most of these psychiatrists, social workers, and activists also referred to Lacanianism, British therapeutic communities, and, albeit 'with some reservations', American models (Antoine, 2010, p. 104). Third, structural and cultural characteristics challenged the survival of these innovations. In the United States, in the 1970s, free clinics, ex-patient groups, and radical alternatives proliferated outside hospitals (Castel et al., 1982). In France, private non-profitable organizations established therapeutic apartments and other *lieux de vie*. But whereas American structures and governance historically favour bottom–up empowerment of people, in France, innovations are often absorbed back into a centralized system based on the principle of equal access to territorially organized resources (Donzelot et al., 2003; Laval, 2019). Similar experiences to *lieux de vie* flourished in the decentralized territories of Italy; in France, they were criticized for, and even faltered from, the absence of clear regulatory frameworks.

By the end of the decade, Basaglia's influence was felt in other networks and organizations. These included the newly formed union, Syndicat des Psychiatres en Formation, mentioned previously, which became the Syndicat de la Psychiatrie in 1977 and took a position to the left of the more established Syndicat des Psychiatres des Hôpitaux. At another level, the intertwining of political and personal friendships between Basaglia and French intellectuals, particularly the sociologist Robert Castel, cannot be understated. Castel's social critique of psychoanalysis, *Le psychanalysme* (Castel, 1973), resonated with the distance Basaglia and many of his collaborators were taking from psychoanalysis, which they viewed at the time as a bourgeois science unable to affect the material reality and misery of patients' lives. Castel and his spouse Françoise Castel, a chief psychiatrist in Corbeil-Essonnes, nourished a network of psychiatrists, self-defined anti-psychiatrists, mental health workers, researchers, philosophers, journalists, and students. The network included David Cooper, Jacques Donzelot, and others who debated the transformation of Italian psychiatry and the larger political issues it touched in real time.

French psychiatrists borrowed few specific ideas or ways of practicing psychiatry from Basaglia, beyond simply critiquing psychiatric hospitals. However, they were particularly influenced by the political framework within which he analysed mental health. Similarly, some familiar with Basaglian mental health experiences in Trieste and elsewhere noted how Basaglians sought to 'hear' the person in the 'patient', inspiring a practice focused on more humanistic relations with patients and staff alike, even within the institution (Amieux-Orsini, 2018). Basaglia also visited La Borde, the clinic where Jean Oury was practicing a radical form of *psychothérapie institutionnelle* and Félix Guattari was developing ideas for his *Anti-Oedipus*. In personal conversations, Basaglia criticized La Borde for being a private clinic, and for not addressing the social reintegration of people with mental illness.

Not all French psychiatrists, however, expressed enthusiasm for Basaglia's work. Like Françoise Castel and others, the psychiatrist Jean-Charles Pascal sent staff to Trieste and invited Basaglia to his *secteur* in Suresnes, near Paris. In retrospect, Pascal viewed Basaglia's practice as adding little more than the absence of harm, justified on the grounds that the neurosciences had yet to find adequate treatment for mental illnesses (Hanon and Sicard, 2014). Other French practitioners were frustrated by what they saw as Basaglia's lack of a theoretical approach to psychopathology (Pascal, 2018) and 'naïveté' regarding the symbolic and the imaginary (Castel, 1980, p. 15). Many considered the French *secteur* far superior to Basaglia's radical anti-institutional critiques and community efforts. This is the flavour of a posthumous tribute in *Le Monde* to the psychiatrist Marie-Rose Mamelet, as an unsung founder of the *secteur*. Noting that in 1944, Le Guillant, Ey, and Bonnafé were already calling for 'the [asylum] walls to be torn down', the tribute concludes: 'It is well before Basaglia, and with far more caution [*prudence*], that, thanks to Marie-Rose Mamelet, those walls really fell. Alongside the introduction of psychotropics, that was a revolution, and a humane one' (Hommage, 1987). As Castel himself remarked, French psychiatrists had history on their side: Pinel, the Law of 1838, Lacan, the *secteur*. Hospital psychiatrists shunned ideas imported from abroad and maintained a 'hexagonal tropism'. Finally, their corporatist interest in preserving the hospital and their own roles, while developing community services, remained deeply anchored (Castel, 1980).

1980–2000: Law 180 and French debates over deinstitutionalization

After Basaglia's death in 1980, discussions in France over his legacy continued well into the 1980s. In particular, the Italian Law 180, passed in 1978, stimulated strong interest among mental health professionals and policy makers, although after it was passed, it had curried only one brief piece in French psychiatric journals, by an

Italian psychiatrist working in France (Del Pistoia, 1979). In 1981, however, Edoardo Balduzzi, a regular Italian correspondent for *L'Information psychiatrique*, edited a special issue on the Law, with articles by several Italian psychiatrists (1981).

In 1982, professionals from various components of the French reform movement, including Lucien Bonnafé, members of ASEPSI, and the Syndicat de la Psychiatrie, met representatives of Psichiatria Democratica in Nice, to discuss connections between the respective statuses of psychiatric reform in France and in Italy. The Italians included Franco Rotelli, who had succeeded Basaglia as director at Trieste; Paolo Tranchina, a Basaglian psychologist based in Florence and editor of the pro-Basaglian bulletin, *Fogli d'Informazione*; and Agostino Pirella, one of the original Gorizia psychiatrists (*Transitions*, 1982).

In 1982 and 1983, *L'Information psychiatrique* followed with a debate between Balduzzi and Max Bellufi, an Italian opponent to the Law (Beluffi, 1982; Balduzzi, 1982). Several French psychiatrists returning from trips to Italy contributed their evaluations of the reform to the journal. Journals such as the ASEPSI's *Transition,* and *Synapse,* also devoted special issues to the Italian reform. Moreover, at least three French research and policy monographs were published on Italian psychiatry (Metge, 1980; Legrand, 1988; Louzoun and Stylianidis, 1987), one of which was commissioned by the French Ministry of Health. The Italian reform movement also entered cultural domains, from events organized by the Italian Institute of Culture in Paris to cultural events organized throughout France by Le Cheval Bleu association, with funds from the socialist Ministry of Culture.

While most of these publications and actions were sympathetic to the reform, the reactions of the French psychiatric establishment, represented by the leader of the Syndicat des Psychiatres des Hôpitaux and university professors, were far more cautious. This is illustrated by the position taken by the editors of *L'Information psychiatrique* who, in several editorials, admitted agnosticism regarding the merits of the Italian reform (e.g. Noël, 1984). The journal's official line was the *secteur* policy, which for the Board included the need for strong institutions, in contrast with the Basaglians' anti-institutional stance. Psychiatric debates over these issues also took place in other forums, including the more interdisciplinary ones of the ASEPSI.

In fact, the context of reform in France exacerbated French debate about the Italian reform. In the early 1970s, a chain of ministerial decrees had provided new impetus to the *secteur* policy by promulgating a series of new norms, along with financial rewards to psychiatrists who would apply the reform. In the next few years, however, French psychiatrists increasingly denounced the lack of support from the conservative governments of Presidents Pompidou and Giscard d'Estaing (Ayme, 1995). In particular, they strongly criticized the 1975 law on disability, which created a whole array of services beyond the *secteur*, and thus beyond psychiatrists' jurisdiction, for people with mental illness (Henckes, 2012). At the end of the decade, the Minister of Health announced that the number of psychiatric hospital beds would be reduced by 40.000. This, along with the simultaneous lack of explicit support for creating community services in the *secteurs*, generated an outcry within psychiatry (Ayme, 1995).

Psychiatrists advocated for a new mental health law to secure *secteur* psychiatry and provide guidelines for professionals and local administrations.

In 1981, the election of a socialist government for the first time in 20 years raised hopes among psychiatrists that psychiatric reform could finally go forward. The nomination of Jack Ralite, a member of the Communist Party, as Minister of Health, reinforced those hopes. In 1981, Ralite appointed a commission to advise on the reform and tap the range of positions on that question. The commission's hearings highlighted divisions within the profession. While young psychiatrists from the Syndicat de la Psychiatrie advocated for a law modelled after the Italian one, explicitly planning for the closure of psychiatric hospitals, the Syndicat des Psychiatres des Hôpitaux took a much more guarded position. Unions representing other mental health professionals also firmly defended psychiatric hospitals, reflecting their corporatist interests. Ralite himself held no strong opinion. After he was replaced by the socialist Edmond Hervé, in 1983, the debate edged even more towards keeping hospitals at the centre of the mental health system.

The law that finally passed in 1985 provided a clear definition of *secteur* policy but organized funding for its services through psychiatric hospitals. In other words, psychiatric hospitals were now required to devote part of their budget to community services, and mental health professionals working in *secteurs* were to be paid by hospitals. A reform of hospital budgets relying on the allocation of an annual block grant (*budget global*) for hospitals, as opposed to funding based on the number of days of patient service over the fiscal year (*prix de journée*), aimed to facilitate the transfer of care to community facilities. However, it was clearly insufficient to really foster change.

Although the Minister and his administration defended the idea that psychiatric hospitals should organize the relocation of their services in communities, the law and subsequent regulations provided few guidelines concerning their future. Their fate would remain a contentious issue in France well into the 2000s. On the one hand, the number of psychiatric beds decreased significantly during that period, from more than 100,000 beds in the mid 1970s to 60,000 in the early 2000s. Although there were significantly fewer beds in public hospitals, the number in private clinics grew. On the other hand, a number of initiatives within the framework of the disability law created a range of services for mentally ill patients that provided alternatives to psychiatric hospitalization. However, these changes were barely monitored by health authorities, and *secteur* policy gave mixed results. Community psychiatry was unevenly developed across France, and two neighbouring *secteurs* could offer widely different types and quality of services (Coldefy et al., 2009). Disparities in available psychiatric services between urban and rural regions exploded.

Even more problematic was the absence of strong leadership by the Minister of Health, who took few measures to resolve this situation of highly disparate levels and types of care among *secteurs* and between geographical regions. Ministerial reports during this period concurred in calling for the development of *secteur* services and resources and the transformation of hospitals (Zambrowski, 1989; Massé, 1992).

However, these recommendations had little direct effect. Aggravating this situation, a reform of the 1838 law which regulated involuntary hospitalization had resulted in an increase in the total number of such hospitalizations. These limitations would lay the ground for the revival of debates in psychiatry in the 2000s, albeit in a new form, to which we now turn.

The limits of deinstitutionalization and the French return to Basaglia in the 2000s

By the 2000s, the debate over the closure of psychiatric hospitals in France had clearly receded. Whilst the *secteur* policy still remained the official line of successive governments, its content had become more and more elusive. No guidelines had been published by the Ministry of Health on the content of *secteur* practices since the early 1990s, and, as we have already seen, several new laws had actually weakened community-based practices. On the one hand, some psychiatric hospitals (notably in Paris) had been closed down, but most remained, albeit with far fewer beds. Moreover, some hospitals transformed part of their sites into nursing homes, resulting in patients being transferred from the old hospital inpatient services to homes that were often within the same facility. On the other hand, the generation of psychiatrists who began to emerge in the 1990s and 2000s expressed interests clearly distinct from those of their predecessors. Both the psychoanalytical and the political perspectives that had dominated the post-1968 generation were receding, in favour of a biologically oriented psychiatry. Whilst some psychiatrists remained interested in social psychiatry, in practice, that field came to be dominated by new rehabilitation practices inspired, in part, by cognitive behavioural theories. At the political level, a conspicuous debate arose on two themes: the coordination between psychiatric and social services for people with mental illness, and the promotion of patients' rights.

In this configuration, Basaglian ideas found new ground among new groups. In northern France, the psychiatrist Jean-Luc Roelandt developed his *secteur* into a showcase of community psychiatry. After a series of visits to Trieste in 1996, he adapted some of the innovations he had observed there, including the cooperatives that provided work to patients and unemployed people from Trieste (Roelandt, 2018). Beginning in the 2000s, young mental health professionals and sociologists attracted to his approach joined him, the Ministry of Health showed interest in his work, and his *secteur* became the only WHO Collaborating Centre for Mental Health in France.

At the national level, Basaglian ideas also entered a renewed debate over the transformation of the psychiatric system, thanks to a report in 2000 by psychiatrists Eric Piel and Roelandt himself, commissioned by Lionel Jospin's Socialist government (Piel and Roelandt, 2001). The Italian model directly inspired two major propositions in the report. The first concerned creating synergy among services through the formal organization of a series of territorial networks uniting psychiatric and social services.

The second was a moratorium on investments in psychiatric hospitals, with the aim of closing them down. The report also included numerous propositions inspired by other sources, including psychiatry's relationship to the judiciary and user representation on local boards. More generally, the report's originality lay in its proposed framework for mental health policy: the delivery of not only psychiatric services to people with mental health problems, but, more broadly, of the whole range of social services they needed.

The Piel–Roelandt report attracted criticism from all segments of psychiatry. It ignited a debate, that would last for over a decade, on the supposed decline of psychiatry's status in French health policies. Entitled 'From Psychiatry to Mental Health', the report was understood by most of its critics within psychiatry as an attack on their discipline. They feared that psychiatry and psychiatrists would become diluted in a sociomedical and social ensemble of all mental health professionals. The very concept of 'mental health' acquired a connotation of managerialism and anti-psychiatry, which it maintains today. Following the Piel–Roelandt report, a new one was commissioned by the conservative government that replaced the Jospin government in 2002. This one toned down the debate by putting psychiatry centre stage, but it shared most of the philosophy of the Piel–Roelandt report on the organization of psychiatric care. In fact, most of the ideas contained in the Piel–Roelandt report still influence French mental health policy, with the notable exception of the moratorium on psychiatric hospital funding.

The limits of Basaglian influence: patients' rights and the contestation of forced hospitalization in the 2010s

An even more striking transformation within French psychiatry concerns the promotion of patients' rights, a movement in contemporary French medicine more generally. Mental health advocacy organizations have existed in France since at least the 1960s, radical anti-psychiatry groups since the 1970s, and psychiatric service user groups since the 1990s. Not until 2002 did a law establish patients' rights to free and informed consent over their treatment and to consult their medical files. This law also allowed 'qualified patients' to represent service users on administrative boards and regional and national consultative bodies.[2] However, it is perhaps the 2005 law on disability that provided the most impetus to patients' rights and user-centred organizations, by financing a type of psychiatric service-user self-help organization— the GEM (Groupe d'entr'aide mutuelle)—which, in practice, has materialized in varying degrees of member participation and decision making.[3] Since then, peer-support

[2] Law no. 2002–303 of 4 March 2002 'on the rights of patients and the quality of the health system'.

[3] Law no. 2005–102 'for the equality of rights and equal opportunity and the participation and citizenship of people with disabilities'. (The French term for the latter is 'handicapped persons').

and other models have been implemented throughout France and have developed around the experience-based expertise of users. Some are peer-run, but wide differences exist in the degree of member autonomy and participation (Lovell, 2012; Lovell et al., 2009).

The extent to which these organizations were influenced by Basaglian psychiatry remains to be seen. The initiators of the 2005 law, who came from civil society organizations rather than the psychiatric profession, do not refer to Italy. However, the more interesting question is the contradiction between the development of regulatory measures to assure patients' rights and promote health democracy, and the greater use of modern forms of confinement and involuntary treatment. These latter include the expansion of involuntary commitment (Coldefy et al., 2015), the rise of special units for 'difficult patients' (Velpry and Eyraud, 2014), and the debates around forms of constraint applied to psychiatric patients in France. In recent years, national and independent reports have brought attention to violence and abuses committed against psychiatric inpatients, and the degradation of conditions in institutions (Lalande and Lépine, 2011). The French Controller General of Places of Deprivation of Liberty has reported an increase over the past 20 years in the use of seclusion (isolation rooms) and physical constraints (straightjackets, packs, bed attachments, etc.), 'with no formal therapeutic basis' (2016). More recently, France's High Authority on Healthcare has proposed measures regulating seclusion and involuntary procedures in psychiatric inpatient units.

Though small activist networks have opposed involuntary hospitalization and psychiatric inpatient conditions since Michel Foucault's post-1968 anti-institutional activism (at that time, the Groupe d'Information sur les Asiles [GIA] was particularly vocal), the two forms of psychiatric hospitalization established by the Law of 1838 have remained more or less in place until recently. Those procedures were so-called voluntary hospitalization (i.e. at the request of a family member or other third party) and forced hospitalization (*placement d'office*, ordered by a public official). In general, French psychiatrists tend to oppose the judiciarization of commitment procedures, despite the decisions of the European Court of Human Rights. In France, only hospital directors, prefects, or mayors (or their delegates)—and not a judge or other legal member—has had the authority to deprive persons of their liberty through involuntary hospitalization.

A major reform of the 1838 law appeared in 1990[4], when voluntary hospitalization (at the request of the patient) was becoming the norm, thereby formalizing decades of practices that had made this procedure the source of most psychiatric hospitalizations. The national climate shifted at the turn of this century, when violence committed by people with psychiatric disorders became a focus for media attention. The presidency of Nicolas Sarkozy, from 2007 to 2012, later politicized the issue. Security

[4] Law no, 90–537 of 27 June 'concerning the rights and protection of persons hospitalized for mental disorders and their conditions of hospitalization'.

measures increased. Some of Sarkozy's proposals, such as required registration of all involuntarily committed patients and their subsequent surveillance by prefects, and certain security measures within psychiatric hospitals, were eventually found to be unconstitutional and abandoned.

The reform that was ultimately legislated in 2011 and implemented in 2013[5] makes three crucial changes. First, it shifts to *judiciarisation*: judges must now approve hospitalization within 12 days of commitment. Nevertheless, the judge intervenes only *after* the individual has been involuntarily committed. Second, it further medicalizes the commitment procedure: the prefect's evaluation as to whether or not commitment 'without consent' is necessary no longer holds primacy over that of the physicians. Third, '*treatment* without consent', including outpatient commitment, now replaces '*hospitalization* without consent': the law essentially expands involuntary treatment beyond inpatient settings.

A major outcome of the legislative reform has been an overall increase in involuntary commitments (with a stabilization of voluntary hospitalizations). The number of people receiving treatment without their consent has more than doubled, as has the number of days of treatment, although the number of hospitalizations has decreased on average (Coldefy et al., 2015). Generally, French mental health practitioners consider these changes to be positive, claiming that they facilitate further deinstitutionalization by expanding treatment settings for patients who are unable or unwilling to provide consent for treatment. Others, however, condemn the limitation of judiciary intervention to the period after the patient has been committed and decry the extension of involuntary treatment beyond the hospital. The risk of a rise in 'exceptional' measures (*dispositifs dérogatoires*) in the case of 'imminent danger' is also of concern (Coldefy et al., 2015).

This continuity of institutional practices outside the institution must be balanced by numerous local innovations (Lovell, 2010), including the gamut of low-demand, mobile services; user-run alternative housing; peer-specialist services; and 'Housing First' models focused on harm reduction, for which accepting psychiatric care is not an eligibility criterion for obtaining housing. Housing First is now an experimental model in four French cities, with ministerial funding (Estecahandy, 2019; Laval, 2019). Individual actors behind some of the innovations—Marseille psychiatrist Vincent Girard and Jean-Luc Roelandt for the integration of peers into psychiatric services, for example—recognize Basaglia's importance and, in Roelandt's case, implemented Trieste-like services. However, these innovations are mostly, and more directly, influenced by North American user-/survivor-centred programmes and harm reduction as they have been practiced in North America, the United Kingdom, and the Netherlands.

Despite increasing attention in other domains of French life to the rights of people with psychiatric disorders, the propensity towards expansion of constraint and the

[5] Law no. 2011–803 of 5 July 'concerning the rights of protection of people under psychiatric treatment and their care'.

translation of involuntary treatment into 'softer' forms raises interesting questions about Basaglia's legacy in France. The success of his anti-institutional movement in Italy was shaped by what might be called an organic, bottom–up organization for change, albeit with a leadership that was originally professional and open to self-criticism. This movement constantly analysed the transformational process in which it was engaged, in political terms, and within a broader context. It demonstrated a willingness to put psychiatric power/knowledge into question. Seen against this backdrop, mainstream French psychiatry never really questioned, in the widest sense, the daily practices and justifications that constitute characteristics—or the residues—of total institutions. Nor were French psychiatrists willing to question the sources of their power. Despite reforms, the psychiatric system in France encompasses a type of social organization whose functioning depends, ultimately, on controlling the responses to the needs of those who are contained within it. Attention to the subject behind the patient, present in Basaglia and Ongaro Basaglia's writings (Lovell and Scheper–Hughes, 1987), rekindled by recent reanalyses of Basaglia's legacy and rereadings of Foucault (Colucci and Di Vittorio, 2005; Sforza Tarabochia, 2013), and further developed in current practices, finds little counterpart in French institutional psychiatry, although it is theorized in psychoanalytically inflected practices.

Conclusion: the paradox of contemporary French psychiatry

Basaglia always warned against assuming that the Italian (or any) anti-institutional model could simply be transferred to a new context (Basaglia, 1987): each 'local' contains its own conditions and contradictions. Within the specificity of the French context, a central reason for its failure to combat the segregation of the asylum, even through new forms, lies in France's rigidly controlled government bureaucracies and in the strong, centralized form of state government, in which reforms are top–down and reinforced by a historical and cultural defiance of intermediary instances. Furthermore, historically and structurally, French forms of governance do not favour bottom–up innovation. When local initiatives arise and transformations are sought, they tend to be poorly, if at all, integrated and replicated. This has resulted in a paradox: the centrality of the psychiatric hospital, on the one hand, and the marginality of exemplary innovations, on the other hand. Psychiatric reforms have existed alongside the logic of the institution, which Basaglia warned against. Hence, not unexpectedly, innovative turns, such as intermediary community structures in an earlier era, or service-user organizations today, always risk adding another organizational layer to a still hospital-centred system. Nor is it surprising that the shift from involuntary hospitalization to involuntary treatment simply extends the steadfast historical logic underlying the psychiatric institution (Lovell and Rhodes, 2014).

References

Amieux-Orsini, M.-C. (2018). Interview by Anne M. Lovell, June 2018.

Antoine, J.-M. (2010). Une histoire, une vie. Deuxième Partie: bouillonnements et conflits. *VST—Vie Sociale et Traitements* 108:103–8.

Ayme, J. (1995). *Chroniques de la psychiatrie publique à travers l'histoire d'un syndicat.* Ramonville-Saint-Agne: Erès.

Balduzzi, E. (1982). A propos de l'article de M. Beluffi: '180 . . . et une nuit. L'homme de Dronero et les écuyers tranchants'. *L'Information Psychiatrique* 58(4):577–80.

Basaglia, F. (1965). Corps, regard et présence. L'énigme de la subjectivité en psychiatrie. *L'Evolution psychiatrique* XXX(1):11–26.

Basaglia, F. (1966). La 'communauté thérapeutique' base d'un service psychiatrique, réalités et perspectives. *L'Information Psychiatrique* 5:413–28.

Basaglia, F. (1978). Le théâtre de la folie c'est encore l'asile. *L'Information Psychiatrique* 54(8):913–14.

Basaglia, F. (1987). Letter from America: the artificial patient. In: N. Scheper–Hughes and A.M. Lovell (eds), *Psychiatry Inside Out: Selected Writings of Franco Basaglia.* New York: Columbia University Press, pp. 127–34.

Basaglia, F. and Ongaro Basaglia, F. (1987). The problem of the incident. In: N. Scheper-Hughes and A.M. Lovell (eds), *Psychiatry Inside Out: Selected Writings of Franco Basaglia.* New York: Columbia University Press, pp. 87–91.

Bec, C. (1977). *Vers une psychiatrie normalisée, histoire d'une stratégie professionnelle: 1945–1970.* Thèse de 3e cycle: EHESS.

Beluffi, M. (1982). '180' . . . et une nuit. L'homme de Dronero et les écuyers tranchants. *L'Information Psychiatrique* 58(1):81–5.

Blanchard, S. (2017). Raymond Depardon: 'J'ai toujours le regret de ne pas avoir photographié mon père'. *Le Monde*, 8 October 2017.

Bonnafe, L. (1980). Franco Basaglia: La rupture. *VST—Vie Sociale et Traitements* 131:4–6.

Carrino, L. (2018a). Un lungo viaggio tra psichatria e sviluppo umano. Presentation at the Scuola Estiva di Salute Mentale, Servizi e Societa, Comeglians (Udine), 27 August 2018.

Carrino, L. (2018b). Personal communication with Anne Lovell, 3 September 2018.

Castel, F.O., Castel, R., and Lovell, A. (1982). *The Psychiatric Society.* New York: Columbia University Press.

Castel, R. (1973). *Le Psychanalysme.* Paris: François Maspéro.

Castel, R. (1980). Préface. In: J.-L. Metge (ed.), *Psichiatria Democratica. L'expérience italienne.* Paris: Editions du Scarabée, pp. 15–27.

Coldefy, M., Le Fur, P., Lucas-Gabrielli, V., and Mousquès, J. (2009). Cinquante ans de sectorisation psychiatrique en France: des inégalités persistantes de moyens et d'organisation. *Questions d'Economie de la Santé* 145:1–8.

Coldefy, M., Tartour, T., and Nestrigue, C. (2015). De l'hospitalisation aux soins sans consentement en psychiatrie. Premiers résultats de la mise en place de la Loi du 5 juillet 2011. *Questions d'Economie de la Santé* 205:1–8.

Colucci, M. and Di Vittorio, P. (2005). *Franco Basaglia. Portrait d'un Psychiatre Intempestif.* Ramonville-Saint-Agne: Erès.

Daumézon, G. and Koechlin, P. (1952). La psychothérapie institutionnelle contemporaine. *Anais Portuguese de Psiquiatria* 4:271–311.

Del Pistoia, L. (1979). Nouvelle législation en Italie. *Psychiatrie Française* X(3):31–5.

Donzelot, J., Mével, C., and Wyvekens, A. (2003). *Faire société : la politique de la ville aux États-Unis et en France.* Paris: Éd. du Seuil.

Escoffier-Lambiotte, C. (1971). 'Antipsychiatrie' ou naufrage de la psychiatrie? *Le Monde* 16 February 1971.
Estecahandy, P. (2019). Avant Propos. Housing First. Au delà du sans abrisme et de la psychiatrie. *Vie Sociale* 23–24:7–10.
Ey, H. (ed.) (1965). Hommage à la psychiatrie Italienne. *L'Evolution Psychiatrique* XXX:1
Ey, H. (1972). L'antipsychiatrie ou les progrès de la science psychiatrique. *L'Evolution Psychiatrique* XXXVII:I
Ey, H., Sivadon, P., Tosquellès, F., Le Guillant, L., and Daumézon, G. (1952). Symposium sur la psychothérapie collective. *L'Evolution Psychiatrique* 3:531–92.
Foot, J. (2015). *The Man Who Closed The Asylums: Franco Basaglia and The Revolution in Mental Health Care*. London: Verso Books.
Foucault, Michel ([1975] 1977) *Discipline and Punish: The Birth of the Prison*. New York, NY: Pantheon Books.
Fourquet, F. and Murard, L. (1980). *Histoire de la psychiatrie de secteur*. Paris: Encres.
Guattari, F. (1976). 'Ce film n'appelle pas un débat. Il le clôt.' (A propos du film *Fous à délier*). *Libération* 5 March 1976.
Hanon, C. and Sicard, M. (2014). Interview de Jean-Charles Pascal. *L'Information Psychiatrique* 90(5):387–94.
Henckes, N. (2005). *Réformer la psychiatrie, organiser les pratiques de secteur. La construction de la psychiatrie de secteur dans 'l'expérience du treizième arrondissement'.* Rapport pour le programme Sciences biomédicales, Santé, Société, MiRe/INSERM/CNRS, Paris, CERMES
Henckes, N. (2007).'Le nouveau monde de la psychiatrie française. Les psychiatres, l'Etat et la réforme des hôpitaux psychiatriques de l'après-guerre aux années 1970' Thèse de sociologie, Ecole des Hautes Etudes en Sciences Sociales.
Henckes, N. (2012). Entre maladie et handicap: repenser la critique psychiatrique de la loi du 30 juin 1975 d'orientation en faveur des personnes handicapées. *ALTER, European Journal of Disability Research* 6:242–54.
Henckes, N. (2016). French deinstitutionalization or the irony of success. Psychiatrists, the state and the transformation of the French psychiatric system, 1945–2010. In: D. Kritsotaki., V. Long, and M. Smith. (eds.), *Deinstitutionalisation and After. Post-War Psychiatry in the Western World*. London: Palgrave Macmillan, pp. 115–33.
Humblot, C. (1997). La folie asilaire selon Raymond Depardon. *Le Monde* 30 May 1997.
Humblot, C. and Devarrieux, C. (1976). Pour la socialisation des handicapés mentaux. Fous à délier par un groupe de cinéastes italiens. *Le Monde* 3 April 1976.
Jaccard, R. (1984). Les hôpitaux psychiatriques italiens menacés de reouverture. *Le Monde* 4 March 1984.
Jakubowicz, A. (2006). Psychiatrie de campagne à Montceau-les-Mines. *Esprit* 329(11):168–73.
Lalande, F. and Lepine, C. (2011). *Analyse d'accidents en psychiatrie et propositions pour les éviter*. Paris: Inspections Générale des Affaires Sociales.
Laurenceau, C. (1972). Inventaire des moyens psychiatriques existant en France. *L'Information Psychiatrique* 48:975–80.
Laval, C. (2019). Genèse du 'Un chez soi d'abord'. *Vie Sociale* 23–24:175–85.
Le Contrôleur Général des Lieux de Privation de Liberté (2016). *Isolement et contention dans les établissements de santé mentale*. Paris: Editions Dalloz.
Legrand, M. (1988). *La psychiatrie alternative italienne*. Toulouse: Privat.
Le Guillant, L. (1947). Une expérience de réadaptation sociale instituée par les événements de guerre. *Hygiène Mentale* 6:85–102.
Le Monde (1971). Le psychiatre italien Franco Basaglia bénéficie d'un non-lieu. 26 May 1971.
Le Monde (1971). Un 'antipsychiatre' italien risque d'être inculpé d'homicide par imprudence. 26 May 1971.

Le Monde (1987). Hommage. Une pionnière de la psychiatrie de secteur. 15 December 1987.

L'Information Psychiatrique (1981). La loi italienne sur la psychiatrie trois ans après. *L'Information psychiatrique* 57:5.

Louzoun, C. and Stylianidis, S. (1987). *La nouvelle psychiatrie italienne*. Paris: La Documentation Française.

Lovell, A.M. (2010). Santé mentale. In: D. Fassin & B. Hauray (eds), *Santé Publique. L'état des saviors*. Paris: La Découverte, pp. 161–72.

Lovell, A.M. (2012). Quels modèles d'expertise pour les usagers en psychiatrie? Vers une notion tri-partite. In: A. BATTEGAY, O. COEHLO, and H. VAZ (eds), *Prendre soin, prendre part, vivre avec. Enjeux et défis de la citoyenneté profane dans les rapports santé-société*. Porto: Livpsic, pp. 47–62.

Lovell, A.M and Rhodes, L.A. (2014). Psychiatry with teeth: notes on coercion and control in France and the United States. *Culture, Medicine, and Psychiatry* 38(4):618–22.

Lovell, A.M. and Scheper–Hughes, N. (1987). The utopia of reality: Franco Basaglia and the practice of a democratic psychiatry. In: N. Scheper_Hughes and A.M. Lovell (eds), *Psychiatry Inside Out: Selected Writings of Franco Basaglia*. New York: Columbia University Press, pp. 1–50.

Lovell, A.M., Troisoeufs, A., and Mora, M. (2009). Du handicap psychique aux paradoxes de sa reconnaissance: Éléments d'un savoir ordinaire des personnes vivant avec un trouble psychique grave. *Revue Française des Affaires Sociales* 63:209–27.

Marmande, F. (2005). Autistes, artistes, à une lettre près. *Le Monde* 25 May 2005.

Masse, G. (1992). *La psychiatrie ouverte. Une dynamique nouvelle en santé mentale. Rapport au Ministre de la Santé et de l'Action Humanitaire*. Rennes: Editions de l'Ecole Nationale de la Santé Publique.

Mauri, D., Gallio, G., Giannichedda, M.G., and De Leonardis, O. (1983). *La Liberta' e' terapeutica? L'esperienza psichiatrica di Trieste*. Milano: Feltrinelli.

Metge, J.-L. (1980). *Pschiatria Democratica ou l'optimisme de la pratique. L'expérience italienne*. Paris: Editions du Scarabée.

Ministère de la Solidarité, de la Santé et de la Protection Sociale. (1990). Service des statistiques des études et des systèmes d'information. Paris 1990. Psychiatrie et Santé Mentale. Paris: La Documentation Française.

Noel, P. (1984). Avant-Propos. *L'Information Psychiatrique* 60(9):987.

Parizot, S. (2013). Rencontre avec Luciano Carrino. *L'Information Psychiatrique* 89(6):453–64.

Pascal, J.-C. (2018). Interview, by Nicolas Henckes, July 2018.

Piel, E. and Roelandt, J.-L. (2001). *De la psychiatrie à la santé mentale. Rapport de mission*. Paris: Ministère de la Santé.

Pinell, P. (2005). La normalisation de la psychiatrie française. *Regards Sociologiques* 29:3–21.

Pivetta, O. (2018). *Franco Basaglia, il dottore dei matti*. Milan: Baldini and Castoldi.

Psichiatria Democratica et Psychiatrie Sociale (1982). Confrontation Franco-Italienne de Nice, 14, 15, 16 mai 1982. *Transitions. Revue Internationale du Changement Psychiatrique et Social* 11–12.

Roelandt, J.-L. (2018). Interview by Nicolas Henckes, September 2018.

Sassolas, M. (2010). Pour quelle psychiatrie militer. *Sud/Nord* 25:139–49.

Sforza Tarabochia, A. (2013). *Psychiatry, Subjectivity, Community: Franco Basaglia and Biopolitics*. Bern: Peter Lang.

Turkle, S. (1978). *Psychoanalytic Politics: Freud's French Revolution*. New York: Basic Books.

Velpry, L. and Eyraud, B. (2014). Confinement and psychiatric care: a comparison between high-security units for prisoners and for difficult patients in France. *Culture, Medicine and Psychiatry* 38:550–77.

Von Bueltzingsloewen, I. (2007). *L'hécatombe des fous. La famine dans les hôpitaux psychiatriques français sous l'Occupation*. Paris: Aubier.
Zambrowski, F. (1989). *Moderniser et diversifier les modes de prise en charge de la psychiatrie française. Rapport au ministre de la solidarité, de la santé et de la protection sociale*. Paris: La Documentation Française.

18

Borderline deinstitutionalization

Yugoslav resonance and dissonance with Basaglia

Vito Flaker, Vladimir Jović, Nataša Cvetković Jović, and Andreja Rafaelič

Periods and topics

Basaglia's work, the Trieste experience, and the 'Italian model' were, and remain, a major inspiration for deinstitutionalization in (former) Yugoslavia. Basaglia's personal and actual impact during the 1960s and 1970s, however, was minimal. It consisted of a few cross-border encounters with Slovene psychiatrists (while Basaglia was in Gorizia) and one presentation in Belgrade just before his death. The Trieste experience, however, remained a source of inspiration to Yugoslav anti-institutional movements in the 1980s, and these have maintained lively contacts with Basaglia's co-workers. These intensified and took on an institutional character in the transition and war period of the 1990s. In the deinstitutionalization endeavours from 2000 onwards, the Italian model was seen as its prototype. This division into decades is marked by Basaglia's and Tito's deaths in 1980, as well as the demise of Western socialism and the onset of neo-conservatism and neo-liberalism. The 1990s were marked by the transition and wars, which ended around 2000. A period of relative stability marked by (pre)accession to the European Union has followed.

Basaglia's geographical position and his impact in Yugoslavia was *borderline*, as was Yugoslav deinstitutionalization. His reception was mixed—ranging from enthusiasm to total rejection. Yugoslav psychiatrists were initially interested in what he was offering, but refuted his message in the 1980s, when faced with domestic anti-institutional movements and the increasing impotence of their social psychiatry project. This remains so, with some exceptions, to this day. The anti-institutional movements in Yugoslavia were born from his legacy, and his ideas contributed to the rise of anti-authoritarianism and democratization. Many community services were established from the 1990s on, and some deinstitutionalization attempts from 2000. However, what used to be Yugoslavia still presents a predominantly institutional landscape, for the last two decades hovering on the edge of real, systematic deinstitutionalization.

These four distinct periods reflect epochs in global as well as ex-Yugoslav history (see Table 18.1). The story of Basaglia's impact in what used to be Yugoslavia needs to be read in such a frame. This chapter also describes Basaglia's resonance through

Table 18.1 Periods of Basaglian influence in (former) Yugoslavia

Period	Agency	Partners	Activity of impact	Global epoch	National politics
1967–1980	Direct Basaglia's impact	(Social) Psychiatry	Social psychiatry, critique and defence	1960s' movements, 'lead' years	Liberalization, self-government
1980–1990	Trieste and Réseau	Social movements	Camps, conferences	Onset of neo-liberalism	Democratization
1990–2000	International projects	NGOs	First community services, war experiences	Post 'Cold War' politics	War and transition
2000–	Supranational bodies	Government institutions	'Hiccups' of deinstitutionalization	Onset of crises	(Pre)accession stabilization

ever widening circles of agency, the emergence of different audiences and partners in action, and his increasing impact on the transformation of services. We have also structured it by the reaction of official psychiatry, followed by the resonance with anti-authoritarian and anti-institutional movements, and, finally, on their impact as 'hiccups' of deinstitutionalization in the region. The sections in this chapter broadly correspond to these periods but extend beyond them to provide an insight into the local social psychiatry movements and deinstitutionalization.

Basaglia was a Renaissance man, combining theoretical discourse, political engagement, reorganization of the services, and new approaches in working with people. Yet, he was neither philosopher, politician, nor manager, and not a therapist. His ability to consistently connect thought and action with organization and contact with people, enabled him to remain human in inhuman conditions. He could construct a humanist utopia overarching the (rationalist) pitfalls of each of these activities; deinstitutionalization as not only a complex but also, essentially, a unitary process. We will analyse Basaglia's resonance (and dissonance) along these dimensions (of theory, politics, organization, and methods), hopefully to show how inseparable they are in reality.

Being on the border

Basaglia began and ended his journey on the Yugoslav border in the cities of Gorizia and Trieste. At that time, this was not only a border between two states, but between two political systems. Yugoslavia was not a part of the Soviet bloc and was developing a democratic socialism based on workers self-government. From both the Yugoslav and Triestian perspectives, the 'iron curtain' lay on the Hungarian border. The Italian–Yugoslav border was an open one, with intense commercial and cultural exchange. In the collective memory of all the ex-Yugoslav nations, Trieste still figures as a prime shopping destination. There were daily shopping buses from most major

Yugoslav cities. Trieste was a synonym for cheap jeans, new records, and fine tiles, and was generally a consumer Mecca. The attraction in the opposite direction was holidays on the East Adriatic and cheap food, cigarettes, and petrol. There was also some political nostalgia on both sides. For Yugoslav right wingers, Trieste was the exit to the West. After 1968, it became an important link to the New Left and student movements across Europe. For Italian left wingers, Yugoslavia was the place of utopia (especially just after the Second Word War). This was beautifully depicted in Pasolini's early novel (1959) *Una Vita Violenta* (*A Violent Life*). This period of Berlinguer's Eurocommunism in the 1970s was also marked by Basaglian experiences. For right wingers, Yugoslavia was the enemy—presenting an imminent threat of Slavic (i.e. communist) invasion. This mutual attraction existed in matters related to Basaglia, albeit only partially; Yugoslav psychiatry chose to be repelled.

Being on the border is an important dimension in understanding Basaglia's work. Trieste after the Second World War remained almost as an enclave, butting into the Yugoslav Eastern Adriatic coast. Gorizia was, like Berlin, a divided city. The Gorizia asylum was right on the border; a friend of ours could watch the unexpected developments from her kitchen on the Yugoslav side. San Giovanni Hospital in Trieste was on the slope extending from the city towards the border. Being on the border equates to being on the periphery (of political interest); in the case of the Yugoslav border, the utter periphery. Deinstitutionalization seems never to have started in a metropolis.

Being on the border also engages minority issues and perspectives. The Slovene minority had an important role in Basaglia's effort. When Basaglia took over the San Giovanni Hospital, the only doctors who stayed on were of the Slovene minority (Jogan and Fonda, psychologist Sedmak, later to be joined by Bavdaž and Ravbar). These minorities had been subject to genocide under fascism, and, still struggling for their rights, more easily understood deinstitutionalization and the concept of the deviant majority (*maggioranza deviante*).

Border has become the metaphor for deinstitutionalization in Trieste. Psychiatry was an institution that set and maintained the border between normality and madness. The new psychiatry made this frontier permeable, transgressive. The place of the new psychiatry becomes 'no man's land' (*terra di nessuno*) which, ideally, should be expanded. Mental health workers and users are the border (tres)passers—'Confinandanti' as Toresini (2011) entitled his novel depicting the complexity of life in the area—allowing the free movement from madness to normality, and from ordinary to uncommon. However, it was not so easy for Basaglia to pass the state border.

Non-practical utopia of social psychiatry

Failed encounter of two psychiatries

At least two meetings between Basaglia and Slovene psychiatrists are known to us, one in Gorizia and one in Ljubljana. After hours of dynamic discussion, in the middle of the night, Basaglia was asked if he would allow a person to commit suicide. At this point, the discussion was finished. Later on, when the then leading Slovene psychiatrist Kobal was challenged to explain why Slovene, Marxist psychiatry did not follow Basaglia, he answered: 'It is enough to do one revolution in one's lifetime. We do not need to go through another one' (Sedmak, personal communication). Leading psychiatrists then came mainly from the ranks of partisans (as was Basaglia), who indeed had achieved a revolution during the war.

These episodes illuminate various features of Basaglia's contact with Slovene psychiatrists. One is the earnest attempts of cross-border collaboration. Basaglia and Slovene psychiatrists shared a common ideological basis—a mixture of Marxism and existentialism. However, the leap Basaglia was taking was too great. Hence the reason for the ultimate failure of such collaboration. On the one hand, Italian psychiatry at the time was quite backward, giving Slovene psychiatrists a sense of superiority. The Italians were also too busy with their own processes, based on *aggiornamento* rather than radical reform. On the other hand, suicidology was becoming a high profile subdiscipline of Slovene psychiatry at that time, and there was no scope to abandon the 'guardian position' which psychiatry traditionally assumes and is constituted upon (Castel, 1976).

Social psychiatry reform based on transinstitutionalization

Since the 1960s, Yugoslav psychiatrists have been engaged in reforming psychiatry. The Institute for Mental Health in Belgrade was established in 1963 with the first day-care hospital. The first Yugoslav Congress of Social Psychiatry was held in 1971 (Peršić, 1971) and regular seminars of social psychiatry started in 1972. At the end of the 1970s, many innovations were in place—both inside the institution (psychotherapy, therapeutic communities, occupational therapy, etc.) and outside (suicide register and lifeline, a club for drug prevention, etc.). Some long-stay hospitals were transformed into modern clinics based on psychotherapy and social intervention—containing crisis units, day and night hospitals, psychotherapy units, etc. However, the former long-stay patients were not resettled in their homes or in any other community setting; mostly, they were transinstitutionalized to social care homes. By such transinstitutionalization, the average hospital stay in Slovenia was halved from 89 days in 1971 to 54 days in 1985 (Milčinski andNovak 1987, p 21). The average stay in a special social care home was over 13 years (Flaker and Urek, 1988, p 27). This transinstitutionalization resulted in approximately 3,000 beds in social-care institutions compared to 1,200 in psychiatric hospitals.

Modernization also meant establishing psychiatric departments in general hospitals, as 'active' psychiatry (reintegration into medicine), whilst retaining asylums on the periphery (there were two on the islands in Croatia). A five-tiered mental health system emerged. This comprised:

1. outpatient services within ordinary community health centres;
2. some outdoor facilities;
3. prestigious 'centres for mental health'—psychiatric clinics with a high concentration of highly educated therapists (often professors at universities);
4. short-term facilities (usually in general hospitals); and
5. long-stay institutions in the health and social-care system.

These last are often neglected in discussions and presentations, but in fact are the hard core of the system.

Offensive defence of the official psychiatry

The rather benign initial reaction to Basaglia turned into outright hostility in the 1980s. In the 1970s, 'anti-psychiatry' (Foucault, Laing, Szasz) was used to establish the basis of social psychiatry as a critique of organic orientation, whilst 'warning' against its excesses as 'counterfeiting the nature of mental disorder and the relationship between mental disorder and society' (Kecmanović, 1978) or as a 'danger of political engagement . . . an attack on authorities' (Kaličanin, 1974, p. 27). In his pamphlet against critical psychiatry, Kecmanović (1986) refuted its theses, one by one. He asserted the existence of mental disorders and biological markers, the validity of genetic theories, and the positive effects of ECT; he praised the humanization of mental hospitals—pointing to how therapeutic communities had flattened the hierarchical pyramid, to the reduced length of hospital stays, to the introduction of intermediate services, and so on. Even if Basaglia was not the prime target of the pamphlet, his analogy of psychiatric institutions and violence and crimes against humanity is used to support the main thesis of the book. By defining psychiatry as an instrument of power, 'critics' were unable to 'recognise the specificity of mentally disturbed man, and that is why he is—*used*' (Kecmanović, 1986, p. 178).

Accusing someone who denounces the *use* (i.e. reification and commodification) of mental health users of exploiting them (for ideological or political reasons, or even personal gains) is a striking inversion of the proposition. Such an inversion diverts attention from the content of the original criticism, without any valid counterargument, and discredits the utterer. It combines three ideological operations of authoritarian power. First, borrowed from psychiatry, axiomatically postulating the real existence of something that needs not be proved—in this case, proving the actual use or exploitation; second, akin to psychoanalytical interpretation, assuming a hidden motive that transcends the obvious—the motive of the critique is not what it seems to be; third, as used in any witch hunt, ascribing personal gain as opposed to common good in the acts of the accused—critics of psychiatry are getting money, fame, and power. Common in all these three operations is that the accusations are uttered from a position of unassailable power, that the victim remains defenceless, and that arguments are made *ad personam*.

Yugoslav politics were pronouncedly anti-Stalinist in essence, but Stalinist qualities remained. Mental health activists had their phones tapped, and their bosses were approached by national security agents, wanting them to covertly investigate anti-socialist behaviour. The leading (social) psychiatrists in Yugoslavia, although not hard-liners of the Communist League, were part of the 'nomenclatura'. They had access to power and could prohibit a users' association, or ban the showing of a documentary on an asylum, or expel 'intruders' from an institution, even if not in their jurisdiction. Above all, they led hierarchical institutions in an authoritarian manner. The need for a common enemy, represented by movements at home and anti-institutional psychiatry abroad, reflected the dwindling prospects for social psychiatry, which sustained the hierarchical power structure of psychiatry in the 1970s.

Decline of social psychiatry

No matter how the conditions improved *within* the hospital, the overall system was still geared for exclusion of the mentally ill. A typical 'moral career of a mental patient' was a downward spiral through ever-stricter circuits of control. From outpatient treatment in primary care or a community facility, to psychiatric departments in general hospitals, to an institution (asylum). For a huge number of psychiatrists, the asylum was the only 'real choice' and, most were honestly convinced, the only humane one. Letting patients out of institutions would be equated with abandonment (with a strong presumption of homelessness). This position was regularly repeated, even as late as 2011:

> Abolishment of hospitals is not the only and real solution to the problem, as 'lunatics' free of strait jackets and the psychiatric hospital would still roam the streets, would still be ridiculed or avoided by passers-by, which implies that these people would not gain benefit substantially from the abolition of psychiatric hospitals.
>
> **(Rašković-Ivić, 2011, p. 10)**

In essence, the model of 'social psychiatry' had failed (Tore, 2014). After initial enthusiasm, it had, by the 1980s, become devoid of real content, with no contribution to constructing new services. Currently, approximately 30–40% of inmates of psychiatric hospitals (data is for Serbia) have no medical indications for hospital treatment (Jović, 2014). The wars in former Yugoslavia brought further decline and deterioration of conditions in psychiatric hospitals. In one, a man's hand had to be amputated due to extended and uncontrolled physical restraint. The director of the hospital denied journalists entry into some departments, explaining 'that there were patients who for "reasons related to their mental state" were left naked' (Hedges, 1997). From 2000, there is almost no trace of the systematic activities which were praised in previous decades of social psychiatry. Psychosocial rehabilitation activities were closed or hugely reduced; patients were still being abused, humiliated, and restrained either physically or chemically without proper control (Council of Europe, 2018). Social psychiatry had been reduced, by neo-liberal policies, to simply the procurement of medication (as agents of psychopharmaceutical corporations) and the monitoring of the ever-rising numbers of social misfits.

Deinstitutionalization versus authoritarianism

The students' revolt of the late 1960s was as intense in Yugoslavia as in many other countries. The interest of the New Left in subjectivity and psychological oppression was consonant with anti-psychiatry. Simultaneously, there was a revived interest in Wilhelm Reich, and the cult Yugoslav film *WR: Mysteries of the Organism* (1971) contained vivid parallels between Stalinism and psychiatric oppression. In 1975, a joint issue of two Slovenian New Left journals (Dolar, 1975) presented a selection of basic 'anti-psychiatric' texts (Laing, 1959) and timely translations of current writings (Szasz, 1971, 1974; Cooper, 1974). Basaglia's contribution, 'L'utopia della realtà', was submitted as a manuscript through Sedmak (Basaglia, 1973/1975). This publication was the first collection of anti-psychiatric texts in Yugoslavia. It received an ambivalent appraisal by Yugoslav psychiatrists, characteristic for the 1970s. This compilation was followed by a series of classic editions on the topic (Laing, 1977; Jervis, 1977; Cooper, 1980; Foucault (Fuko), 1980; Szasz, 1980). These translations resulted out of increased public interest, manifest in popular culture (e.g. *One Flew over the Cuckoo's Nest*), and were not, as the joint issue of the journals, an expression of multi-party interest by the New Left student activists and psychiatrists with support from Trieste. The first and only selection of Basaglia's papers was published in 1981, by a group directly linked to Trieste; this time not only as a publishing venture, but as an expression of the interest in change.

In the transition from the 1970s to the 1980s, two groups with anti-institutional programmes appeared, one in Belgrade and one in Ljubljana. Their emergence mirrored the transition from the universalistic project of the New Left to the particularistic issues of the 1980s (feminism, gay rights, disability, ecology, peace). These groups were initially closely allied to the new humanistic therapies, which seemingly had many 'anti-psychiatry' traits. They denounced psychiatric rigidity, were against labelling, were democratic, and promoted the normalizing of mental distress. The relationship between the two groups was, at the onset, mutually reinforcing; however, in the second half of the 1980s, they grew apart because of differences in goals, activities, and structures.

The Ljubljana group, a splinter of the student activist movement, had a history of anti-institutional practice. From 1976, child psychiatrist Anica Kos and social work lecturer Bernard Stritih engaged the group in action research. This involved simultaneously developing new forms of volunteer work, for the inclusion of children with various labels into mainstream activities. The most important was long- lasting action in the scouts organization, as a means of transforming institutions, of creating a new professional culture and democratic relationships in both organizations and in the community (Stritih and Mesec, 1977; Stritih and Kos, 1978; Stritih, 1979). This practice was based both on the emerging tradition of anti-authoritarianism (anti-psychiatry, anti-pedagogy, new criminology, radical social work) and on the new therapeutic approaches already mentioned. It presupposed that the Yugoslav system of self-government needs micro processes of democratization, and that these can be introduced by action research. In formulating this action research, the work of Gilli (1977)—a sociologist and Basaglia's co-worker in Gorizia—was very important.

The two groups engaged in publishing and publicizing, and in practical activities. The first feat of the Belgrade group was to publish selected Basaglia papers (1981). Probably not by coincidence, virtually the same selection was published six years later in English (Basaglia, 1987). The group had organized a meeting of the Réseau (Network) of the Alternatives to Psychiatry in 1983 (with Cooper, Guattari, Rotelli, Carino, and others present), and published its proceedings in 1987 (Petrović and Mlađenović, 1987) and 1988 (Mlađenović, 1988). The Ljubljana group organized a new meeting with the Triestians, with Guattari as a guest. They published an abridged version of Goffman's *Asylums* (Flaker and Urek, 1988, pp. 73–137) and a selection of papers including Rosenhahn's experiment, reports from Trieste, Szasz's idea of the psychiatric will (advance directives) (Urek, 1991). Members of both groups regularly visited Trieste as participants in events or as volunteers. Through the Réseau, they were internationally connected to activists and users' groups such as Irren Offensive in Berlin, L'autre Lieu in Belgium, and Runaway Houses and Mental Patients' Union in Holland. With their cooperation, they staged a number of events in Belgrade and Ljubljana. In 1988, on the tenth anniversary of the Law 180 conference in Trieste, the Alpe Adria Network for the Promotion of Mental Health was established to address formal institutions. This was to prove instrumental in developments of the next decade.

The practice of the groups ranged from impromptu mental health work such as counselling, organizing crisis support, and advocacy for users, through to more organized activities and prolonged efforts. The Ljubljana group, with its action research tradition and links to the university, had more resources available and greater skills for organizing volunteer work and camps. In the second half of the 1980s, the group was supported by the Socialist Youth Organization, which by then had become an umbrella organization for diverse new social movements and the focus of the democratization process in Slovenia. This support enabled the Ljubljana group to stage international volunteer camps in the long-stay social care home of Hrastovec, the last stop in the Slovene institutional system.

The goal of the first camp, very much inspired by the Trieste experience, was to draw public attention to the problem of institutions and to provide the stimuli for better working and living conditions in institutions through everyday, civilian activities. During the second camp, it was realized that continuous action was needed, and the Committee for Social Protection of Madness was formed. The name was a provocation, a paraphrase of the Committee for Protection of Human Rights, formed at the time to defend political activists arrested by military police. The group continued to organize camps (outside the institution, after being expelled from it by established psychiatry). It advocated for change and organized public events and happenings. In the 1990s, it became the first mental health NGO in former Yugoslavia and started to provide community services.

These movements played an important part in the democratization process in Yugoslavia in the 1980s, the main political issue being that of fighting authoritarianism. Their importance was not only as a part of an ensemble of diverse social movements. They put the issues of madness, total institutions, professional oppression, and deinstitutionalization on the agenda for change. They attracted massive attention by positioning deinstitutionalization as a way to, and prerequisite of, democracy. By the example of Trieste, and their own activities, they showed that dismantling oppressive structures is possible. Even more, they were developing, on the basis of Basaglian tradition, a social technology of skills and organizational knowledge that produced democratic solutions and new ways of living together. As such, they contributed to the hope, in the 1980s, that a more democratic, humanized socialism was possible. This hope was soon to be hijacked by the neo-liberal agenda.

The war in the 1990s disrupted the Belgrade movement. Its activists became engaged in the peace and feminist movements (Women for Peace). In Slovenia, the war was brief (10 days), and the movement had a chance to implement some of their ideas in the new framework of governance. They formed new associations, group homes for people with long-term mental distress, day centres and clubs, mutual support and self-help groups, advocacy services, social enterprises, users' associations, and so on.

The major resource and the hub for these developments was the interdisciplinary post-graduate programme 'Community Mental Health Studies', established by the leading members of the movement at the School for Social Work. In an EU-funded project (Tempus), with help from the Alpe Adria Network and Basaglians, a consortium was constructed. This consisted of the Trieste services, the London School of Economics (Shula Ramon, David Brandon, MIND), and the Richmond Fellowship, with some input from Austria, Germany, and France (Félix Guattari of the Clinic de La Borde) and participation of the Ljubljana Psychiatric Hospital (!). This diversity and variety enabled the programme to provide a triangular synthesis of Anglo-Saxon and Italian approaches, coupled with its own tradition and knowledge (with some Gallic and Teutonic flavour) (Ramon, 1995). For reasons of cultural hegemony and higher academic standing, the British impact was probably stronger. It also provided some solutions that were not present in Trieste at the time (advocacy, users' run services, personal planning and direct payments, etc.). Triestian input lay in the knowledge of how to organize services and to stage successful conversion of the services, of power distribution (in the line of Gramscian analysis), and of the collective way of working. Besides this, the geographical and cultural proximity of Trieste was helpful, and differences regarding some issues (individual versus collective, health versus social, cultural versus technical, etc.) enabled participants to form their own polyvocal syntheses. They did not need to copy or just transfer know-how from one milieu (Zaviršek and Flaker, 1995).

Despite all the achievements of the 1990s—the creation of new services, enrichment of the social care system, new methods and techniques, and establishing the basis of a unique Slovene school of social work—there are misgivings about the results of this process. One is that it caused the dilution of the movement—its 'NGOization'. Members of the movement became preoccupied with the functioning of their organizations, with the institutional division of labour; they lost their 'advocacy' edge and necessary activism. A second is that the process took place almost exclusively in the social-care sector, while psychiatry remained more or less as it was. The reasons for this lay both in the antagonism that psychiatry had developed, and also in the preoccupation that activists had with maintaining their own territory, busy with their innovations and forgetting the need for change. A third misgiving was that all these new services failed to diminish institutional capacities at all. The process of deinstitutionalization, the closure of the institution, remained a challenge for the future.

The movements did resurface, in a different form, in Slovenia in the following decades. In the wave of successful deinstitutionalization in the first decade of this century, there was an air of change among the staff working in the institutions. When this process subsided, a 700-km march (the 'Walkout') from one institution to another was staged by a group of activists in 2010 (Flaker and Rafaelič, 2012). The following year, they joined others, in the Occupy Movement, to bring the issues of mental health oppression and deinstitutionalization back onto the agenda. Their actions included occupying the mental hospital and ministry for social care for a day (Rasza and Kurnik, 2012; Flaker, 2012). In deinstitutionalization, especially in the Basaglian tradition, there is an imperative for movement—internal commotion and new consciousness, and linking with external social movements. All over former Yugoslavia, such movements have appeared in periods during the last decades, when deinstitutionalization acquired some momentum.

'Hiccups' of deinstitutionalization

The history of deinstitutionalization in the former Yugoslavia is quite long, but there is not much to tell. Its beginning could be dated back to 1967, with the first attempt to change a youth home in Logatec, as in Gorizia, by introducing democratic relationships and style of working. The experiment in Logatec was the beginning of new practices and action research in Slovenia (Vodopivec, 1974). Again, as in Gorizia, the experiment encountered its 'natural limits', resulting finally in wholescale reform—the deinstitutionalization of child and youth homes in Slovenia (Skalar, 1986). Although there are some institutional remnants (causing child protection issues), this was the only systematic attempt at deinstitutionalization in former Yugoslavia, and probably in any socialist country.

Most of the modernization of psychiatry in the 1970s was achieved through transinstitutionalization. However, there were two brave attempts at a thorough transformation of mental health facilities. In Varaždin, Croatia, a long-stay facility was transformed, and attempts made to construct an 'extended' therapeutic community involving the community itself (Brajša, 1986). In Modriča, Bosnia, the institution was transformed along the lines of socialist self-government. Residents moved into the immediate community and achieved all their civil rights by virtue of employment. Both attempts were the result of independent, solitary action of the institutions' management. They were influenced by social psychiatry ideology, but were met with criticism rather than recognition from the psychiatric elite.

While the war meant disruption for some movements and processes, it also presented challenges and opportunities. These were of two kinds. There were instances when institutions in the war zones emptied, and alternatives needed to be sought (often in community settings). Also, mental health professionals engaged in many projects with victims of war (violence, trauma, refugees) began working in a completely new way. The war experience also brought a different perspective on the demarcation of normal and crazy—'Is it normal to hide at home or walk through sniper fire?'; 'Can a traumatised professional assess the trauma of the other' (Loga, 2004, pp. 79–84). However, these opportunities and experiences were, with the exception of Bosnia and Herzegovina, seldom used to change services. A schizoid division of the professional working self arose: one job was temporary but well paid, in an internationally supported NGO; the other job paid next to nothing but offered steady employment in the public service. Such a divided professional identity was supported experientially and institutionally—the experience of the institution and the community, of seeing oneself as helping or controlling the other, remained on parallel lines that never met.

Bosnia was different in a few ways. The devastation of hospitals was massive, war was total. The presence of Mario Reali from Trieste, an enlightened WHO official, reminded the leading psychiatrist Cerić of his youthful admiration of Basaglia. The plan was forged not to rebuild hospitals but to install a network of community mental health centres (Cerić et al., 2001). This plan was enacted with funds from the World Bank and international support, including from the Alpe Adria Network, which also replicated the Ljubljana Tempus programme (Flaker, 1999, 2004).

The Bosnian experience was to be replicated throughout the peninsula via the South East Europe (SEE) Mental Health Project (Maurer and Murko, 2008), implemented by the Stability Pact in collaboration with the WHO. Mario Reali was the consultant specifically responsible for Serbia and Albania. The goals were ambitious—a general reform of mental health service provision and establishment of national mental health bodies and pilot community mental health centres (CMHC). Most of the countries involved developed a mental health strategy, and some adopted new mental health laws, but there was no real change to the system. Although ambitious and well-funded, the project had little impact, except for some local transformations (most of which ceased after termination of the project) such as a community mental health centre in each participating country. The pilots were short-lived because of the limited time in which funding was available and because of resistance from the main institutions (or a lack of determination to close them). The result was a return to the institutions.

In Slovenia, realizing that the new community services did not result in reduced institutional capacities (Flaker et al., 1999), the active deinstitutionalization of Hrastovec began. Almost 300 out of 650 residents were resettled in just a few years, and the quality of community services was improved (Cizelj et al., 2004). Other special social-care homes followed the example, which resulted in 1,259 resettlements (equivalent to more than a quarter of the total capacity of long-stay institutions in Slovenia). However, the process eventually stopped, owing to a lack of political will and of new legislation and new ways of funding, and, also, partially because of burnout amongst the actors. This arrest resulted in an expensive two-tiered system, with the demise of the earlier utopia. What was meant to be an alternative to institutions became their accessory (Flaker et al., 2015b).

In the last decade, either on the initiative of international NGOs and agencies or as a requirement of EU pre-accession, there have been many attempts to embark on systematic deinstitutionalization across former Yugoslavia (Croatia, Serbia, Macedonia, and Montenegro). Usually, there have been good results, not only in the strategies drawn up but also in actually resettling residents from the institutions, training staff to work in the community, and establishing community facilities. The most successful were attempts in children's homes (with support from UNICEF); results were also substantial in social-care homes for those with intellectual disabilities and long-term mental distress. Results were less successful in psychiatric institutions and old-age homes. However, most of these initiatives were not fully implemented, resulting, as in Slovenia, in a two-tier system of care and reinstitutionalization—both in regard to residents returning to the institution and community services developing the properties of institutional care.

What became obvious was that there were 'hiccups' in the process— it would start, stop, start again, only to stop again, and so on. One obvious cause of such 'hiccupping' lies in the design process for projects, which fragments time, will, and resources. It is also a top–down process: when local activity is eventually stimulated, the project stops. Another disruptive feature is the lack of either prolonged engagement or continuity of presence of international experts. Even when their work is successful and they are willing to continue, another team may be chosen. Local experts are put aside and underestimated. Even without the project dynamic, as in Slovenia, hiccups can be caused by exhaustion of resources, usually secondary to a lack of political will.

Despite the ill effects of such hiccups (projects ending, loss of hope, resources misspent, increased costs of the two-tier system), there are productive aspects to them. They enable regrouping, rethinking, and the use of obstacles as new opportunities (e.g. expulsion from the institution creates group homes). Such hiccups might be necessary for the leap from quantity to quality—to proceed from local experience and experiments to system change. Accumulation of experience, sharpening your tools, and creating a common vision are necessary to progress. Antidotes to hiccupping include continuity on the ground (secured by movements, and preferably including users), dedicated professionals and domestic leaders, along with strong coordination. The Italian experience and presence (e.g. the Alpe Adria Network, the engagements of Lorenzo Toresini and Mario Reali, the annual meetings in Trieste and Dubrovnik) provided some of this, plus mutual support and continuity in the region. The main virtues were closeness (both geographical and cultural), comradery, and a focus on people and not just institutions.

Decoding the Basaglian legacy

Theoretical triangulation

Basaglia provided the most complete and consistent conceptualization of deinstitutionalization at the time. Although it may seem cumbersome today, it is still valid and useful. From his major influences—existentialism, Marxism, and interactionalism (Goffman, Lemert)—he built a triangle that allowed informed navigation. This was through aspects of structural oppression and the division of labour, the dynamics of exclusion and identity formation in everyday life, and the reading of the human experience of these. He glued the triangle together with the Foucauldian theme of the productive role of madness. Basaglia's theoretical construction never gained the status of a dominant discourse, even less of a dogma in Yugoslavia, not even in the anti-institutional movements. It allowed a polemic stance—against the institutions and over possibly failing future developments. It had a programmatic edge in envisaging the 'practical utopia': an ethically valid and pragmatically viable development. His works were used not as textbooks but, rather, as handbooks, as manuals to consult when in doubt. His work and engagement also strengthened the interest in important authors previously not well known in Yugoslavia (e.g. Guattari and Deleuze, Goffman, Castel).

Three concepts were particularly useful in Yugoslavia: the practical utopia, the role of the professional, and the importance of contractual power. All three concepts have critical–analytical properties and simultaneously serve as guidelines for action. Empowerment, although a post-Basaglian term originating from the South African struggle against apartheid, is progressively being diluted into a psychological concept (becoming assertive). Basaglia's conception of power as contractual power, an ability to enter into economically and socially meaningful relationships, is not only an antidote to this psychologization but a crucial tool in deinstitutionalization and post-institutional settings. Working with deprivileged people raises the issue of how to use the power invested in (delegated to) the profession so that power is redistributed, and that those initially without power acquire some. Deinstitutionalization is the distribution of power. The practical utopia is empowering, enabling both users and professionals to head towards common goals and to engage in a continuous challenge.

Riddle of deinstitutionalization politics

Basaglia's politics were more difficult to comprehend from the Yugoslav angle. What was obvious was that his political engagement was a pragmatic one. Purists on both sides of Yugoslav politics looked at this with dismay. For party liners, it was hard to swallow that he was integrating student radical movements into his practice and that he sometimes entered into conflicts with the Communist Party. For the student activist, it was that he was dealing with institutionalized politics. For both, cooperation with the right (DC) was scandalous. For those of us who accepted that pragmatism is a necessity and admired his ability to use the interinstitutional space, the practical side of it was the problem; the art of such politics still remained a riddle. Former Yugoslav anti-institutional activists never mastered this art. Even continuous cooperation with Basaglians was not much help. It appeared that the practical politics of former Yugoslavia were too complex, and the politics even more context-bound than deinstitutionalization itself. In addition, the Yugoslav protagonists were reluctant to step into politics, since this would mean 'dirty business' and 'selling your soul to the devil'. Perhaps it is just a question of good and bad luck. Was Basaglia simply lucky to be invited to Trieste by Zanetti? Was the 'perfect storm' (Hester, 2012) of an unseemly marriage between Thatcher's cost-cutting agenda and radical professionals a coincidental event combining diverse forces of the epoch or a historical necessity? Either way, the Balkans are an area where luck is singularly lacking.

Conversion versus substitution

The Trieste model of deinstitutionalization was one we have termed *conversion* (Flaker et al., 2015b), as the transition to community services involved converting the assets and resources of the institution for community use. In deinstitutionalization, conversion is less about space and more about usingthe resources belonging to the institution (e.g. using the same staff, the same financial sources, the power of the agency). In the Anglo-Saxon tradition, *substitution* is more frequent, and involves shutting down the institution and substituting it with completely new services, often provided by NGOs or by statutory services formed by local authorities (Ramon, 1992). Both models have their merits and flaws, and are seldom enacted as pure models, but rather as a mix or hybrid venture. Even in Trieste, some responsibilities passed to social cooperatives to bypass public-sector budgetary constraints and to develop new types of services. The conversion model seems more appropriate for the Balkan situation. It does not present the danger of loss of jobs; it is a collective, and precludes the loss of resources already invested in care.

However, international agencies, dominated by an Anglo-Saxon outlook, often impose reform on the lines of 'substitution'. This can include a British expert insisting that he never saw a successful conversion of an institution (in his words, 'an institution to transform itself!'). The substitution model is a top–down operation—a political decision must be made in order to perform it. This, too, is in line with the logic of international agencies, and it strengthens their already 'neo-colonialist' position and their perception on the ground. Resistance is an inevitable consequence and has happened on several occasions. The common Balkan legacy is of the semi-colonial status that various countries had in the Habsburg and Ottoman Empires. This mentality is that they obey the master to his face, but do it in their own way and in their own interest, but, if necessary, rebel. This may produce Potemkin villages to satisfy the master instead of achieving real change, which should be bottom up. On the other hand, conversion needs political support in crucial moments of transformation. This did not happen in the two most promising developments in Hrastovec and Osijek. Knowledge of the Italian tradition and the presence of Triestian colleagues on the ground, however sporadic it was, enabled deinstitutionalization in former Yugoslavian countries to withstand this prevailing top–down approach and enact at least some elements of the conversion model.

For bottom–up conversion, approaching democratization of the institution while it is still functioning is of a crucial importance. Introducing community assemblies, intensified teamwork, and other small symbolic changes (e.g. giving people knives and forks, opening up spaces to residents that were previously the staff's preserve) can be skipped in the substitution model. In the conversion model, such changes are vital in producing the 'practical utopia' (in managerial slang, 'creating the vision of the organization'). They mobilize the staff and the residents, enabling the conversion of their roles as they prepare to leave the institution. They help create a vision of a common future. This is what is badly needed, not only in deinstitutionalization but also in society at large, especially in the Balkans. What deinstitutionalization contributes is a vision of new solidarity.

Basaglian impact on Yugoslav deinstitutionalization

None of the deinstitutionalization attempts in the former Yugoslavia were led directly by Basaglia's former co-workers. Replication and diffusion (in Euro-slang, 'dissemination') of the deinstitutionalization occurring in Italy was, in great part, performed by Basaglia's co-workers (from Gorizia and Trieste). They assumed posts in other hospitals, which then started to transform into community services. When Pinel's disciples took up positions in regional hospitals, they resembled Charlemagne's 'comites' (who had spread the king's authority across a vast kingdom and diffused 'alienism'). This seems possible within a unified political area. There were practically no such instances of a Basaglian assuming at least a temporary resident position in some other country. There were examples of people 'learning the craft' in Trieste and then replicating it in their own country (Brazil and Argentina, to a lesser degree in Austria and Germany) (e.g. the 'Basaglia house' in Linz). This process was present in Yugoslavia, but to a very limited extent (e.g. the first group home in Slovenia).

More often, the general idea (conversion) was adopted (along with some practical solutions) and applied in a politically, culturally, and socially different setting (Hrastovec, Bosnia). In these instances, there was usually some mentoring support from Italian colleagues (Toresini, Reali, Mezzina, and others), but the ideas were integrated with other concepts, methods, and organizational solutions. These were partly imported from other countries with deinstitutionalization experience (in the early days, mostly from Britain) and partly invented on the spot, based on domestic traditions and local necessities.

This led to a 'second generation' of Basaglian influence, now merged with other sources of inspiration. Protagonists with new experiences were invited to support attempts at deinstitutionalization starting anew (e.g. activities of Flaker and co-workers in Bosnia, Serbia, Macedonia, or of Pfeiffer in Serbia and Albania). A number of projects were fuelled by expertise and inspiration from the Anglo-Saxon experience of deinstitutionalization (mostly in Britain, but also in Ireland and the USA). However, the 'spirit' of Basaglia and Trieste was still present. This was partly because of Yugoslav embeddedness in the culture and vicinity of Trieste, and partly because, by now, the deinstitutionalization praxis had become more or less an integrated whole, a body of theoretical and practical knowledge.

Some early attempts (Varaždin, deinstitutionalization of youth and children's facilities in Slovenia) were quite autonomous. The experience in Modriča was as autonomous as can be, built solely on the propositions of Yugoslav self-government and very general ideas of social psychiatry and therapeutic communities. Some of the deinstitutionalization was accidental, caused by war (Vrlika, Bosnia) or lack of space in an institution, but later integrated into a conceptualized practice and reorganization.

Camps were a consistent part of Yugoslav (Slovene) deinstitutionalization. In engaging volunteers in collective action—bringing a fresh, civilian attitude (e.g. taking residents out, staging cultural events)—they were directly influenced by the Basaglian tradition. They were also part of a tradition of voluntary work, usually with an action research component. The camps were used as the main tool in the first phases of transformation of an institution—stirring things up, enhancing democratization, and introducing new methods of working. They were also an important source of mutual learning, facilitating change as a process of such learning.

Open-coded approach

Basaglia had created a new and unique approach to people in distress. However, this was never coded as a special method—there is, for example, no Basaglian therapy, protocol, procedure. Yet, thousands of young people and professionals swarmed to Trieste to learn it, and among them many Slovene, Serbian, Bosnian, and Croat students. So what did they learn? If we were to ask them, they would probably reply that it was not the method, but the Basaglian or Triestian *style of working*.

This, among other things, means that the method developed was (by intention) left open. This has two advantages. One is that it can be developed and enriched according to the local situation, as had happened in Trieste. The other is that the approach to another human being does not become reified and decontextualized. The original Triestian approach had elements which we have elsewhere named and coded as advocacy, open dialogue, family conferences, whole-life planning, strength perspective, risk taking, crisis intervention, and so on. An obvious advantage of coding a method—giving it a name and making it a package—is that it becomes a commodity ready for distribution. Yet, Triestian colleagues never had workshops presenting such specifics. The hidden trap of coding is that closed-circuit methods, even if practiced in an open fashion, have a reductionist effect, losing the original force that derives from deinstitutionalization and empowerment. In Slovenia, there was a consistent effort to integrate and develop the received methods of personal planning and risk analysis. The aim was to enable users to express their desires, to be enabled and empowered by resources available to them or to professionals. By this, they could resist institutionalization or leave institutions and lead an independent life, and take risks, by knowing how to reduce harm and enhancethe benefits of their actions.

What was especially attractive for Yugoslav students was the Triestian insistence on the ordinary—a perspective of everyday life complemented by the critical stance to deviance. Giving a person an ordinary existence— money, a flat, a possibility to enjoy the companionship of other people—instead of therapy, was a major epistemological breakthrough: providing a person with a 'normal' situation, rather than making a person normal. Ordinary life, and not the clinical observation of normalcy of behaviour, became the criterion of the successful intervention. Only in the early 1990s (through David Brandon, 1991) do we come across the tradition of normalization, based on Nirje's work and the spectacular elaboration of Wolfensberger (1983). A deviant social role cannot be corrected—it has to be supplanted by enabling, by providing the resources and means to lead an ordinary life. Even if the Basaglian practical approach to deviance was not as methodically coded as Wolfensberger's, it had an edge that 'normalization authors' were struggling in vain to master: that deviance (madness) can be productive in problematizing normality, the liberating effect that real inclusion into society brings. Deviants pose riddles about what is mind (madness), what is property (theft), and what is pleasure (drugs). In the Triestian praxis (not just practice), it was neither a Foucauldian theoretical nor cultural issue. It was the practical everyday riddle—solved in many different ways. How will the community, relatives, neighbours, and friends re-evaluate their experience with the other? How can a person condemned to the role of 'mental patient' acquire as many valued social roles as possible? Will they dilute, and eventually obliterate, his or her *master deviant role*?

What was fascinating was the complete, unconditional faith in humanity; of everybody's ability (including that of the most 'disabled patients') to be human, to engage in contractual relationships, and to be him or herself. Students have learned that risks are to be taken. The fear of something happening (in Yugoslav services, the professional's responsibility for the patient's or user's behaviour) is the user's responsibility, his or her way of being human. They have learned also that when people are free to be human, nothing 'much' is going to happen. Basing one's professional role on the fear of eventual danger becomes redundant. In Trieste, they became free of worry and were able to set up the first group home, almost with a click of the fingers. Beforehand, they had discussions about how to make the group home work (e.g. to provide care and security). Then, it was just an ordinary thing to do.

We can conclude that Triestian and Italian experiences, and the Basaglian body of thought and style of working, were a major source of inspiration for Yugoslav attempts of deinstitutionalization. However, they were far from being exclusive, and were never fully replicated. Bits and pieces have molecularly surfaced in the 'hiccups' of Yugoslav deinstitutionalization attempts (e.g. Cerić remembering Basaglia). Our analysis could well lead to the conclusion that deinstitutionalization, as a scheme of action, cannot be exported from one place (where it has been successfully accomplished) to another (where it has to (re)start); that, as a whole package, it is not an easily transferable technology. The reason arises from both sides—its origin and its destination. There are intricacies to a singular experience of deinstitutionalization and its development that cannot be understood, sometimes even by the actors involved themselves, let alone from the perspective of recipients. The contextual contingencies at the receiving end always differ greatly from the source. In the case of Basaglia's proper work, it is also about receiving material from quite another epoch.

Ideology or technology?

Today, Basaglia's texts read as quite archaic and even cumbersome. Marxism and existentialism have been in demise; the politics have quite another face. The logic of service provision has changed for the better (rights-based, person-centred, holistic) and for the worse (bureaucratization, managerialism). Methods of working with people are much more eclectic. Deinstitutionalization now appears as a technology free (or devoid) of ideologies. The fact that 'it has survived the demise of its generative ideologies can be seen as point of its validity—the ideologies have fallen but the deinstitutionalisation is still standing' (Toresini, personal communication). This contention is partly true and partly false. It is an accurate description of what has happened, but it must be understood also as an effect of a neo-liberal ideology and regime, which professes, in post-modern fashion, the 'absence of ideologies'. Nevertheless, deinstitutionalization is still a highly ethical and value-based *praxis*. It is based on the moral imperative that everybody has the right to live with others, in a community, according to the ethics of non-exclusion; the right to live a life of our own and be a productive member of society and the community (United Nations Convention on the Rights of Persons with Disabilities: UNCRPD). The original notions of emancipation, contractual power, new professionalism, and so on, have not only been renamed (into empowerment, user and strength perspectives, participation, etc.) but have also been incorporated, embodied into the actual and tangible apparatus ('dispositif' in Foucault's terminology) or machines that deinstitutionalization installed on the ground. What we have witnessed has been a move from *theory* to *praxis* (in an Aristotelian sense), from discourse to apparatus, to concrete assemblages guided by real abstract machines.

There have been recent attempts to make a conceptual synthesis of deinstitutionalization (of which this book is probably one) (Flaker, 2015). The most well-known and widely distributed is probably the *Common European Guidelines of the Transition from Institutions to Community Care* (Expert Group, 2012). As a semi-official document, it is excellent, and it prescribes necessary action components for such a venture. It is most useful for planning action, for constructing a strategy at both national and institutional levels. When applying it to a concrete context, it has to be adapted and modified. For this, not only research but also theory is needed, a critical ground-level consciousness. Deinstitutionalization must be always alert and polemic, with the remnants and reoccurrences of institutionalization in everyday practice. Such a critique is needed to avoid returning to the original point of departure.

However, the required contextualization should not only be local or national; it has also to be global. Deinstitutionalization has been one of the very few achievements of contemporary social policy that has actually improved people's lives. That said, it has remained detached from the present social, cultural, and economic context, as a self-standing item. To link it to the (ever)-present crisis of financial capitalism, the rise of populism, and other dimensions of the present situation, a robust theoretical apparatus (and elegant platform of action) is needed. This means going back to its roots and reviving some of its conceptual basis, whilst also manufacturing new concepts that go beyond the narrow definition of deinstitutionalization. It means addressing the issue of what the new solidarity should be, how people can live together and exist on this planet. In this, deinstitutionalization has a lot to offer, and also a lot to receive.

Finally, whilst institutions were seen sometimes as a 'final solution', deinstitutionalization is an infinite solution, both temporally and spatially, and has many solutions to single problems to offer. Deinstitutionalization is a sublime process, creating a sublime community of humanity (as opposed to delineated communities based on exclusion). It moves the borders (limits) of human existence to ever-fuller living.

References

Basaglia, F. (1973–1975). L'utopia della realtà. Congrès de la Société Suisse de Psychiatrie, Geneva, May 1973. Published (1974) in: *Schweizer Archiv für Neurologie, Neurochirurgie und Psychiatrie*, no. 114/1974; and (1975) in: *L'Altra Pazzia*, L. Forti (ed.), Milano: Feltrinelli.

Basaglia, F. (1987). *Psychiatry Inside Out: Selected Works of Franco Basaglia*. New York: Columbia University Press.

Bazalja, F. (1981). *Negacija institucije*. Beograd: Vidici br. 5.

Brajša, P. (1986). *Bajnski dvori—neobičan razvoj jedne obične psihijatrije*. Varaždin: NIŠRO.

Brandon, D. (1991). *Increasing Value: The Implications of the Principle of Normalisation for Mental Illness Services*. Manchester, UK: Salford University College.

Castel, R. (1976). *L'ordre psychiatrique*. Paris: Minuit.

Cerić, I., et al. (2001). Rekonstrukcija službe za zaštitu mentalnog zdravlja u federaciji Bosne i Hercegovine [Reconstruction of mental health in federation of B&H]. *Medicinski Arhiv* 55(1, suppl. 1):5–25.

Cizelj, M., Ferlež, Z., Flaker, V., Lukač, J., Pogačar, M., and Švab, V. (2004). *Vizija posebnih socialnih zavodov.* Ljubljana: Skupnost socialnih zavodov Slovenije in Fakulteta za socialno delo.

Cooper, D. (1974). *The Grammar of Living*. New York: Pantheon Books.

Cooper, D. (1980). *Psihiatrija i antipsihiatrija*. Zagreb: Naprijed.

Council of Europe: Committee for the Prevention of Torture (2018). *27th General Report of the CPT*, 19 April 2018. Available at: http://www.refworld.org/docid/5ae2df814.html

Dolar, M. (ed.) (1975). Nova pota psihiatrije [New ways of psychiatry]. *Problemi* 13(10–12):154–6 and *Časopis za kritiko znanosti, domišljijo in novo antropologijo* 3(11). [Joint issue of journals on anti-psychiatry]

European Expert Group on the Transition from Institutional to Community-Based Care (2012). *Common European Guidelines on the Transition from Institutional to Community-Based Care*. . Available at: deinstitutionalisationguide.eu/wp-content/uploads/2012/12/2012-12-07-Guidelines-11-123-2012-FINAL-WEB-VERSION.pdf

Flaker, V. (1999). Proposed developments in Sarajevo. *Out Loud* Summer/Autumn:6–7.

Flaker, V. (2004). Il progetto Tempus. In: V.A. Lallo and L. Toresini (eds), *Il tunnel di Sarajevo: il conflitto in Bosnia-Erzegovina: una guerra psichiatrica?* (Dossier, 2). Portogruaro (Ve): Nuova Dimensione, pp. 115–20.

Flaker, V. (2012). *Direktno socialno delo*. Ljubljana: Založba /*cf.

Flaker, V. (2015). Deinstitutionalisation as a machine. *Dialogue in Praxis* 4(1–2):1–22. Available at: http://dialogueinpraxis.fsd.uni-lj.si/index.php?id=5&a=article&aid=45

Flaker, V. and Leskošek, V. (1995). The impact of a Tempus community mental health training programme on Slovenian mental health social work. In: S. Ramon (ed.), *International Perspectives of Health Social Work in the 1990s*. London: ATSWE, pp. 19–29.

Flaker, V. and Rafaelič, A. (2012). 'Walkout', Dialogue in Praxis, vol. 1–2, no. 1–2, pp. 119–131, [Online] Available at: http://www.dialogueinpraxis.net/index.php?id=5&a=article&aid=19

Flaker, V. and Urek, M. (eds) (1988). *Hrastovški anali za leto 1987*. Ljubljana: RK ZSMS.

Flaker, V., Rafaelič, A., Ratajc, S., and Toresini, L. (2015a). Ideas on deinstitutionalisation in Slovenia: report on the workshop in Dubrovnik. *Dialogue in Praxis* 4(1–2):1–22. Available at: http://dialogueinpraxis.fsd.uni-lj.si/index.php?id=5&a=article&aid=51

Flaker, V., et al. (1999). *Oblike bivanja za odrasle ljudi, ki potrebujejo organizirano skrb in podporo: analiza in predlog ukrepov*. Ljubljana: Visoka šola za socialno delo.

Flaker, V., et al. (2015b). *Izhodišča dezinstitucionalizacije v Republiki Sloveniji (Končno poročilo, verzija 3.2).* (študija po naročilu Ministrstva za delo, družino, socialne zadeve in enake možnosti, omogočila EU z uporabo Evropskega socialnega sklada). Ljubljana: Fakulteta za socialno delo.

Fuko, M. (1980). *Istorija ludila u doba klasicizma*. Beograd: Nolit.

Gilli, G.A. (1977). *Kako se istražuje*. Zagreb: Školska knjiga.

Hedges C. (1997). Gornja Toponica Journal: written on these faces, the torment of Serbia. *New York Times* 13 December 1997. Available at: https://www.nytimes.com/1997/12/13/world/gornja-toponica-journal-written-on-these-faces-the-torment-of-serbia.html?pagewanted=2

Hester, R. (2012). The perfect storm—a moment for decarceration. *Dialogue in Praxis* 1(1):27–39. Available at: http://dialogueinpraxis.fsd.uni-lj.si/index.php?id=5&a=article&aid=11

Jervis, G. (1977). *Kritički priručnik psihiatrije*. Zagreb: Stvarnost.
Jović, V. (2014). Psihijatrijske bolnice u Srbiji: Rezime. In: S. Biserko (ed.), *Briga o mentalnom zdravlju: Po meri ljudskog dostojanstva*. Beograd: Helsinški odbor za ljudska prava u Srbiji, pp. 44–9.
Kaličanin, P. (1974). Psychiatric protection in community psychiatry. In: S. Morić-Petrović (ed.), *Psihijatrija u društvenoj zajednici [Psychiatry in Social Community]*. Beograd: Zavod za mentalno zdravlje, pp. 11–35.
Kecmanović, D. (1978). *Društveni korijeni psihijatrije*. Beograd: Nolit.
Kecmanović, D. (1986). *Upotreba duševnog bolesnika*. Beograd: Prosveta.
Laing, R.D. (1959). *The Divided Self—An Existential Study in Sanity & Madness*. London: Tavistock.
Laing, R.D. (1977). *Podeljeno Ja. Politika doživljavanja*. Beograd: Nolit.
Loga, S. (2004). Appunti di guerra. In: A. Lallo and L. Toresini (eds), *Il tunnel di Sarajevo: il conflitto in Bosnia-Erzegovina: una guerra psichiatrica?* (Dossier, *2*). Portogruaro (Ve): Nuova Dimensione, pp. 79–84.
Maurer, D. and Murko, M. (2008). *Approaching Mental Health Care Regionally: The Mental Health Project for South-Eastern Europe*. Sarajevo: South-Eastern Europe Health Network and WHO Europe.
Milčinski, L. and Novak, M. (1987). *Duševno motene osebe v socialnih domovih SR Slovenije*. Ljubljana: Univerzitetna psihiatrična klinika Ljubljana.
Mlađenović, L. (ed.) (1988). *Alternative psihijatriji: materijali sa međunarodnog skupa 'Psihijatrija i društvo' u Beogradu od 1–7 decembra 1983*. Beograd: Lila ulica.
Peršić, N. (ed.) (1971). *Socijalna psihijatrija [Social Psychiatry]*. Zagreb: Pliva.
Petrović, A. and Mlađenović. L. (eds) (1987). *Mreža alternativa*. Kragujevac: Svetlost.
Ramon, S. (ed.) (1992). *Psychiatric Hospital Closure: Myths and Realities*. London: Chapman Hall.
Ramon, S. (1995). Slovenian social work: a case study of unexpected development in post-1990 period. *British Journal of Social Work 25*:513–28.
Rašković-Ivić, S. (2011). Deinstitutionalization of psychiatry in Serbia—arguments in favour and against. *Engrami 33*(4, Suppl. 1):2–10.
Rasza, M. and Kurnik, A. (2012). The Occupy Movement in Žižek's hometown: direct democracy and a politics of becoming. *American Ethnologist* 39(2):238–58. DOI: 10.1111/j.1548-1425.2012.01361.x
Skalar, V. (1986). Načrt prenove zavodov za usposabljanje v srednjeročnem obdobju 1986–1990. *Iskanja* 4(5):61–5.
Stritih, B. and Mesec, B. (1977). *Prostovoljno preventivno in socialnoterapevtsko delo z otroki. Rakitna—akcijskoraziskovalna naloga: socialnoterapevtska kolonija*. Ljubljana, Inštitut za sociologijo.
Stritih, B. (in Kos, A.) (1978). *Nepoklicno in prostovoljno delo pri varstvu duševnega zdravja*. Ljubljana: Inštitut za sociologijo in filozofijo.
Stritih, B. (1979). *Nepoklicno prostovoljno preventivno delo z mladino v krajevni skupnosti in OZD: 2. del*. Ljubljana: Inštitut za sociologijo.
Szasz, T.S. (1971). From the slaughterhouse to the madhouse. *Psychotherapy: Theory, Research and Practice* 8(1):64–7.
Szasz, T.S. (1974). Medicine and madness. Special report. In: *Encyclopaedia Britannica Yearbook*. Chicago: The Encyclopaedia Britannica, pp. 454–5.
Szasz, T.S. (1980). *Ideologija i ludilo*. Zagreb: Naprijed.
Tore, R. (2104). *Prava istina o psihijatriji*. Zagreb: Profil.
Toresini L. (2011). *Confinandanti*. Merano: Alpha & Beta.

Urek, M. (ed.) (1991). Subpsihiatrične študije. *Časopis za kritiko znanosti* 19:138–9.
Vodopivec, K. (ed.) (1974). *Maladjusted Youth: An Experiment in Rehabilitation.* Lexington, Mass: Saxon House.
Wolfensberger, W. (1983). *PASSING: Program Analysis of Service Systems Implementtation of Normalization Goals.* Downsview: National Institute on Mental Retardation.
Zaviršek, D. and Flaker, V. (1995). Developing culturally sensitive services. *Social Work in Europe 2* 2:30–6.

19
The Trieste model

Obstacles to replication in San Francisco

Robert Okin

Introduction

Franco Basaglia, the father of the Italian mental health revolution, has had influence on mental health systems far beyond the borders of Italy. In the United States, however, he has had almost no influence, and indeed no name recognition. Unlike certain countries that rejected his views, he was not snubbed or discredited, or even debated in the USA. He has simply remained unknown. In an effort to introduce his contributions to the USA, the Department of Anthropology at Berkeley hosted a two-day seminar in 2005 at which his ideas were presented by Peppe Dell'Acqua, director of the Trieste Mental Health Department, and Roberto Mezzina, director of one of Trieste's community mental health centres, In 2006, Dell'Acqua, Mezzina, several academics at Berkeley, and myself (as Chief of Psychiatry at San Francisco General Hospital) established a collaboration involving mutual site visits, seminars, and discussions to determine the feasibility of replicating the Trieste model in San Francisco or, at least, introducing some of the elements of that model (Portacolone et al., 2015).

This chapter traces the process of deinstitutionalization as it occurred both in Trieste and the United States, and discusses the mental health systems that developed in their wake. The Italian and American participants concluded that, currently, wholesale replication of the Trieste model would not be feasible in San Francisco and cities similar to it (Portacolone et al., 2015). The chapter however raises the question as to whether other American cities have conditions more conducive to the introduction of at least some of the principles espoused by Basaglia.

The results of Basaglia's advocacy were dramatic and can be seen today in Trieste. The mental hospital is closed; the stigma that so often accompanies clients, wherever they live, has been dramatically reduced; and clients are truly integrated as full citizens into the life of society. Many participate in the creation of life projects, jobs, and social relationships, and are actively engaged in public life. People with mental illness work and live alongside the rest of the community, almost never requiring acute hospitalization or long-term medicalized care (Mezzina, 2014; Mezzina and Danbiuea, 1995).

Demographic contrasts between the two cities

San Francisco and Trieste could not be more different. Trieste is a homogeneous, largely middle-class city, with virtually no poverty, very limited drug abuse, almost no poverty or crime, a tight family structure, a universal right to healthcare and housing, and a healthy supply of affordable housing. San Francisco, in contrast, is a city with an ethnically diverse population of 850,000, a large number of poor and disabled people, and stark disparities in the income and wealth of its residents. In the last eight years, San Francisco has surpassed New York as the city with the highest income gap between rich and poor residents. The existence of such a large class of extremely poor and disabled people creates a situation in which the demand for human services is intense, and in which the large number of mentally ill people are forced to compete for these services with other disadvantaged groups.

Contrasts in the process of deinstitutionalization

To a great extent, the obstacles to replication of the Trieste model, or at least some of its features, can be traced to the way deinstitutionalization was carried out in the USA compared to the process in Italy. Deinstitutionalization in the USA both preceded and occurred independently of that in Italy. However, deinstitutionalization processes in the two countries had a defining influence on the kind and quality of care, or lack of it, that clients experienced after discharge.

Deinstitutionalization in the USA was made possible by the discovery of antipsychotics, but was promoted by three forces, each advocating deinstitutionalization (but for different reasons). Firstly, clinicians were appalled by the conditions of state hospitals and recommended community treatment, but failed to recognize the extent of support and the kinds of services people with mental illness would need in order to flourish in the community. Secondly, civil rights lawyers were troubled by the unregulated authority of psychiatrists to involuntarily commit people on the basis of very loose criteria. They were able to persuade state legislators to enact more stringent commitment legislation. Many of these attorneys were almost exclusively concerned with preventing involuntary admission and fostering discharge of patients, regardless of their ultimate fate. Lastly, state legislators sought the closure of their mental hospitals with the expectation that vast sums of money would be saved, regardless of the human cost. Because of their interest in cost containment, state legislatures refused to reallocate sufficient hospital funds to create a community system. They persisted, even when it became clear just how many discharged patients were struggling, often for their lives. While deinstitutionalization improved the quality of life for people who were less disabled, others were discharged to communities that had no prior connection to them, were unprepared to accept them, were actively hostile to them, and were unwilling to finance services for them. Unlike in northern Italy, the services that were ultimately developed in the USA, with notable exceptions, were usually fragmented, underfunded, overwhelmed, and forced to cope even in the absence of a robust social safety net (Okin, 1978, 1982).

The predominance of fiscal motivations for deinstitutionalization in the USA was totally unlike the process in Trieste, where the goal of improving and transforming the lives of patients was determinative. The underlying principles of this process were far less radical in the United States where the values of the hospital, the primacy of the medical model, and the hierarchical staff structure were never challenged, but largely transferred to those services that eventually developed in the community.

Another crucial difference between the Italian and American process of deinstitutionalization was the political context. Advocates for the mentally ill in the United States never developed political allies, until very late in the process, when families developed the National Alliance for the Mentally Ill. This lack of broad-based support from American society had a profound influence, then and now, and largely accounts for the lack of funding from state legislatures to develop a community system.

By the time that deinstitutionalization had taken its course in the United States, the census of mental hospitals showed that numbers had declined from 550,000 in 1955 to 40,000 today. Deinstitutionalization was one of the largest social experiments ever carried out in the United States. Arguably, this along with its negative outcomes for so many, was only possible because its subjects were a poor, disenfranchised, politically and economically powerless group of people, with no capacity to object. Replicating the Trieste model (or any of its elements) would require confronting the entire legacy of deinstitutionalization in the American context. As described by the participants in the Trieste–San Francisco collaboration, this seemed highly improbable (Portacolone et al., 2015).

Contrasts in the social and economic infrastructure

Along with other cities, San Francisco felt the impact of state hospital closures. As the census showed a decline in the number of Californian mental hospitals, the number of people with mental illness living in abject poverty in San Francisco increased. The condition of their lives was grim before discharge, and was arguably more so after. A major reason for this was, and continues to be, the great inequality in wealth, along with the poor social safety net in the USA in contrast with Italy. There is no right to housing and no universal right to healthcare, much less mental healthcare. Any attempt at replication of the Trieste model would have to overcome this problem (Portacolone et al., 2015). The lack of affordable housing in San Francisco is particularly intense. This shortage has become even more severe in recent years, largely due to the changing economics of the city, and particularly the recent expansion of high-paying jobs in the technology sector. The San Francisco metropolitan area has added 400,000 new jobs in the last few years, but only 50,000 new housing units. Driven by the resulting demand, the average monthly rent in the city skyrocketed by 38%, from

$2,900 to $4,000 between 2012 and 2017. The average monthly rent for one-bedroom apartments in San Francisco is now $3,363 (Cote, 2014; San Francisco Planning Department, 2018). To put this in perspective, the average monthly Supplemental Security Income (SSI) on which most mentally ill people depend and pay their rent is approximately $800. The only form of housing that is available for this paltry amount is dilapidated single-room cccupancy (SRO) hotels in the poorest part of the city. In these rooms, usually with no kitchen and with a shared bathroom, residents with mental illnesses live alone, impoverished, cut off from their families, with minimal staff supervision, and almost no personal possessions. Nothing in their rooms reflects their individual identities. Most live in these settings for years, subsisting on a level of government support that barely covers the cost of these rooms, much less anything else. Faced with the choice of paying for rent, food, or drugs, some people choose the latter and often are forced to give up their rooms, no matter how inadequate. With no right to housing in the United States, many poor people living on marginal incomes or vulnerable for other reasons find themselves squeezed out onto the street (Hogan, 2017).

It is not only the dearth of affordable housing and the subsistence level of SSI that explains the degree of homelessness in San Francisco and would have to be solved by any attempts at Italian replication. Other factors include the lack of adequate services including hospital beds, the refusal of judges to involuntarily admit many disturbed people to acute care beds, the extent of substance abuse among individuals with mental illness, and their social isolation. San Francisco has the dubious honour of having the highest per capita homeless population in the United States, although many other cities share the problem to a lesser degree. There are now 7,500 people in San Francisco who are homeless. Of this number, 4,500 are completely unsheltered each night, with only 1,200 shelter beds to 'accommodate' them (Hogan, 2017). Of those shelters that do exist, some are cramped, poorly staffed, and sparsely appointed. Many clients refuse a bed even when one becomes available because of these conditions. People are afraid of having their few possessions stolen or contracting a disease from the person sleeping a few feet away from them. Others feel both humiliated and mistreated by staff and by the policy of shelters that leads to their eviction each morning. Where do they go? Back to the streets for another day of tedium, the elements, and the struggle to survive.

Unlike other people who become homeless for financial reasons, and who find their way back into some form of housing within several months, people with mental illness tend to become chronically homeless. This is partially because their functional limitations and symptoms often make it insuperably difficult to master the complicated application process for housing and SSI. Living for years on the streets aggravates peoples' symptoms, intensifies their suffering, increases their vulnerability to criminalization, and shortens their lifespans by an average of 25% (O'Connell, 2005). A proposal to levy a 0.5% tax on wealthy businesses with revenues in excess of $50 million was opposed by the Mayor for political reasons, but passed by the voters in November 2018 (Keeling and Brinklow, 2018). This would have added 4,000 new supported housing units and 1,000 shelter beds for chronically homeless people, but is being actively thwarted by the corporations. They are fighting the measure in court, despite benefitting massively from the city's resources and that it would make only a trivial dent in their profit margins. Any attempt at replication of the Trieste model, we concluded, would have to face the power of these corporations as well as the more general lack of political support for people with mental illness.

Contrasts in the mental health systems

San Francisco is not devoid of mental health services, despite the grimness of the housing situation. In fact, the mental health system has many of the same kinds of services as Trieste, but the values that drive this system, and the funding available to support it, are very different. The mental health system in San Francisco consists of a public general hospital with 40 acute beds, two 20-bed long-stay units, a very busy and crowded psychiatric emergency service, and several intensive case-management programmes that serve thousands of disabled people. In addition, there are several private general hospitals with psychiatric beds, five long-term locked facilities with hundreds of patients, a number of drug-treatment programmes, a crisis intervention house, several long-term supported apartments, a patient-operated cafe, a mental health court, and a team of outreach workers who provide limited support for people living on the streets.

Notwithstanding this array of services, every one of them is completely overwhelmed by clients with multiple medical, mental, social, and economic needs. Staff have neither the mandate, time, or space to care for people in ways that routinely occur in Trieste. Staff can spend only a limited amount of time with each client. They are consequently forced to limit their aspirations to helping them meet their most basic needs for survival, monitoring their medications, stabilizing their symptoms, helping them find or manage their housing, and assisting them with the very complicated process of securing SSI. Staff have almost no time to deal with the crucial issues of how to include their clients into San Franciscan society, how to help them develop life projects, and how to assist them in developing work skills or in finding other ways of spending their time. This is compounded by the lack of separate funding for vocational or day services. The vast majority of the vocational funds that the state provides are targeted to people with acute physical disabilities, who are likely to use vocational services to return to full or partial employment, which is the metric the state uses to measure success. Severely mentally ill people, whose disorders are often chronic, are routinely passed over when state vocational funds are distributed. As a result, clients spend their time in their rooms watching television or sitting on the sidewalks, often in a state of inebriation or drugged on methamphetamine, pot, or crack. The mentally ill in San Francisco may have an existence, but not a life.

In addition to the limited staff time, and the absence of a real social safety net, staff are also constrained by the medical model within which they work and the fee-for-service reimbursement system which supports this model. In most cases, the recovery model is accepted in name only. Services must be deemed 'medically necessary' to qualify for reimbursement and be directed by a physician who is at the top of the staff hierarchy and whose authority, after deinstitutionalization, was simply transferred from the mental hospital to the community system. This makes it almost inevitable that staff see their clients through the lens of symptoms and diagnoses. That clients are also suffering from isolation, grim poverty, and empty lives tends to be less appreciated, largely because the reimbursement system will not pay for interventions to address these problems. Integration into the fabric of society, rehabilitation, and the creation of life projects tend not to fit so easily into the medical model and the financing system which reinforces it. Consequently, staff are forced to limit their aspirations and interventions to narrower medical interventions. Helping clients live and work alongside others in society is often simply not economically feasible, constrained both by the amount of funding available and limits on the services it can pay for. An ironic and self-defeating characteristic of the system is that once clients have made progress in achieving the limited goals staff have for them, they are discharged to a much lower level of care, to make room for other, more disturbed clients. This imposes a ceiling on clients' lives that keeps them poor, dependent, and barely surviving, since the system entitles them to nothing more. The contrast with Trieste could not be more dramatic.

If the case-management and outpatient system in San Francisco is overwhelmed, the acute-care system is even more so, largely due to the lack of acute hospital beds. Patients who decompensate in their rooms or on the street are forced to wait, sometimes for days, in a crowded, noisy psychiatric emergency department with no design elements to soften its barren walls, and with no privacy barriers between the beds. The lack of inpatient beds has become even more severe in the last 10 years, since the Department of Public Health cut 25% of its original 80 acute beds (Nevius, 2016). There are, as a result, simply not enough beds on inpatient units to accommodate all of the acute patients who need them. Many people are simply discharged from the emergency department without admission, often back to their barren SRO hotels or the streets from which they came, and usually without any realistic plan for aftercare. Many return within a few days, only to be held briefly in the emergency room and then discharged again, often with the same outcome. Patients who are able to secure an inpatient bed are also often discharged prematurely, without any realistic plan, in order to make way for other patients pressing for admission (Nevius, 2016). The streets or a shelter bed have become acceptable discharge sites simply because of the lack of alternatives.

Compounding the lack of bed availability is the restrictive manner in which the courts interpret California's involuntary commitment law. Although the commitment law, as written, allows courts to involuntarily admit patients who are a danger to themselves or others, or are so disabled as to be unable to care for themselves, judges interpret the last criterion very narrowly. If patients are clothed (albeit in rags) and are living on the streets, but are able to find food in garbage cans or soup kitchens, they are deemed to be capable of taking care of themselves. The police, in frustration, sometimes take people with mental illness to jail simply to give them time off the streets.

The substance abuse epidemic in the United States

Added to all this is the substance abuse epidemic. This has changed the face of mental illness in the United States to a degree that never occurred in Trieste, and that would greatly complicate attempts to replicate its model. Many people in San Francisco turn to drugs in an attempt to deal with the harshness of the conditions in which they live and to assuage their symptoms. But this strategy usually backfires, for it dramatically worsens their lives, aggravates their symptoms, often increases their tendency to violence, and makes treatment of their mental illness more difficult. Addicted for years to drugs, many people present to the service system in San Francisco in a much more disturbed state than those in Trieste. The scale of the problem and the city's refusal to address it can be measured by the 1,200 methadone treatment slots for 22,000 injection drug users (Sorensen et al., 2007). It is not that the city does not see the problem or cannot figure out a solution. Rather, it has chosen to do almost nothing about it. If people with severe mental illness are marginalized and abandoned by San Francisco, those who abuse substances are even more so.

Criminalization in the United States

The same factors that lead to the prevalence of homelessness among the mentally ill also lead to their criminalization. This phenomenon exists throughout the United Sates. People sometimes commit serious crimes or, more frequently, minor trivial nuisance crimes as a result of their psychiatric symptoms, their drug addictions, the harsh conditions of their lives, absence of necessary care, and isolation from the fabric of society. Their SSI and Medicaid are lost as a result of their incarceration, and they are released with no provision for housing or services, and with only a few dollars to restart their lives. Obviously, many end up homeless again, only to be returned to jail when they commit another trivial crime. This is not just a problem in San Francisco. There are ten times more mentally ill people in jails and prisons throughout the United States than in state hospitals, and three times more than in state and general hospitals put together (Johnson, 2016). A study in 2006 by the Department of Justice reported that 64% of local jail inmates, 56% of state prisoners, and 45% of federal prisoners have symptoms of serious mental illnesses (Bureau of Justice Statistics, 2006). The Los Angeles jail houses more mentally ill people than any hospital in the country, and the largest 'mental health facility' in San Francisco is the county jail, where 15% of the population has a psychotic disorder (Hwong, 2016). For mentally ill people in jail and prison, the process of deinstitutionalization is more accurately described as transinstitutionalization. Many mentally ill people gain freedom from one institution only to lose it in another, much harsher institution—an illusory victory indeed. Data supporting this claim, while needing adjustment for population growth, demonstrates how much this is in fact the case. In 1955, there were 550,000 people in mental hospitals. Today, there are 40,000 people in mental hospitals, but 350,000 mentally ill people in jails and prisons (Torrey et al., 2014).

The criminal justice system, besides serving the purposes of punishment and refuge, serves another, darker purpose. It has become the latest way of segregating the mentally ill and excluding them from society, a purpose previously served by the mental hospital. Unlike the experience of Trieste, the segregation of the mentally ill has never been successfully challenged in the United States. This is clearly a major problem, and yet it is completely hidden from view—which, of course, is the idea. For mentally ill people in jails and prisons, the stigma of criminalization has been added to that of mental illness, poverty, and differentness. In contrast to the United States, Trieste has very few mentally ill people in forensic institutions. Those who do end up in jail or prison trigger intensive efforts by the mental health system to bring them back into society. Attempts at replication of the Trieste model in San Francisco would have to confront all of the factors, including the demographics of the city and lack of a real social safety net, that contribute to this use of jails and prisons to segregate the mentally ill.

Cultural values

The cultural values of the society in which a mental health system is embedded have a profound influence on the system developed. It is not only the structural elements in American society, and San Francisco in particular, that would make replication of the Trieste model difficult, but the values embraced by American culture. It is these values that largely stand in the way of creating the kind of service system that exists in Trieste.

The United States, despite its diversity, which contributes to its greatness, is quite ambivalent about the differences that exist among us. In certain important respects it places a premium on homogeneity as a value. This can be seen in our intolerance of differences based on race (e.g. slavery in the nineteenth century, segregation in schools and neighbourhoods even today), religion (e.g. stiff immigration quotas for Muslims), intellectual prowess (or lack of it), national origin (e.g. Vietnamese people during the Vietnamese war, people from Guatemala approaching our borders, illegal immigrants), and people with physical and sensory disabilities (Portacolone et al., 2015).

When we observe mentally ill people, what we see are the ways we are different from them, rather than the fundamental ways we are the same under the skin. We see their differences, not their underlying humanity. These differences blind us to the ways we are similar and make it difficult for us to identify with, connect to, and empathize with the mentally ill. This, in turn, greatly interferes with our willingness to share our own resources and those of the rest of society with them. In the political arena, we deprive them of the funding they need to do anything but survive. In what becomes a vicious cycle, starving mentally ill people of a decent life, keeping them symptomatic, impoverished, and isolated, reinforces how differently they appear. This makes us feel even more distant, different, and disconnected from them, more unwilling to provide the funding they need to escape their empty existence.

American culture places a very high value on the medical model. We tend to medicalize the mentally ill person's suffering, which often blinds us to the other causes of his suffering—poverty, isolation, exclusion from the fabric of society, social and economic problems, and failure to aspire to and pursue life projects in the vocational, social, and political realms. Even if we recognize these as problems, our exclusive adherence to the medical model causes us to minimize their importance and saps our urgency in addressing them. This occurs despite the fact that, in many cases, the person's medical symptoms are either expressions of, or are intensified by, the problems in these other areas. Supporting the medicalization of services is the fee-for-service reimbursement system which limits payment to interventions that are deemed 'medically necessary'. There is no stable source of funding for services that are 'socially necessary' or required for rehabilitation. The use of this medical model in the United States also has implications for the role and authority of the psychiatrist, for it is this professional, in his role as medical practitioner, who is anointed by society as the expert on the treatment of the client's medical symptomatology. While of crucial importance, this devalues the contributions of other staff who might have more expertise than the psychiatrist in addressing the challenges of integrating the client into the life of the community, developing life projects with the client, and so on.

For all these reasons, Basaglia argued that the person's diagnosis be 'set aside' or 'bracketed' so that the suffering person could be truly seen, first and foremost, as a human being, notwithstanding his symptoms (Scheper–Hughes and Lovell, 1984). The client's illness does not define him, and this being the case, the medical model, which operationally reduces the person to a collection of symptoms, is not particularly useful as the exclusive framework for understanding the aetiology of his problems, nor in planning and financing interventions for their solution. Basaglia did not advocate debunking this model. Instead, he regarded it as only one way of conceptualizing the client's suffering and argued that it needed to be complemented with a recovery model that more accurately and comprehensively described the totality of his needs, along with the planning and financing of interventions to address them (Scheper–Hughes and Lovell, 1984).

American culture tends to place a high value on self-reliance, independence, self-sufficiency, and economic productivity, whereas Italian culture seems to accept the fact that some people, for whatever reason, do not have the capacity to meet their own needs and have to depend on others, the family, the government. In the United States, these values became idealized, possibly because they were so important for survival in a young country whose westward push into unsettled territories had no structures available to help and protect them. People were forced to live or die by their own work, talents, and decisions. Having pulled themselves up by their own bootstraps, people came to believe that they deserved what they had made of themselves and that others, regardless of their personal, sometimes inborn limitations, had to follow their example. Helping others, except in certain restricted ways, was viewed as infantilizing and likely to create an unwarranted state of dependency, for which people deserved censure and blame, not compassion. The legacy of this is ubiquitous in American society. We tolerate and in fact accept the misery of people who cannot make it in our society: they deserve the life they are leading. Conversely, wealthy people believe they are entitled to their wealth, and this belief inspires only barely concealed resentment against those who need wealth shared for their survival, and who are considered undeserving precisely because they need it. The question asked by many is why should American society help those whom it holds in contempt for their dependency. As the terrible and impoverished foster-care system in the United States demonstrates, even the dependency of abused or neglected children reflects this hostile stance against those who cannot make it on their own. In fact, the entire economic structure of American society is based on these values.

Unlike Italy with its more progressive system of taxation, the United States has a tax structure that is designed not only to permit but to protect vast disparities of wealth. Though graduated to some extent, it is far less so than European democracies. Equality of opportunity has largely become an empty phrase and is contradicted by many of society's policies and institutions. It is no longer held as a real value, except perhaps in name. An important example of this is the way public schools are financed. They depend largely on local funding which, because of the de facto economic segregation of neighbourhoods, ensures that wealthy children go to the schools with the best financing and highest quality (Bidde and Berliner, 2002; Payne and Bidde, 1999). Over the last 50 years, America has become increasingly polarized between rich and poor. Democrats and Republicans voted to keep peoples' wealth within their families, primarily benefitting those who have the most wealth to retain, and their descendants. People have to earn the right to the most basic of society's fruits on which their survival depends, rather than deserving them just because they are human. If some people suffer, then too bad—they must be to blame. The idealization of an economic system that both tolerates and keeps a large proportion of its population in poverty contributes to the grim conditions of life that many mentally ill people are forced to endure. This is simply the price that must be paid to protect peoples' property rights, however irrelevant and empty these are to those who have no property.

San Francisco has a particularly strong tradition of ignoring the plight of people who are suffering, as evidenced in the protracted struggle to create and pay for a suicide net under the Golden Gate Bridge. One person jumps to his death every two weeks from this bridge. People in the United States, as part of their 'right to freedom', have the right to suffer, even die. The debates about paying for solutions to homelessness also reflect this. While Americans, in the abstract, believe that homelessness is a societal problem, it is often because people lying on the street offend our sensibilities rather than because they are suffering. Further evidence for this cynical conclusion can be found in the laws that San Francisco and many other cities have passed, making it a crime for homeless people to sit or lie on sidewalks, even though these cities have not provided sufficient beds to give them an opportunity to sit or lie anywhere else. In contrast, in Italy, sharing is an important aspect of what it means to be a nation and community, and the highly graduated nature of the tax structure makes this a reality. As evidenced by the universal right to housing, healthcare, and income, Italy embraces an obligation to care for its most vulnerable citizens. The mental health system can therefore concentrate on helping people deal with issues beyond those of mere survival.

While, in theory, the family structure is considered important in the USA, the degree to which it actually assumes responsibility for its most vulnerable members is often questionable. This is aggravated by the degree of social, economic, and geographic mobility in this country. This may have had its origins in the immigration of people from other countries to the United States, as well as in the separation of families that occurred when some family members struck out for the west early in our history. Economic factors have contributed, and continue to contribute, to this phenomenon as well. The result of this level of geographic mobility is that many very disabled, mentally ill people have lost contact with their families. Some families are desperate to find and help their mentally ill relatives, but the lack of societal support for these families makes this very challenging. Everyone is left to cope for themselves—families as well as their mentally ill relatives. Families in Trieste, in contrast, generally house, help, and support those of their relatives who do not fit in and lack the internal resources to become self-sufficient. This is facilitated by the relative lack of geographic mobility, and made easier by a social and economic policy that recognizes that such families deserve financial support.

American society is ambivalent about the value it places on choice and political freedom. Most 'normal' people are seen as having rights to choice and freedom. But those who are stigmatized, like the mentally ill, much less so. The need for coercion at various points in their lives is seen as mildly unfortunate but not a form of violence that challenges society's fundamental principles. Imprisonment, involuntary commitment for perceived dangerousness, forced medication, and seclusion and restraint are all used liberally against people with mental illness, and are often seen as legitimate and reasonable interventions. In these situations, violent interventions are used in the name of safety and are not only permitted, but seen as obligations of those whom society has entrusted with official power and authority. The large number of mentally ill people in jail, and the number of mentally ill people who are wrongfully shot and killed by the police 'because they look dangerous' are examples. Involuntary commitment, imprisonment for nuisance crimes, and seclusion and restraint are much less common in Italy. Every attempt is made to use interpersonal efforts to persuade people, calm them down when they are agitated, and give them real choices about their lives.

The United States places a value on the segregation, isolation, marginalization, and social exclusion of people it views as different. Segregation has a long and cherished history—whether it be directed towards the separation of the races, or the isolation of mentally ill people in jails, shelters, and nursing homes. It is viewed as an acceptable means of dealing with deviance and differentness. The inclusion and integration of mentally ill people into public life, where they can work and live among other people, are important guiding principles of the Italian community system. The closing of the mental hospitals was, in large part, promoted by Basaglia precisely because they were used to segregate people from society. Inclusion in all spheres of life was necessary as a first principle of the new community mental health system. Basaglia recognized that segregation and isolation were among the reasons for people's symptoms, and unless active measures were taken to prevent it, the phenomenon was likely to recur outside the hospital. Integrated living situations and work within social cooperatives were designed to ensure that this did not happen. Without these kinds of radically new social structures, people with mental illness could not be fundamentally helped, even if some of their symptoms could be ameliorated. What was the point of freeing them from segregation in mental hospitals if the new system simply recreated it in some other form, whether it be in sheltered (i.e. 'segregated') workshops or in mental health ghettos?

Model treatment programmes

The values of American society would seem to make whole-scale replication of the Trieste model extremely challenging. Notwithstanding this, San Francisco has developed several model programmes: case-management teams, mental health and drug courts, a client-run cafe, and a trauma recovery centre, amongst others. Some have won national prizes. Other cities also host model programmes created by local enlightened leadership, though in isolation from, and unaware of, the mental health revolution that occurred in Italy. Examples include Fountain House, which was developed first in New York City (Anderson and Fountain House, 1999; Doyle et al., 2013; Flannery and Glickman, 1996), the Village in southern California (Chandler et al., 1997), various programmes of supported employment (Drake, 1996; Drake et al., 1996), and the service system in western Massachusetts that led to the closure of Northampton State Hospital (Okin, 1984). The Program for Community Living, which utilized assertive community treatment (ACT) teams (Stein and Test, 1980), was first created in Wisconsin and then generalized to other cities and towns throughout the country. But even these programmes are limited in scope, and have not been as successful as Trieste in promoting the inclusion of mentally ill people into society. Nor have they been able to eliminate the need for acute and long-term hospitalization, or prevent the incarceration of people with mental illness. In Wisconsin, the birthplace of the ACT model, 10% of the general prison population are mentally ill, with mentally ill people accounting for 46% of those held in solitary confinement (Wade, 2009).

Even if San Francisco could be considered an outlier in the extent of the obstacles to replication of the Trieste model, the experience of other cities has proven how challenging it is to develop truly progressive programmes. The values in American society, and the way these express themselves (particularly in the thin social safety net, the use of the medical model, the financing system, and the demographics of the population in other cities), have so far proven too difficult to overcome.

Notwithstanding this limited success, the question remains whether there are any cities or towns with conditions that might be hospitable to the introduction of crucial elements of the Trieste model. Attempts might best be undertaken in cities and towns with very different demographic characteristics. They would need an adequate supply of affordable housing, a lower cost of living, a smaller drug problem, and the predominance of a capitation approach to financing of mental healthcare instead of a fee-for-service system. In addition, they would need a greater sense of community, where families live in closer proximity to their mentally ill relatives, and enlightened and progressive local political and mental health leadership. Whether these characteristics would insulate progressive programmes from the factors described in the body of this chapter remains to be seen, but Trieste, with all its favourable characteristics, may end up being an isolated success story in the extent to which other locations have been able to implement the kind of services advocated by Basaglia.

Conclusions

Basaglia was, and still is, almost completely unknown in the United States. Perhaps the United States, in its transatlantic isolation and, some would say, its arrogance, believes it has nothing to learn from the rest of the world. Or perhaps the differences between the two countries make the Trieste model seem irrelevant to this country. The latter explanation would appear to be the case in the attempted replication in San Francisco. The demographic differences between the two cities, the overriding influence of American values, the structural problems of San Francisco and the United States more generally, the drug epidemic, the thinness of the national social safety net, along with other factors, made it impossible for mental health leaders in the two cities to envision this translation. Although San Francisco has certain excellent services, with radical aims, that have improved the lives of many people, its experience demonstrates that American reforms, though significant, could not alter enough of the crucial structural obstacles necessary to fundamentally transform the experience of people with mental disorders. They may have less symptoms, but most are still living in poverty, deprived of meaning and aspirations.

Other cities have done better. They have provided the context for model programmes, but their lineage was independent of the Italian reforms. Some of these have had wide replication and express many of the same elements advocated by Basaglia. However, even these programmes have not permitted real integration in housing and work, nor have they led to the abolition of various forms of coercion, involuntary commitment to hospitals, criminalization in jails and prisons, and seclusion and restraint in emergency departments. Mentally ill people are still not treated as first-class citizens. It seems clear that a model of care, no matter how progressive, simply cannot be fully implemented in the absence of a hospitable context in which to embed it. This in fact is one of the reasons that Basaglia's model has not been fully implemented in the rest of Italy, beyond Trieste. Despite the robustness of its social safety net, and elements conducive to reform, other factors in Italy, crucial to its translation, have not been fully present. This should not discourage attempts at replication in selected cities in the United States. There may be places that are uniquely conducive to services similar to those of Trieste which could overcome the obstacles that exist elsewhere in the country.

Notwithstanding the challenges to replication in San Francisco, the Trieste model has much to teach us. It can serve as an important source of inspiration and validation of American experiments with model programmes. It reminds us that any progressive mental health system must be based on a belief that mentally ill people are, first and foremost, human beings with social and economic rights, not just civil and political rights. They have a right to flourish, not simply be free of overt forms of coercion. In many cases, their problems are not simply biological but are aggravated, and sometimes caused, by the society in which they live. Providers must be responsible for addressing the totality of their needs, not just their symptoms. The Trieste model is inspiring precisely because it demonstrates what people with mental illness are capable of when they are helped to lay claim to their economic, social, political, and civil rights; and when they are given access to mental health services that include a vision of mental health as part of life itself (Portacolone et al., 2015).

References

Anderson, S.B. and Fountain House (1999). *Fountain House, 1948–1998: A Transforming Vision.* New York: Fountain House.

Bidde, B. and Berliner, D. (2002). Unequal school funding in the United States. *Educational Leadership* 59:48–59.

Bureau of Justice Statistics (2006). *Mental Illness of Prison Inmates Worse Than Past Estimates.* Washington, DC: US Department of Justice.

Chandler, D., Hu, T. W., Meisel, J., McGowen, M., and Madison, K. (1997). Mental health costs, other public costs, and family burden among mental health clients in capitated integrated service agencies. *Journal of Mental Health Administration* 24:178–88.

Cote, J. (2014). Sneak peek: Mayor Ed Lee has a housing solution. *San Francisco Chronicle* 17 January 2014.

Doyle, A., Lanoil, J., and Dudek, K.J. (2013). *Fountain House: Ccreating Community in Mental Health Practice.* New York: Columbia University Press.

Drake, R.E. (1996). Substance use reduction among patients with severe mental illness. *Community Mental Health Journal* 32:311–14.

Drake, R.E., McHugo, G.J., Becker, D.R., Anthony, W.A., and Clark, R.E. (1996). The New Hampshire study of supported employment for people with severe mental illness. *Journal of Consulting and Clinical Psychology* 64:391–9.

Flannery, M. and Glickman, M. (1996). *Fountain House: Portraits of Lives Reclaimed from Mental Illness.* Center City, Minn.: Hazelden.

Hogan, C. (2017). Why SF's homelessness problem is still complicated. *The Bold Italic.* Available at: https://thebolditalic.com/why-san-francisco-s-homelessness-problem-is-still-complicated-c4b16e0a7107

Hwong, A. (2016). SF largest mental health facility—the jail. *San Francisco Chronicle* 30 November 2016.

Johnson, J.K. (2016). Criminal justice reform will fail if we don't fix mental health care too. *San Francisco Chronicle* 8 July 2016.

Keeling, B. and Brinklow, A. (2018). Proposition C, SF's homeless service tax explained. *Curbed SF.* Available at: https://sf.curbed.com/2018/10/18/17965810/proposition-c-sf-homeless-tech-tax-election-2018

Mezzina, R. (2014). Community mental health in Trieste and beyond. *Journal of Nervous and Mental Disease* 202:440–5.

Mezzina, R. and Danbiuea, V. (1995). Beyond the mental hospital: crisis intervention and continuity of care in Trieste: a four-year follow-up study in a community mental health centre. *International Journal of Social Psychiatry* 41: 1–20.

Nevius, C.W. (2016). Hospital services for mentally ill suffer drastic cuts. *San Francisco Chronicle* 2 March 2016.

O'Connell, J. (2005). *Premature Mortality in Homeless Populations: A Review of the Literature.* Nashville: National Health Care for the Homeless Council.

Okin, R.L. (1978). The future of state mental health programs for the chronic psychiatric patient in the community. *American Journal of Psychiatry* 135:1355–8.

Okin, R.L. (1982). State hospitals in the 1980s. *Hospital & Community Psychiatry* 33:717–21.

Okin, R.L. (1984). Brewster v Dukakis: developing community services through use of a consent decree. *American Journal of Psychiatry* 141:786–9.

Payne, K. and Bidde, B. (1999). Poor school funding, child poverty and mathematics achievement. *Educational Researcher* 28:4–13.

Portacolone, E., Segal, S.P., Mezzina, R., Scheper–Hughes, N., and Okin, R.L. (2015). A tale of two cities—the exploration of the Trieste public psychiatry model in San Francisco. *Culture, Medicine and Psychiatry* 39:680–97.

San Francisco Planning Department (2018). *SF Housing Needs and Trends Report, July 2018.* San Francisco Planning Department.

Scheper-Hughes, N. and LOVELL, A. (eds.) (1984). *Psychiatry Inside Out: Franco Basaglia.* New York: University of Columbia Press.

Sorensen, J.L., et al. (2007). Access to drug abuse treatment under Treatment on Demand policy in San Francisco. *American Journal of Drug and Alcohol Abuse* 33:227–36.

Stein, L.I. and Test, M.A. (1980). Alternative to mental hospital treatment. I: conceptual model, treatment program, and clinical evaluation. *Archives of General Psychiatry* 37: 392–7.

Torrey, E., Zdanowicz, M., and Kennard, A. (2014). *The Treatment of Persons with Mental Illness in Prisons and Jails: A State Survey.* Arlington, VA: Treatment Advocacy Center.

Wade, K. (2009). *Inmate Mental Health Care 2009–2010.* Washington, DC: Department of Correction, Department of Health Services.

20
Deinstitutionalization, the welfare state, and social engineering

Basaglia in the Swedish context

Alain Topor

> I have not created a new theory, but a self-critical practice and I do believe that we have to live in a kind of culture revolution. I think this is the only way to live.
>
> **(Basaglia, 1978, unpublished interview in Stockholm)**

Introduction

It would be quite easy to argue that the work of Basaglia and his colleagues had no influence on mental health policy, thought, or practice in Sweden. However, at the same time, the mental hospitals have been closed, and laws have been passed which guarantee mental health service users' basic citizens' rights. How is it that Sweden is one of the few countries, besides Italy, to have taken the radical step of closing all its mental hospitals? How can the Swedish way of deinstitutionalization be understood, and what was the impact of the work of Franco Basaglia and his colleagues on this development? Finally, we will look at how Basaglia's analysis of the mental health field can be applied in the present institutional situation in Sweden, and also in other high-income countries.

The Swedish context

Basaglia always stressed the importance of the context in order to understand and analyse the possibilities and consequences of changes in the mental health field (Basaglia, 1987a), and we will follow his example.

Sweden is one of the Scandinavian welfare states. Development of the welfare state started in the 1930s and is commonly called the 'folkhemmet' ('the people's home'). The material basis of this home project was the huge natural resources located in the country, and the engineering culture this created. In addition, Sweden remained (officially if not in practice), neutral during the Second World War, and so started the post-war period with its production capacity intact. A feature of this engineering culture is a social engineering view of how social and political problems and conflicts should be understood and solved. The main component of this worldview is that problems should be managed through rational analysis and negotiations between the involved partners, leading to reasonable compromises.

The Scandinavian welfare model includes a comprehensive welfare state, with a high percentage of the workforce unionized. It is based on the economic foundations of free-market capitalism. Some common traits include support for 'universalist' welfare aimed specifically at enhancing individual autonomy and promoting social mobility. Sweden is recognized to have a high standard of living and quality of life, and safe, solid systems in education, working life, and health and welfare services.

In the 1930s and 1940s, individuals who remained on the margins of society were considered as a threat to this 'home'. Because of their various personal problems or genetic make-up, they were unable to contribute to the common good through participation in the labour market. Here, we can see the downside of social engineering. People with different ethnicities (e.g. Lapps, Roma) were studied and catalogued, from 1931 onwards, in Europe's first Race–Biological Institute, at the University of Uppsala. Sweden developed a policy of encouraging individuals from the lower levels of society, showing 'problematic behaviours', to 'agree' to be sterilized. During parliamentary debates in 1941, the Minister of Justice took a stand on sharpening the old law from 1934 in the following terms:

> The aim of the law is to sanitise the Swedish tribe; to free it from the reproduction of heredity that could mean that in future generations there would be individuals who are not desirable members of a sound and healthy people.

There was broad parliamentary support for this move. In 1958, the Race–Biological Institute was renamed as the Institute for Medical Genetics, but the sterilization policy went on into the 1970s. Over 60,000 individuals (a great majority women) were sterilized and, remarkably, most of them after the end of the Second World War.

Starting in the 1950s, the welfare state became more inclusive. General reforms directed at improving the living conditions of the elderly, children, and different marginalized groups were adopted. The 'people's home' also built psychiatric institutions. In the middle of the 1960s, there were an impressive 36,000 beds in psychiatric institutions, for a general population of about seven million. Whilst new mental hospitals were built during the post-war period, it became clear that this was both an expensive and ineffective solution. However, it was not until the mid 1970s that the number of inpatients in psychiatric institutions started to slowly decline.

The Swedish way of closing mental hospitals

Deinstitutionalization in Sweden had four sources:

1. the total institutions' lack of efficiency,
2. the growing part of the population who were regarded as at risk and in need of psychiatric interventions,

3. civil rights, and
4. the desire to make psychiatry medical again.

There was no formal decision to close mental hospitals in Sweden: no parliamentary vote, as in Italy and its Law 180, for their closure. It seems rather that there was a political consensus that mental hospitals were not adequate, in the sense of being effective instruments to take care of people with mental illnesses. However, the closing of total institutions was also part of the social democratic people's home project. Its main goal was to secure both formal civil rights and also decent living conditions for all citizens, including the different marginalized groups who had been excluded from the welfare state's initial construction.

Total institutions for those with intellectual and physical disabilities, and the elderly, were closed prior to the start of the discussion about closing mental hospitals. This may have contributed to the lack of public debate when the turn came for mental hospitals. A new law on social services was adopted in 1978 and applied from 1982. This law stated the responsibility of the municipalities for taking care of housing and daily activities of individuals with 'handicaps', including those with psychiatric diseases. The efforts of most municipalities focused on individuals with intellectual and physical disabilities, leaving aside those with mental health problems. However, the Social Service Law sanctioned a division of labour between psychiatry and social work which, at least formally, made the downsizing of the mental hospitals possible.

The National Board of Social Affairs (NBSA) estimated that one third of the entire population was in need of support for psychological distress (Socialstyrelsen, undated). Thus, building more institutions, separated and separating from local communities, could not be a solution. Swedish administrators, psychiatrists, and politicians started to look for new answers to manage a growing population in need of psychiatric and psychosocial interventions. In 1982, the NBSA issued a report entitled *Psychiatric care without mental hospitals* (Socialstyrelsen, 1982). In this report, a panel of 'experts' discussed, rationally, the pros and cons of mental hospitals and the slow ongoing downsizing of these institutions. The experts developed an argumentation based, on the one hand, on a need for psychiatry to reconnect with other medical specialties to develop further its knowledge base and its practice and, on the other hand, on the risk that hospitals were 'hindering the possibility to find the best treatment, rehabilitation and care for the patients' (Socialstyrelsen, 1982, p. 15). They also held that psychiatry had no special competence concerning such aspects of everyday life as housing, daily activities, social life, and participation in cultural events (Socialstyrelsen, 1982, p. 115). Thus, responsibility for aspects of the social life of patients should be transferred to the social services, organized at a municipal level.

The potentially revolutionary thought of closing the mental hospitals was thus put in a context of saving psychiatry from responsibility for what were presented as the social consequences of biomedical illnesses. The argument was that social problems concealed psychiatry's original medical mission to treat the illnesses of the soul. Existing socially oriented services in mental hospitals and community-based services (day hospitals, rehabilitation services, supported housing, etc.) should be outsourced to social services in municipalities.

In an international overview included in the report, five pages were dedicated to experiences in the USA, to where two of the experts had made a study visit. The American experience was described as interesting but difficult to implement in Sweden because of the deficiencies of the American welfare model. The Italian experience was mentioned in 13 lines, and Law 180 (about the closing of the Italian mental hospitals) was described as 'the most radical decision about de-institutionalisation' (Socialstyrelsen, 1982, p. 94). However, the application of the Law was considered to have led to severe problems, even though it had reduced the number of inpatient beds. The report also mentioned that despite these negative aspects, networks of small community-based institutions had been rapidly created as a consequence of the Law. These integrated inpatient and outpatient care in the same structure. Despite a generally negative attitude to the changes in Italy, there was some interest in the construction of concrete alternatives to inpatient care. However, this recognition of aspects of Italian deinstitutionalisation was not developed further in the report.

Different reports from the NBSA published during the 1980s opted for a sectorized model, with preventive and early interventions, acute inpatient services in general hospitals, and community-based services for treatment and rehabilitation. Their administrative boundaries were to match those used in the municipalities, to facilitate cooperation between the two organizations. In reality, the sectorization of psychiatric care was used by staff with different orientations to conquer parts of the psychiatric field. At the end of the 1980s, it was possible to see a division between a psychodynamic-oriented, community-based organization and a more traditional biomedical orientation in inpatient care. This resulted in a 'revolving door' experience for individuals with severe mental health problems. Simultaneously, community-based services attracted a new clientele to psychiatric care.

Independent of these problems, downsizing of the mental hospitals progressed and, in 1987, five years after the publication of *Psychiatric care without mental hospitals*, the first Swedish mental hospital was closed (Figure 20.1). By 1997, all hospitals had been closed. The 36,000 beds have now (as of 2018) been reduced to about 3,000 located in psychiatric services in general hospitals. But, as mentioned earlier, there has been no official proposition or decision, on a national level, to close these institutions. They just faded out and were slowly replaced by community-based social and psychiatric services and psychiatric wards in general hospitals.[1] It is important to note that all psychiatric inpatient care was, and is, publicly financed. The dismantling process did not result in the creation of new, privately financed inpatient institutions.

To address problems caused by the gap between psychiatric inpatient and community-based services and the lack of initiatives from the municipalities, a new parliamentary committee was established. In its final report, it proposed just to 'clarify' the responsibility of the municipalities, already stated in the Social Service Law, by stipulating that it concerned both people with physical and mental handicaps

[1] The move from psychiatry to municipalities/social work can be found in other Scandinavian welfare countries, such as Denmark and Norway.

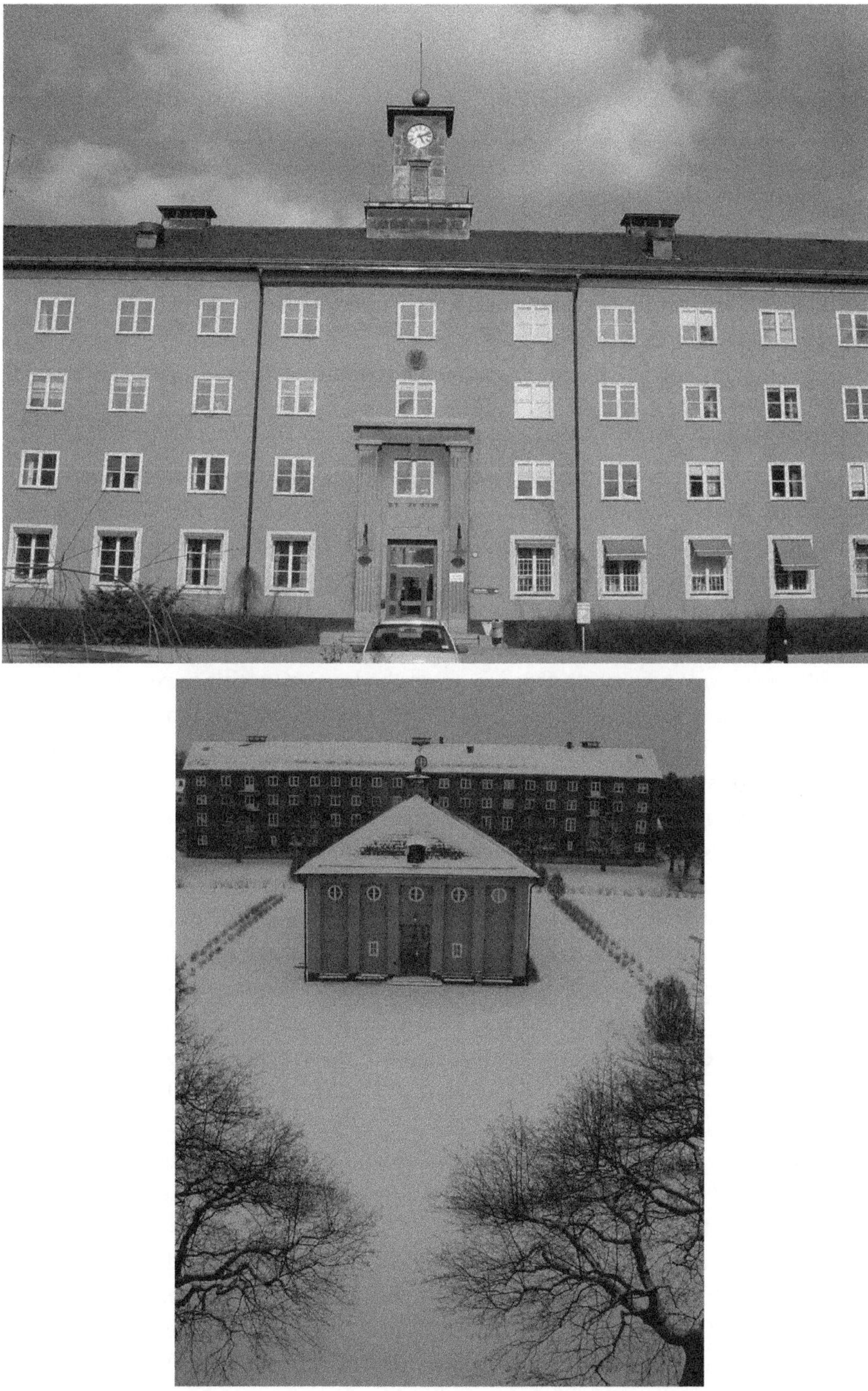

Figure 20.1 Beckomberga Hospital in Stockholm, one of Europe's largest psychiatric hospitals (with 2,000 patients in the mid twentieth century), closed in 1995.
© Alain Topor

(SOU, 1992; Markström et al., 2004). Thus, the committee did not propose any important changes but, of far greater importance for the development of specialized social services, tax income was moved from the regions (psychiatric care) to the municipalities (social care) to finance the creation of new services. In addition, about one billion Swedish crowns (about 100 million euros) were allocated from the state to support this development.

During this process, there were a few references to the Italian experiences, probably motivated by articles published in the English-speaking journals (Foot, 2014). The difficulties for different actors in the Swedish mental health field in studying the Italian experiences requires acknowledging the profound cultural differences between the two countries. The social engineering tradition characterizing Swedish culture had many features that help us understand this lack of interest.

Social changes were part of the social democratic project, and party officials were not interested in being challenged by representatives from the mental health field. To characterize mental health problems as consequences of the modernization of production and everyday life conditions in the 'people's home' was perceived as an attack on the dominant vision of Swedish society. To emphasize psychiatry's social and political roles was perceived as 'ideological' and, thus, contrary to the scientific credo.

Another difference between Italy and Sweden was the latter's existence of an influential users' movement. In Sweden, from the late 1960s, this movement held the closing of mental hospitals as one of its central goals. It managed to build bridges to both the Social Democratic Party and social-liberal groups in the bourgeois parties. It did this by stressing a civil rights' perspective and the need to go through the political parties to change psychiatry, without questioning the social role of psychiatry.

There was also a difference between the two countries on a broader cultural level. Basaglia's proposition to put mental illness into brackets could not be understood by mental health staff. In the social engineering model, there is an absolute belief in rationality and truth, and in the linear growing of knowledge. In Sweden, changes in the mental health field were never connected to a fundamental questioning of mental illness and diagnosis. Even as late as 1999, a leading psychiatrist, Heilig, continued to make use of the anti-psychiatry straw man as he wrote about 'Szasz, Laing, Basaglia and others who claimed that mental illnesses do not exist' (Heilig, 1999).

Neither phenomenology nor existentialism were taught in Swedish universities until the 1980s, even though Sartre was awarded the Nobel Prize in literature in 1964. Foucault could not even present his doctoral thesis in Uppsala, where he stayed between 1955 and 1958, because it was judged to be full of speculative generalizations. Another illustration of the cultural differences between Italy and Sweden can be seen in the translation into Swedish of only one of the books written by Basaglia and his colleagues (Basaglia, 1971). It was published in a collection focusing on critical Marxist literature studies, and its original title *The Negated Institution* (*L'Istituzione Negata*) became *Down with Institutional Psychiatry!*

Were there only incompatibilities between the two cultures, however? In reality, there was also a curiosity in some radical circles about diverse Italian experiences and political thinkers. The practical democracy practised in Bologna, with its Conselli di quarteri—holding popular meetings about local political questions in different parts of the city—was a source of inspiration. So was the historic compromise between factions of the centrist parties and the Communist Party, discussed by Enrico Berlinguer and Aldo Moro.

In search for practical solutions, Swedish psychiatrists, politicians, administrators, and members of the users' movement visited Arezzo, Trieste, and other Italian experiences. Foot has a point when he writes that 'Trieste became a "concrete utopia", a place where transformation could be touched, experienced, seen with your own eyes' (2014, p. 241). This utopian aspect, as well as the discourse around the institutions, was ignored by Swedish visitors. Instead, they concentrated their attention on the concrete aspects of the organization of care and the legislation.

An example of the complex relationship between the two cultures may be seen in the work of the Swedish psychiatrist of Portuguese origin, Filipe Costa. He wrote a critical, but far from negative, article about Franco Basaglia, entitled 'Franco Basaglia; a courageous reformist at the service of the state' (Costa, 1979), before becoming head of a psychiatric sector in Stockholm. He then sent all his staff away for one week to Trieste, to see the accomplished utopia. In this way, he wanted them see and feel that his own ambition to close the wards of his organization was not utopian.

Social engineering in practice

In a democratic state, a positive aspect of social engineering is that the technicians of knowledge execute what they have been told to do by their hierarchy. Whereas the application of Law 180 in Italy met local resistance, and change took a long time, the closing of mental hospitals throughout Sweden was accomplished quite rapidly.

Once the process of closing the mental hospitals was well advanced, the debate then centred around two issues: crime and homelessness. The risks of transinstitutionalization from psychiatric hospitals to prisons have been discussed internationally (Priebe et al., 2008; Konrad, 2002). This transfer seems to be the case in parts of the USA where 'in 2012, approximately 356,268 inmates with severe mental illness were in prisons and jails, while about 35,000 severely ill patients were in state psychiatric hospitals' (Lithwick, 2016). Abandonment and homelessness connected to the downsizing of psychiatric hospitals have also been noted in a North American context (Dear and Wolch, 1987; Knowles, 2000). Neither developments were systematic problems in Sweden. Although individual tragic incidents, including the murder of the foreign minister, have occurred, all citizens are guaranteed a basic income (besides having their rent paid) and access to public healthcare, lowering the risks both for criminality and for homelessness.

According to the latest statistics from the NBSA (2008), 8,200 people are living in group homes and different forms of supported housing. These homes might show institutional characteristics, but the persons living there have their own apartment and their own key. They are able to come and go as they wish. Over 15,400 are receiving social support in their own home. The trend is to provide more support in people's homes and less supported housing. Social clubs do not register their visitors, so we only know that most municipalities offer possibilities for social activities and for more goal-directed rehabilitation, such as Individual Placement and Support. Most people receiving different support from social workers have also community-based mental health treatment.

To understand the Swedish experience necessitates also giving attention to the question of civil rights.

Not only about mental hospitals

Most attention to the work of Franco Basaglia and his colleagues and Law 180 has focused on the closing of the mental hospitals. However, the Law was about voluntary and involuntary treatment (Parlamento Italiano, 1978), and introduced a cultural revolution in the decision process for involuntary treatments and, thereby, in our understanding of mental 'illnesses'.

Usually, with some variations between different countries, the decision to initiate involuntary treatment was taken by psychiatrists. These were considered experts on the needs of mentally ill persons and on when such persons posed a risk to others and/or their own life or well-being. The decision was presented as a purely medical one. After such a decision, the person could be forced, against his or her will, to spend an indeterminate period of time in a psychiatric institution and to follow certain treatment interventions. Thus, responsibility for a person's loss of their most fundamental right had been transferred from the state and the justice system to a purely medical figure (see Castel, 1976).

Law 180 changed this, and the change had important repercussions for the very status of psychiatric knowledge and, formally at least, for the status of the person/patient as a legal subject. According to Law 180, a decision on involuntary psychiatric treatment has to be made by a psychiatrist but has also to be submitted to a tutelary judge and confirmed by the local mayor. In this way, political power was placed in a superior position to medical power and its claims about judging the person and their social environment needs on medical/scientific grounds. The decision about involuntary treatment becomes a social and political question.

In Sweden, the question of civil rights played a central role, beginning during the first years of the 1980s with the abolishment of old laws about incapacitation and legal guardianship. A parliamentary committee was appointed to present a proposal for a new law about involuntary psychiatric treatment. The solution proposed by the committee (SOU, 1984), and adopted by the parliament, was to submit the decision of two psychiatrists about psychiatric treatment against the person's will to an 'administrative court', where a lawyer assists the person/patient. Thus, the patient is recognized as a person/citizen. Members of the committee made visits to Italy, and especially to

Trieste, where they could see the work accomplished shortly after the reform and discuss it with service users and representatives from the psychiatric care services, the municipality, and the police. It might be argued that, in many cases, neither mayors nor administrative courts are really acting as defenders of the service users' civil rights, but that they have been colonialized by mental health professionals and their ideology (Zetterberg et al., 2014). As Basaglia consistently argued, the application of a law is not built in the law itself, but depends on power relationships on a societal level, in this case outside the mental health field (Basaglia, 1987a, pp. 290–1).

Italy—Sweden: two roads to deinstitutionalization?

It is possible to see a parallel between the shifting of power from medicine/psychiatry/psychiatrists embodied in Law 180 and the restriction of biomedical psychiatry in regard to persons/users/patients. The central theme in these changes in Sweden was 'normalization'. However, it was not the person with mental health problems who had to be normalized, but their living conditions. As with any citizen experiencing problems finding a place to live or support to maintain it, these problems had to be managed by social services, without intervention from psychiatric services. In Italy, the mental health services often took the initiative to create cooperatives and different collective housing solutions. However, this entailed the risk of expanding the psychiatric field outside its formal competence. Efforts were made in these initiatives to integrate both individuals who had had contact with mental health services and those who had not, thus lowering the risk of segregation and marginalization (De Leonardis et al., 1994).

Differences between the Italian and Swedish approach include the role of psychiatry and psychiatrists in the mental health field. Basaglia and his colleagues wrote about how institutions were agents of the construction of what was usually understood as mental illnesses. Through a reconstruction of the patient as a citizen, they initiated practical experiences around the country, creating deinstitutionalization institutions in parallel to the closing of psychiatric hospitals (Castel, 1981; De Leonardis et al., 1986). They also worked in prisons and forensic institutions to manage the risks of transinstitutionalization (Konrad, 2002; Chow and Priebe, 2013). Despite all this, by keeping the psychiatric organization under the leadership of doctors, Basaglia and his colleagues did not challenge the fundamental power of the biomedical establishment. In an interview with Franco Basaglia that we conducted in Stockholm, he stated,

> Medicine and psychiatry are different forms of social control, but the political and social aspects of psychiatry are often overlooked. The knowledge of psychiatry is very small, but the power of psychiatry is important and expressed through the oppression doctors imposed on the patients.
>
> **(Basaglia, personal communication, 1978)**

The possibility of outsourcing important parts of psychiatry's responsibility to social work never presented itself to Basaglia and his colleagues. Could such a move be considered as part of the normalizing process, part of deinstitutionalizing practice, part even of a deeper shift towards a 'social paradigm' (Priebe et al., 2013)?

This question could be connected to Basaglia's critique of a purely technical solution to the contradictions inherent in psychiatry, which he wrote about in his 'Letter from America' (Basaglia, 1987b). It is at least worthwhile to critically analyse the new institutions/wards in place in general hospitals, and in what ways they differ from the old institutions. It could be possible to argue that most users do not stay any length of time in these wards, and that many of them are able to leave the wards during daytime. Nevertheless, it would be wrong to forget the symbolic power of closed institutions, even on those—both users and staff members—who do not stay in them but are in their margins.

Basaglia in today's context

Basaglia was aware that the consequences of the important changes he and his colleagues had managed to impose on psychiatry were dependent on power relationships outside it, in the political field. The 1970s were a period of societal changes, and Basaglia refers clearly to this potential when he wrote about 'the forces of revolt' against 'the general economic status quo' (Basaglia, 1987b, p. 133). The present period is less clement, and how the neo-liberal states will use the mental health field and its organization is an open question. The important contribution of Basaglia's work in the current situation may be the instruments he and his colleagues developed to analyse the contradictions in the mental health field. New contradictions have emerged that influence mental health. Here, we will mention three of them: the extension of the mental health field; evidence-based interventions and deinstitutionalization; and the new institutional landscape.

Before the 1990s, few people sought help themselves from psychiatric services. To become a 'mental patient' was associated with severe mental illness, stigma, and non-voluntary treatment. Today, we tend to define different human difficulties in individualized, medicalized psychiatric terms. This pathologization of normality has been supported by changes in diagnosis manuals (Frances, 2013). Pharmaceutical companies have spent huge sums of money publicizing their products and friendly biased research results (Whitaker, 2010; Götske, 2013). A culture of permanent self-improvement, reflected in the media and on the web, has resulted in an increasing number both of people being defined as having mental health problems (Kessler et al., 2005) and asking for psychiatric diagnosis and interventions, and of 'at-risk' populations requiring preventive and early interventions. Two consequences of this trend is that a diminishing part of psychiatry's funding and attention is now directed to the traditional users of mental health services and that a new form of self-institutionalization is happening (if we accept that not only buildings constitute institutions) (Brinkman, 2016). Of course, Basaglia and his colleagues could not have imagined such changes. However, the development of accessible community-based psychiatric services has changed the culture around 'mental illness', and not always as Basaglia might have thought.

We can see internal contradictions between the advanced practices developed in the aftermath of deinstitutionalization, recovery-orientated experiences (Davidson et al., 2010; Mezzina et al., 2006), and the bio-medical and new public management guided counter-attack under the banner of 'evidence-based interventions' and national guidelines (Priebe and Slade, 2002). The impact of these policies on deinstitutionalizing practices has not yet been analysed. However, it is clear that if the budgets of health organizations are dependent on the registered use of evidence-based interventions, then the possibility of developing deinstitutionalization's institutions and recovery-orientated practices is threatened.

External contradictions are manifested in the function of structures, practices, and knowledges developed in the community. These interventions were often created in connection and collaboration with the civil society. However, with the development of the neo-liberal state, their capillary presence in the community might be transformed into powerful forms of control of the so-called populations at risk (see Basaglia, 1987b). The tendency in social and health bureaucracies to standardize and centralize the collection of information about marginalized individuals risks transforming liberating practices into instruments of surveillance: a transfer of the panopticon from institutions of bricks and mortar to the community, through networks of micro institutions—a panopticism (Burton-Ernst, 2012).

This self-critical regard must surely be one of the most important parts of the Basaglian heritage. However, it is one of the most difficult to assume, as it asks us to examine even our own and our colleagues' efforts and successes in developing deinstitutionalizations' institutions through the lens of societal transformations outside mental health.

References

Basaglia, F. (1971). *Ned med den institutionella psykiatrin*. Stockholm: Pan/Norstedts.

Basaglia, F. (1987a). Problems of law and psychiatry. The Italian experience. In: N. Scheper-Hughes and A. Lovell (eds), *Psychiatry nside Out. Selected Writings of Franco Basaglia*. New York: Columbia University Press, pp. 271–91.

Basaglia, F. (1987b). Letter from America. In: N. Scheper-Hughes and A. Lovell (eds), *Psychiatry Inside Out. Selected writings of Franco Basaglia*. New York: Columbia University Press, pp. 127–36.

Brinkmann, S. (2016). *Diagnostic Cultures. A Cultural Approach to the Pathologization of Modern Life*. New York: Routledge.

Burton-Ernst, A. (2012). Deconstructing panopticism into the plural panopticons. In: A. Brunon-Ernst (ed.), *Beyond Foucault—New Perspectives on Bentham's Panopticon.* Ashgate: Burligton, pp. 17–42.

Castel, R. (1976). *L'ordre psychiatrique. L'age d'or de l'aliénisme.* Paris: Les éditions de minuit.

Castel, R. (1981). *La gestion des risques. De l'anti-psychiatrie à l'après psychiatrie* [*Risk Management: From Anti-Psychiatry to Post-Psychiatry*]. Paris: Les Editions de Minuit.

Chow, W. and Priebe, S. (2013). Understanding psychiatric institutionalization: a conceptual review. *BMC Psychiatry* 13:169.

Davidson, L., Raakfeldt, J., and Strauss, J. (2010). *The Roots of the Recovery Movement in Psychiatry. Lessons Learned.* Chichester: Wiley-Blackwell.

Dear, M. and Wolch, J. (1987). *Landscape of Despair. From Deinstitutionalization to Homelessness.* Polity Press: Cambridge.

De Leonardis, O., Mauri, D., and Rotelli, F. (1986). Deinstitutionalization, another way: the Italian mental health reform. *Health Promotion* 1(1):151–65.

De Leonardis, O., Mauri, D., and Rotelli, F. (1994). *L'impresa sociale.* Milano: Anabasi.

Foot, J. (2014). Franco Basaglia and the radical psychiatry movement in Italy, 1961–79. *Critical and Radical Social Work* 2(2):235–49.

Frances, A. (2013). *Saving Normal.* New York: Harper Collins.

Götzsche, P. (2013). *Deadly Medicines and Organised Crime. How Big Pharma Has Corrupted Healthcare.* London: Radcliffe.

Heilig, M. (1999). Återskapa den medicinska kulturen inom psykiatrin! *Läkartidningen* 96(41):4427–33.

Kessler, R., Chiu, W., Demler, O., and Walters, E. (2005). Prevalence, severity, and comorbidity of twelve-month DSM-IV disorders in the National Comorbidity Survey Replication (NCSR). *Archives of General Psychiatry 62*(6): 617–27.

Knowles, C. (2000). Burger King, Dunkin Donuts and community health care. *Health and Place* 6(3):213–24.

Konrad, N. (2002). Prisons as new asylums. *Current Opinion in Psychiatry* 15(6):583–7.

Lithwick, D. (2016). Prisons have become America's new asylums. *Slate* 5 January 2016. Available at: http://www.slate.com/articles/news_and_politics/jurisprudence/2016/01/prisons_have_become_warehouses_for_the_mentally_ill.html?via=gdpr-consent

Markström, U., Sandlund, M., and Lindqvist, R. (2004). Who is responsible for supporting 'long-term mentally ill' persons? Reforming mental health practices in Sweden. *Canadian Journal of Community Mental Health* 23(2):51–63.

Mezzina, R., Borg, M., Marin, I., Sells, D., Topor, A., and Davidson, L. (2006). From participation to citizenship: how to regain a role, status and life in the process of recovery. *American Journal of Psychiatric Rehabilitation* 9(1):39–62.

Parlamento Italiano (1978). L. 13 maggio 1978, n. 180—Accertamenti e trattamenti sanitari voluntary e obbligatori. Available at: https://it.wikisource.org/wiki/L._13_maggio_1978,_n._180_-_Accertamenti_e_trattamenti_sanitari_volontari_e_obbligatori

Priebe, S., Burns, T., & Craig, T. (2013). The future of academic psychiatry may be social. *British Journal of Psychiatry* 202(5):319–20.

Priebe, S., et al. (2008). Mental health care institutions in nine European countries, 2002 to 2006. *Psychiatric Services* 59(5):570–73.

Priebe, S. and Slade, M. (eds) (2002). *Evidence in Mental Health Care.* Hove and New York: Brunner–Routledge.

Socialstyrelsen (undated). *Psykisk hälsovård 1. Forskning, social rapportering, dokumentation och information. Arbetsgruppen för psykisk hälsovård.* Stockholm: Liber.

Socialstyrelsen (1982). *Psykiatrisk vård utan mentalsjukhus.* Socialstyrelsen redovisar 1982:8.

Statens offentliga utredningar (1984). *Psykiatri, tvånget och rättssäkerheten*. SOU 1984:64. Available at: https://weburn.kb.se/metadata/054/SOU_7262054.htm

Statens offentliga utredningar (1992). *Välfärd och valfrihet—service, stöd och vård för psykiskt störda*. SOU 1992:73. Available at: https://weburn.kb.se/metadata/188/SOU_8351188.htm

Whitaker, R. (2010). *Anatomy of an Epidemic—Magic Bullets, Psychiatric Drugs and The Astonishing Rise of Mental Illness in America*. New York: Random House.

Zetterberg, L., Sjöström, S., and Markström, U. (2014). *The compliant court: procedural fairness and social control in compulsory community care. International Journal of Law and Psychiatry* 37(6):543–50.

21 Making sense of Basaglia

Cross-cutting themes and unresolved issues

Tom Burns and John Foot

The Oxford symposium

A feature of Basaglian literature, which Foot highlights in Chapter 1 of this book, is that most, if not all, of it has been written by his adherents and those directly involved in the movement. As Foot found, with his historical research, access to sources is often tightly controlled and differing perspectives are strikingly absent (or tend to form separate bibliographies which rarely come into contact with each other). The one exception to this are the writings of Giovanni Jervis. These have generally been seen as the expression of a personality clash, a falling out, or even a betrayal, rather than treated as a source of alternative insights. This should come as no surprise. Individuals who have been inspired and influenced by Basaglia are likely to want to write about him and his achievements. In those countries where his ideas did not take root or directly influence practice, he is either unknown to clinicians or viewed as merely a vaguely interesting or marginal historical figure.

However, as this book bears witness, Basaglia did not go unremarked, even in those countries that did not adopt his teachings. He was a significant cultural figure on the international stage—taken seriously in social debate throughout Europe and beyond (see Figure 21.1). Why his ideas and practice did not become established in different settings tells a varied and illuminating story. What we find is that his message and movement were invariably considered; he was rarely simply overlooked or ignored.

Why and where his approach was rejected deserve examination, as do the reasons for the wide variations in its implementation, from country to country and region to region. Distrust of the 'biomedical paradigm' and anger with 'psychiatric hegemony' were key features of Basaglia's life work, as several of these chapters attest. However, it is not enough simply to blame 'psychiatric conservatism' or 'professional self-interest' for his rejection. Whether or not we agree with the reasons for it, the rejection was often closely argued. Neither was a local position on Basaglia and the Italian question necessarily fixed; it could change over time. Chapters 14 and 16 of this book (looking at the Netherlands and Germany, respectively) demonstrate this particularly clearly. Even if the initial reception did not generate changes in practice, the evaluation of his importance in published documents could change, as shown in Germany. Understanding the varied contexts, and the contents of the reactions and the differing

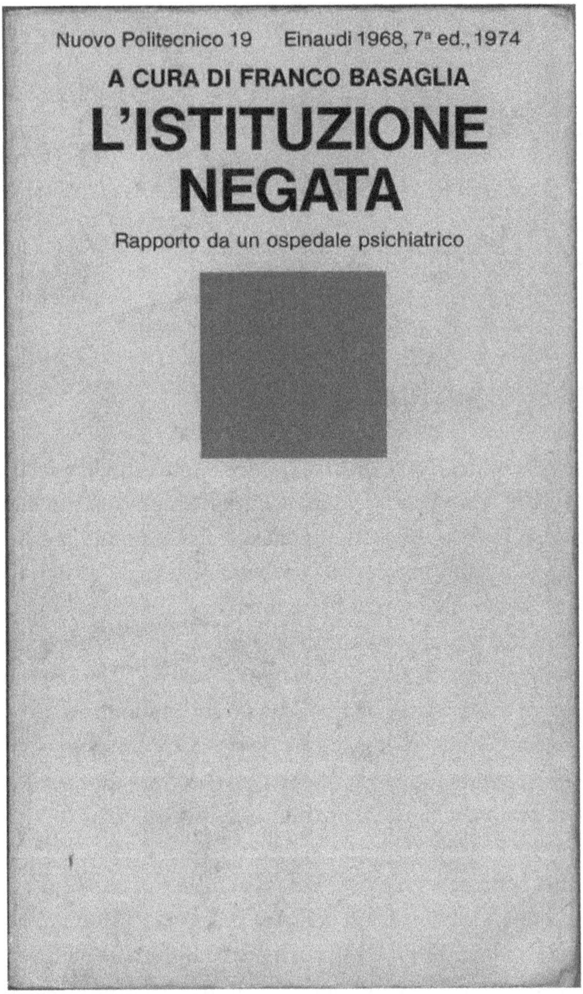

Figure 21.1 Cover of the seventh edition of *L'istituzione negata*, edited by Franco Basaglia.
L'Istituzione negata, a cura di Franco Basaglia, Torino 1974. Courtesy Giulio Einaudi editore.

receptions to his movement, have the potential to deepen our understanding of the man and his message. They also throw into sharp relief the inherent contradictions in his work.

It was for these reasons that we decided on this book and the symposium in Oxford. The chapters here describe these different experiences. Their differences in style give a flavour of these very different approaches. They range from the dry and analytical to the enthusiastic and celebratory. The contrast between a predominantly 'humanist' and predominantly 'rational' approach, the balance between emotion and intellect, and the tensions between the technical and the political are all played out in these pages, as they were in the symposium. All have their part to play in understanding Basaglia's influence and impact, and that of the Italian road to deinstitutionalization.

The format of the symposium was that each presentation lasted 20–25 minutes, followed by 20 minutes of discussion. Time was set aside at the end of each day to address unresolved issues, and informal discussions continued into the evenings. These discussions were cordial and productive, but it would be misleading to overlook the strength of feeling. There were some very real differences of interpretation.

'Adopters' and 'sceptics'

We have used a crude division into 'adopters' and 'sceptics' to help structure our reports of the issues. It should be stressed that this division refers to the content of the chapters—not their authors. Nobody travels to a symposium and writes a chapter about Basaglia without admiring the man and his movement. This binary division is, of course, an oversimplification. There was a range in the forms and degrees of adoption, as there was in the scepticism or rejection. The degree of adoption also varied both within regions, and over time. Each had its own unique character. Basaglia, we are sure, would have been gratified by this. He acknowledged the contradictions inherent in his approach and insisted that his work was not a template to be repeated in other contexts. There is no single metric for assessing the extent of his influence. There is no index of 'Basaglia-ism' to rate his impact on a scale from one to ten. However, we believe any observer of the meeting would have been struck by this division and easily able to allocate the presentations, as the chapters, between two such camps.

During the presentations and discussions, several issues kept recurring and a number of striking absences became obvious. We devoted a session on the last day to focus on these. For most, there is no simple 'yes/no' answer, but we believe they deserve careful attention. Hopefully, by setting them out here, they may receive more detailed and structured investigation by future scholars. We will start with the omissions.

Absent considerations

The role of primary care

Mention of the potential of primary care or family medicine in mental health is strikingly absent from Basaglia's writing and that of his adherents. He simply has no position on this. Nor does it figure significantly in the response to his position or developments afterwards. This would seem to reflect the movement's main concern with severe mental illnesses (psychoses) and with those who had been detained and neglected in mental hospitals. Basaglia wrote little about diagnosis, other than to 'place [it] in brackets'. However, both the literature and service developments suggest that his interest was restricted to severely disabled patients. Indeed, some of his critical comments about the ostensible self-indulgence of the French preoccupation with psychotherapy confirm this.

Strengthening the role of primary care in mental health has become a key priority for the WHO over the last three decades and it features centrally in most regional mental health policy documents. Post-1978 services in Italy have adapted somewhat to this. However, it is striking that these services have the highest rates of direct self-referral in Europe. Mezzina confirmed, during the discussion of this issue, that over 60% of assessments in Trieste were of self-referrals—not via a general practitioner. Similarly, he confirmed that psychiatrists conduct these assessments. Basaglian countries tend to have high rates of medical provision but have fewer highly qualified non-medical practitioners who might otherwise share this function.

Specialist teams

Basaglian psychiatry is characterized by generic services. Other than a clearly critical stance towards forensic services, there is little, if anything, written about specialist services such as drug and alcohol abuse, old age, eating disorder, neuro-development, and personality disorder. A Basaglian resistance to specialist teams is entirely consistent with his thinking. If diagnosis is to be put in brackets and subsumed in importance, then there is little to be gained by organizing teams along such lines. Italy was one of the few European countries that actively resisted the wave of assertive community treatment (ACT) services that swept Europe following Stein and Test's publications from Wisconsin (1980). The highly prescribed and technological ACT approach was described as 'non-Italian'.

In part, the Basaglian indifference to specialization may also stem from the extent of private practice in the countries where his ideas took strongest hold. There has always been a range of local practice, and some parts of Italy (Milan for example) have long been more comfortable with specialization. Italian psychiatry was as famous in foreign psychiatric circles, in the 1980s, for the Milan School's family approach to eating disorders. Maria Selvini Palazzoli was probably more commonly cited in the psychiatric literature during this period than Basaglia.

The model of care espoused by the Mediterranean and South American authors during the symposium was still firmly based on the local, generic community mental health team (CMHT). This was very similar to the early French 'secteur' system and the UK catchment area teams prevalent until the end of the 1990s. Whether the rapid increase in specialization of services since then in North Europe (along with the inevitable fragmentation and loss of continuity of care) is an advance or not is beyond the scope of this book. However, this reliance on generic teams, and indifference to specialism, remains a characteristic distinguishing Basaglian from non-Basaglian services.

Women

Psychiatry has a tortured and, in many aspects, dishonourable history in its treatment of women. It has been, for most of its existence, an exclusively male-dominated profession. This is true of much of medicine; indeed, most professions altogether. Given the nature of its work, however, gender cannot be simply dismissed as an unfortunate, but peripheral, historical concern. Psychiatry, and particularly Basaglian psychiatry, is an endeavour which is focused on human relationships. Among social relationships, gender is surely one of the most powerful influences. We would expect it to be intensively debated and explored. Yet it simply does not feature in Basaglian writings. Indeed, descriptions of the services in Gorizia and Trieste portray a system utterly dominated by male doctors, who make the decisions which are then carried out by female nurses and social workers. They portray a very traditional gender-role division in a very traditional society.

This total male domination of the Basaglian story is particularly surprising given the importance of his wife, Franca Ongara, to all his thinking and writing. Just how influential Franca Ongara was in Basaglia's work may be debated, but that she was immensely influential is not. She was a towering figure who went on, as Senator after his death, to play a crucial role in the protection of his work and legacy.

In the symposium discussions, it transpired that there had been a short-lived women's-only service in Trieste, in response to this situation. It was established against considerable resistance and comprised a team staffed entirely by women, for women. It appears to have faded out after a couple of years and nothing formal has been published about it. As can be seen from the chapters in this book, the Basaglian movement remains largely silent on the gender question.

Contentious issues

Anti-psychiatry

Basaglia insisted that he was not an anti-psychiatrist. In this he is not alone—Thomas Szasz and Ronald Laing also both insisted they were not anti-psychiatrists. Indeed, David Cooper (who coined the term in 1967) seems to be the only well-known anti-psychiatrist to willingly embrace the label. There were strongly divided opinions in our group about whether or not Basaglia is meaningfully considered to be an anti-psychiatrist. There is no accepted definition of the term, so it is inevitably a matter of judgement. Foot has discussed the various definitions of anti-psychiatry, and how these changed over time, in his work on the Basaglian movement (see also Wall, 2018).

The issue has importance as Basaglia was initially dismissed as an anti-psychiatrist by many of his detractors. What many of these critics appear to mean is that he denied the importance of psychiatric knowledge and the value of psychiatric treatments.

His writings are undoubtedly dismissive of the value of diagnosis. It is not clear if he even kept clinical records. In his defence, it is argued that by 'putting the diagnosis in brackets' he was simply emphasizing a holistic approach to assessment and care. Yet this point had already been repeatedly made, before him, by those in the therapeutic community movement. They emphasized the personal and social dimensions of care, without being quite so critical of diagnosis. Maxwell Jones considered diagnosis as only one part of an assessment, but he still insisted it was important and that psychiatrists had an obligation to be well trained in the art (Jones, 1968).

On the treatment front, Basaglia's writing focuses more on what should be avoided, such as hospitalization and ECT, than on what should be done. Medical treatments were, however, not prohibited, and Jones and Poletti comment pointedly on the high levels of antipsychotic prescribing they observed in Italian services (Jones and Poletti, 1985).

Neither diagnostic practice nor treatment practice provide clear boundaries for distinguishing anti-psychiatry. In our discussions, the presence of a radical stance opposing traditional psychiatry emerged as its core feature. Different anti-psychiatrists emphasized different areas of contention—compulsion, diagnosis, objectification, hospitalization. All, however, emanated a disapproval of the status quo and a conviction that psychiatry's errors reflected society's inherent contradictions. The solution to psychiatry's woes could not be found in improvements in the quality of practice but only through a fundamental rethinking of man's place in society and, perhaps, through radically transforming that society.

Oìsin Wall, who wrote on the influence of the British anti-psychiatrists on Basaglia (see Chapter 2 in this book), took the position that it *is* meaningful to call Basaglia an anti-psychiatrist. However, he drew our attention to how the UK anti-psychiatry movement rapidly evolved, during Basaglia's time away from psychiatry, towards an increasingly radical agenda for society. It morphed into a component of the counter-culture rather than a radical psychiatry movement. Basaglia fitted more easily into this earlier anti-psychiatry stage, but even then there were important differences of emphasis. Basaglia was consistently more interested in social and political relationships—not individual emancipation. His emphasis on solidarity finds little echo in other anti-psychiatrists. Basaglia also remained within the system, working to alter public mental health services, while other anti-psychiatrists were content with experimental alternatives. In this respect, it seems particularly unjust to 'dismiss' him with this label, as Sir Martin Roth did in 1972.

Hegemony or planning, versus crisis

A recurring observation by adopters was the resistance they observed from the psychiatric establishment to Basaglia's ideas. Indeed, this was noted in both adopting and rejecting regions. In some presentations, this was attributed simply to medical conservatism –a suspicion of new ideas and a preference for accepted and familiar practice. However, it was more often seen as a defensive reaction to protect privilege and authority, expressed through the language of Gramscian Marxism as 'hegemony'. Whether Basaglia was a Gramscian Marxist, or indeed any form of Marxist, is taken up later. This resistance was the subject of considerable debate. What was clear is that such professional resistance is not entirely cerebral. The language used in these counter-arguments often testified to strong feelings, sometimes hostile, but most often referred to as 'anxiety' or 'fear'.

How convincing is this position? The UK experience was used to explore it. Tom Burns (author of Chapter 11 in this book) was an active clinician at the time of the UK's rejection, and recalled no atmosphere of professional anxiety. There was no strong professional concern other than that expressed in the notorious articles by Jones and Poletti. If anything, the atmosphere was one of irritation or exasperation. not one of professional insecurity. This should come as no surprise after a decade of scathing attacks from the anti-psychiatrists had left the psychiatric establishment essentially intact.

A clarification which arose in this discussion centred on cultural differences in response to crisis. The Italians (and, by extension, Southern Europeans more widely and also South Americans), it was proposed, are quite used to crisis in their political and cultural life. They view it as an opportunity for change and development. Northern Europeans, on the other hand, place a greater emphasis on stability and predictability. They generally view crises with disquiet. An alternative (and more convincing) explanation of the anxiety driving the rejection of Basaglia could be a North European, broadly anglophone, concern with responsibility and order, and technical solutions, and a rejection of overwhelming theory.

Simon Sinclair's anthropological study of medical training in the UK (1997) vividly describes it as a prolonged apprenticeship, occupied with moulding and transmitting values and professional attitudes as much as with transmitting knowledge. A key feature of this training is the need to contain patient's anxieties and shoulder responsibility, even in highly uncertain situations. While the language of modern medicine is couched in terms of partnership and autonomy, core professional values still owe much to paternalism. Such a mindset would recoil at the prospect of simply 'freeing' a patient with longstanding problems and disabilities from hospital. It would demand a carefully considered discharge plan. It would view any failure to do so as an abrogation of the first Hippocratic principle of 'do no harm'. So the anxiety felt by the psychiatric establishment may be more about failing to live up to their internalized professional ethics, rather than any threat of loss of social power and status. What to Basaglians is humane and progressive might look to some North Europeans like recklessness. What to the North Europeans is responsible and rational might look to Basaglians like paternalistic timidity. These cultural and institutional differences need to be explored more widely in order to provide a basis for further research.

Social capital and implementation

All three Italian authors acknowledge the variation in implementation of Basaglia's reforms across their country. Trieste is held up as the example of full and pure implementation, and other northern cities (Bologna, Ferrara) bring their own interpretation and style. In their 1985 paper, Jones and Poletti commented that implementation was far less evident as they moved south and 'problems were more in evidence'. This has generally been interpreted as a reflection of the greater poverty and overall lack of resources in the Italian south compared to the very wealthy north—a recurrent theme in Italian politics.

There was consensus that this is, indeed, a significant aspect of the poorer implementation—but not a full explanation. It was suggested that the differences between such northern regions as Emilia-Romagna and Tuscany and the southern ones of Calabria and Sicily lie as much in their cultures and histories. The northern and central regions, with their historical links to city states, have a tradition of social cohesion and civic solidarity which has evolved over a millennium. In the south, this is not always the case. Here, the culture is more dominated by lower levels of trust and, it has been argued, less commitment to civic organizations and laws. Robert Putnam's seminal work *Making Democracy Work: Civic Traditions in Modern Italy* (1993) describes the failure of local government in much of southern Italy. He argues that this is related not to poverty, or even education, but to the relative lack of social capital.

However, there were important examples of psychiatric reform in southern Italy, which have not received the attention they deserve (including in this volume). One example is the life and work of Sergio Piro who was based, for much of his career, in Naples. The same can be said for the extraordinary success of the movement in Perugia, which is generally unremarked apart from Foot's opinion and in local studies (Foot, 2015). In these two places (and elsewhere in Italy, such as in Arezzo and Ferrara), the practice and theoretical reflections of psychiatrists and activists matched, and often went beyond, that linked directly to Basaglia in Gorizia and Trieste. The international fame of Trieste, and the global reach of Basaglia's writings and experiences, are also linked to specific social and cultural factors, as well as factors related to the media. But Basaglia was by no means the only show in town.

The implementation of closure and deinstitutionalization was patchy, even across much of central and northern parts of Italy. In one northern city, in the 1990s, patients were simply moved, en masse, to care homes, when the final closure date for asylums was set. Social capital provides some of the explanation, but much else—politics, the strength of the movement, resources, and psychiatric traditions—had their impact. Nonetheless, the Basaglian approach does appear to require high levels of social capital in terms of social solidarity, welfare provision, tolerance, plus civic and political activity and engagement. It is unlikely that such an approach would thrive in areas where social capital is lacking. This reliance on strong social capital may have important implications for the continuing impact of his approach in an era of increasing neo-liberalism with its emphasis on individualism, mobility, and competition. Robert Okin's chapter on the USA (see Chapter 19 in this book) vividly demonstrates the impossibility of introducing the Basaglian approach in the absence of even minimal social solidarity or capital.

Ideologue or not?

Whether Basaglia (and the movement as a whole, which was always highly divided internally) was over-ideological or not was hotly debated. The criticism that his approach was too ideological, or indeed too political, was often raised by his opponents as a reason for scepticism. Certainly, his statements about the political nature of diagnosis were taken, by such critics, as reflecting a preoccupation with ideology rather than patient welfare. The alternative view advanced was that Basaglia was intensely pragmatic: he was always focused on process and negotiation, rather than proposing an ideology or model. On many occasions, he insisted that those listening to him should *not* try and emulate what he had done in Trieste: 'the Italian experience is not a model for elsewhere' (Basaglia, 1980). But in reality Gorizia, Trieste, and other places did become models for many. Certainly, the power of Trieste was (and continues to be) in the observation of what went on there. Basaglia exhorted those who were interested to visit and experience it ('viene a vedere'), rather than follow some form of manual. The movement had a complicated relationship with ideology, and with the political left as a whole.

There appears to be a conflict here between the practice of Basaglianism and what was often written and said about it. The practice emphasizes engagement, fluidity, and freedom. The writing is undeniably ideological on the whole, and much appears extremely dated when read today. Those actively engaged in the practice experience the former and consider the criticism of excessive ideology unwarranted. Those observing from outside can hardly avoid the ideology. For many, this moral and ideological stand promoting justice and inclusion is the very attraction of the approach. Much will depend on whether you focus on the 'concrete' or the 'utopia' when judging the impact of the movement.

Was Basaglia a Marxist?

Basaglia's perceived Marxism was undoubtedly a black mark against him in the USA and in some European and South American contexts. His followers use the language of Gramscian Marxism liberally: an attack on psychiatric 'hegemony' is a regular feature of their writings. Yet, remarkably, Basaglia never used the term 'Marxism' in his writings and he was never a member of a Communist Party. He was briefly a member of the Italian Socialist Party, but not politically active in his later years. Communist officials strongly supported the movement in many Italian cities, but in other places they were hostile to Basaglian approaches. By the time Law 180 was passed in 1978, the Communist Party had developed into a strong supporter of reform. Basaglia was certainly a man on the left and—since his death in particular—he has developed into a hero figure for many veterans of the movement.

It is hard to ignore the left-wing tone of most of Basaglia's thinking and action. His emphasis on the social determinants of diagnosis, and his comments at the 1964 London conference (where he characterized patients as those deemed non-productive in economic terms, with exclusion the consequence) are Marxist in all but name. Economic forces, and the use by powerful groups to obtain personal benefit from them at the cost of those without power, are central to the Basaglian movement and the concept of *emarginazione*. While it was contested at our Oxford symposium that he was ever a Marxist, it is undeniable that his message is profoundly left-wing. This was much of its attraction, and particularly so in the context of the movements of 1968 and the 1970s, in Italy and elsewhere. But it should also be underlined that much of Basaglia's practice was borrowed and adapted from experiences elsewhere that he witnessed or read about. Dingleton in Scotland is one example. In addition, his thinking reflected his reading of the literature relating to post-war experiences in France, and Goffman's work on asylums (Goffman, 1961). He also derived much of his thinking from phenomenological philosophy which guided his approach, above all, to patient subjectivity and the asylum.

There is no doubt that, for a time, Basaglia and his circle became attracted by Mao's approach to Marxism. In particular, the emphasis on tolerance for multiple takes on socialism ('let a thousand flowers bloom') appealed, as did the idea of 'barefoot doctors', immersed within society, and the concept of a cultural revolution.

Areas of definition

Therapeutic communities

Two rather technical issues also presented themselves repeatedly in discussion and deserve attention. 'Therapeutic community' is a term much used in Basaglian writings. It is obvious that this term is used rather differently by Italian and anglophone writers. The term also has differing meanings between the UK and USA. In the UK, therapeutic communities are assumed to be 'democratic therapeutic communities'. These were first described by the analyst Tom Main in the late 1940s and developed by Maxwell Jones in the treatment of war neurosis and, subsequently, of personality disorder. These emphasize the group living–learning situation as the central treatment, and are characterized by informality, joint activities, and open reflection on experiences within groups. In the USA, they became widely used in drug and alcohol rehabilitation, and while sharing much of the group ethos and emphasis on joint activities, they are much more rigid and often quite punitive. Italians generally use the term much more loosely to mean any group residential situation that is not coercive (e.g. hostels, group homes). Being alert to these differences in usage should help avoid misunderstanding.

Basaglia adopted the term in Gorizia, after visiting Dingleton, but within his 'therapeutic community' the meetings took on a more radical and patient-run form. Nonetheless, there were many similarities—at least in formal terms—between the therapeutic community of Gorizia and that seen in the UK. In Trieste, Basaglia abandoned this approach to concentrate on the speedy deinstitutionalization of the entire asylum.

What is a mental hospital?

When can one say that all the mental hospitals in a country are closed? This apparently simple question proved to be anything but straightforward. All the countries reported in this book have residential psychiatric establishments, and all allow patients to be compulsorily detained in them. In Italy, there are 15 beds in diagnosis and cure wards attached to district general hospitals. This figure varies greatly in practice as it is set by regional health authorities, who run mental healthcare in Italy. If there were 100 beds instead of 15, would this then constitute a mental hospital? Or if the beds were standalone and separate from the general hospital, but still only 15 in total, would this then be a small mental hospital? What exactly constitutes a mental hospital and distinguishes it from a psychiatric inpatient unit?

Italy and Sweden claim to have closed all their mental hospitals. Yet Sweden has more psychiatric beds and more compulsory admissions per 100,000 population than Ireland, which does not make any such claim. It is clear that there is a range of institutional settings which are linked to contemporary mental healthcare. Practices vary greatly from place to place, within and between countries. The Italian asylums took over 20 years to be finally closed, but wards remain and certain practices—such as mechanical restraints—have returned in many places.

Absolute agreement could not be reached about what constitutes a mental hospital, but a general consensus emerged about some key features, none of which were individually definitive. However, the likelihood of an institution being called a mental hospital increased as each of these features was confirmed.

Firstly, a mental hospital is one that only deals with psychiatric patients. It is not a part (even if a very large part) of a general hospital. This distinction is still far from simple. What about a large psychiatric unit that abuts a general hospital or is in its grounds? What about a predominantly psychiatric hospital that has some medical facilities in its grounds (perhaps utilizing buildings no longer needed)?

Secondly, a mental hospital is big. Small psychiatric units, even if standalone, were unlikely to be considered as mental hospitals. In the UK, it was recommended that new psychiatric units should house no more than a total of about 90–100 patients distributed in up to five wards. Above that it was assumed that they would be increasingly institutional in character. In practice, this is often exceeded; so is a 150-bedded unit a mental hospital? What if those 150 beds included two or three large specialist facilities, such as an eating disorder ward or dementia assessment unit, in addition to the routine beds? Most at the symposium believed that very large institutions of several hundred patients should be called mental hospitals. However, the cut-off point is not straightforward.

Thirdly, a mental hospital is one predominantly housing long-stay patients. When Basaglia arrived in Gorizia and Trieste. a large number of the patients had been there months or years, and many expected never to leave. This situation has changed radically across virtually all of Europe. There is a variation in the provision of long-stay accommodation, but most countries have some for forensic patients. Many also provide for the small group of highly resistant psychosis and developmental disorder patients who seem impossible to support in the community. Does a 30-bedded secure unit with patients admitted for several years constitute a mental hospital?

Psychiatric provision in many countries still retains units which include some of these characteristics. Generally, they do not manifest all three; there are few large, long-stay institutions left. However, whether or not a country has closed all its mental hospitals is likely to remain a point of contention for some time to come. The large, nineteenth-century, forbidding asylums which dominated mental healthcare for so long are, in most countries, a thing of the past. But questions of institutionalization, medication, restriction on movement, locked and unlocked wards, forced treatment, and patient input remain pertinent and relevant.

Final words

Basaglia's desire, and that of many of those working in psychiatry in Italy, to close down the asylum system was radical and highly influential. However, mental healthcare remains a controversial issue in all the countries discussed in this volume. His influence, and that of the Italian movement and Law 180 of 1978, were immense but remain contested. Some nations embraced Basaglia's ideas entirely, some in part, while others were intensely sceptical. Often, there was confusion and debate about what those ideas entailed, and what were the 'lessons' of the Italian story. Some ignored Italy altogether.

The story of what happened in Italian mental healthcare institutions from the 1960s onwards, and its global reach and reception since then, is fascinating, rich, and surprising. This book, it is hoped, tells a set of stories which have not been told before, and certainly never in this way—in dialogue with each other and with the broader Italian story. We have tried to bring together international experiences and understandings, connecting individuals, institutions, and discussions. It is to be hoped that this book will inspire further debate and reflection. This is certainly the spirit in which this work is intended to be read.

References and further reading

Arbex, D. (2013). *Holocausto brasileiro.* Geração Editorial.
Babini, V.P. (2009). *Liberi tutti: manicomi e psichiatri in Italia: una storia del Novecento.* Bologna: Il Mulino.
Barham, P. (1997). *Closing the Asylum: Mental Patients in Modern Society.* London: Penguin.
Basaglia, F. (ed.) (1967). *Che cos'è la psichiatria?* Parma, Italy: Provincial Administration of Parma.
Basaglia, F. (ed.) (1968). *L'istituzione negata [The Institution Denied]*. Turin: Einaudi.
Basaglia, F. (1980). Problems of law and psychiatry: the Italian experience. Report of the Fourth International Congress on Law and Psychiatry. *International Journal of Law and Psychiatry* 3:17.
Basaglia, F. (1981). Breaking the circuit of control. In: D. Ingleby (ed.), *Critical Psychiatry: The Politics of Mental Health.* Harmondsworth: Penguin, pp. 184–92.
Basaglia, F. (2000). *Conferenze Brasiliane,* F. Ongaro Basaglia and M. Grazia Giannichedda (eds). Milan: Raffaello Cortina Editore.
Cipriano, P. (2015). *Il manicomio chimico. Cronache di uno psichiatra riluttante.* Milan: Elèuthera.
Crossley, N. (2006). *Contesting Psychiatry: Social Movements in Mental Health.* London and New York: Routledge.
Foot, J. (2015). *The Man Who Closed the Asylums. Franco Basaglia and the Revolution in Mental Health Care in Italy.* Milan: Feltrinelli.
Giacanelli, F. (2014). *Nascita del movimento antimanicomiale umbro,* Pliniana: Fondazione Angelo Celli per una cultura della salute; Selci-Lama [San Giustino].
Goffman, E. (1961). *Asylums: Essays on the Social Situations of Mental Patients and Other Inmates.* New York: Anchor Books.
Gijswijt–Hofstra, M., et al. (eds) (2005). *Psychiatric Cultures Compared: Psychiatry and Mental Health Care in the Twentieth Century. Comparisons and Approaches.* Amsterdam: Amsterdam University Press.
Jones, K. (1993). *Asylums and After. A Revised History of the Mental Health Services: From the Early 18th Century to the 1990s.* London and Atlantic Highlands (NJ): Athlone Press.
Jones, K. and Poletti, A. (1985). Understanding the Italian experience. *British Journal of Psychiatry* 146:341–7.
Jones, M. (1968). Beyond the Therapeutic Community: Social Learning and Social Psychiatry. New Haven, Conn.: Yale University Press.
Kritsotaki, D., et al. (eds) (2013). *Deinstitutionalisation and After. Post-War Psychiatry in the Western World.* London: Palgrave.
Micheli, G.A. (2019). Not just a one-man revolution: the multifaceted anti-asylum watershed in Italy. *History of Psychiatry* 30(2):133–49.
Piro, S. and Carrino, C. (2010). *Quando ho i soldi mi compro un pianoforte. Conversazioni con un protagonista della psichiatria del '900.* Napoli: Liguori Editore.
Porter, R. and Wright, D. (eds) (2003). *The Confinement of the Insane: International Perspectives, 1800–1965.* Cambridge: Cambridge University Press.
Putnam, R. (1993). *Making Democracy Work: Civic Traditions in Modern Italy.* Princeton: Princeton University Press.
Roth, M. (1972). Presidential address: 'Psychiatry and its critics'. *Canadian Journal of Psychiatry* 17:343–50.

Scheper–Hughes, N. and Lovell, A. (eds) (1987). *Psychiatry Inside-Out: Selected Writings of Franco Basaglia*. New York: Columbia University Press.
Scull, A. (1977). *Decarceration*. New Jersey: Prentice Hall.
Scull, A. (1997). Historical reflections on asylums, communities and the mentally ill. *Mentalities* 11(2):1–19.
Scull, A. (2015). *Madness in Civilisation. A Cultural History of Insanity, from the Bible to Freud, from the Madhouse to Modern Medicine*. London: Thames and Hudson.
Sedgwick, P. (1982). *Psychopolitics (The Politics of Health)*. London: Bloomsbury/Pluto.
Sinclair, S. (1997). Making doctors: an institutional apprenticeship. *London, General Psychiatry* 37:392–7.
Stein, L.I. and Test, M.A. (1980). Alternative to mental hospital treatment. I. Conceptual model, treatment program, and clinical evaluation. *Archives of General Psychiatry* 37(4):392–7.
Taylor, B. (2014). *The Last Asylum: A Memoir of Madness in Our Times*. London: Hamish Hamilton.
Wall, O. (2018). *The British Anti-Psychiatrists: From Institutional Psychiatry to the Counter-Culture, 1960–1971*. Oxford, New York: Routledge.
World Health Organization (1978). *The Future of Mental Hospitals*. Copenhagen: WHO Regional Office for Europe.

Index

Figures are indicated by *f* following the page number.

For the benefit of digital users, indexed terms that span two pages (e.g., 52–53) may, on occasion, appear on only one of those pages.

Adam 31, 35
Alpha Club 26
Amieux, Marie-Claude 279
Andreoli, Vittorino 251
anti-fascism 7–9
anti-psychiatry 23, 83–85, 176, 258–59, 301, 351–52
Anti-University of London 34, 36–37
Appadurai, Arjun 83–84
Arbours Association 29
Argentina 129
  Basaglia Argentina Conference 140
  deinstitutionalization 130–31, 132–35
  desmanicomialización 134
  Legal Unit No. 22 138
  MDRI/CELS report 136
  Mental Health National Monitoring Body 138
  military dictatorship 129–30
  National Directorate for Mental Health 130–32
  National Mental Health Law 26657 136–38
  Río Negro reforms 100, 108, 132–35
  Universidad Popular de las Madres de la Plaza de Mayo conferences 136
assertive community treatment 328, 350
Asylum: the magazine for democratic psychiatry 205

Baillon, Guy 280
Bairaktaris, Kostas 164
Balduzzi, Edoardo 282–83
Balestrieri, Antonia 250–51
Balvet, Paul 276
Bangay, Frank 220
Baremblit, Valentín 134
Barnes, Mary 28–29
Barton, Russel 182
Basaglia, Franco xiii, 6*f*, 50*f*, 57*f*, 120*f*
  anti-fascism 7–9
  death 18–19
  early career 4–5
  father (Enrico) 7
  friendships 13–14
  global mental health 89–91
  ideology 85–86, 183, 355
  implementation of reforms 354
  imprisonment 7–8
  international influence 79
  Marxism 355–56
  misunderstandings of 82–87
  networks 5–6
  personality 7, 10–13
  philanthropic concerns 86–87
  therapeutic dimension 163–64
  university career 5, 9–10
  wife (Franca Ongaro) 1, 4, 8–9, 14, 15–16, 114, 158*f*, 351
Basaglia's Law (Law 180) xiii, 18–20, 55, 70–71, 161–62, 260, 282–83
Basauri, Victor Aparicio 158*f*
Battaglia, Giovanna 208
Belize 103, 107
Bellufi, Max 283
Berke, Joseph 29, 32, 36–37
Berlin, Isaiah 184
Bigwood, Lyn 207
Binswanger, Ludwig 229–30, 231
biomedical model 44, 87
Bollati, Giulio 13
Bonnafé, Lucien 276, 278, 280, 283
Borgna, Eugenio 229–30
Bourne, Harold 196–97
Bracken, Pat 197, 200
bracketing the diagnosis 62, 117, 163, 325, 338, 351–52
Brasilia Principles on the Development of Mental Health Care in the Americas (PAHO/WHO) 101
Braziers Park conference 34–35
Brazil 98, 113
  Barbacena hospital 119
  Belo Horizonte parade 122
  centres for psychosocial care (CAPS) 103–5, 119, 125
  community services 104–5
  conferences 95–97, 114–15
  deinstitutionalization 80, 104–5, 119

Brazil (*cont.*)
epistemological debate 117–19
First International Symposium on Psychoanalysis Groups and Institutions 116
mental health legislation 118–19, 122
Mental Health Workers' Movement (MTSM) 116–17
National Day of Anti-Asylum Fight 117–18, 122
reforms 79–80, 100, 103–6, 119
residential services 105
Returning Home programme 105
Social Movement for a Society Without Asylums 117–18
Unified Health System (SUS) 104, 117
Valuation and Restructuring Programme of the Psychiatric Assistance Hospitals 120–21
Brétécher, Paul 280
Briskin, Sid 28, 29, 38–39
Britain *see* United Kingdom
British Journal of Psychiatry 177–82, 196–97
Browne, Ivor 199–200
Burtson, D. 31–32

Callieri, Bruno 229–30
capability for voice 142
Caracas Declaration 98–100, 134–35
Cargnello, Danilo 229–30
Carrino, Luciano 279
Castel, Françoise 281–82
Castel, Robert 119, 214, 280, 281–82
Cayetano, Claudina 107
Chávez, González de 156–57
Chile 103, 106–7, 123
citizenship 53, 54
civil rights 55–56, 98–99, 340–41
clinical recovery 47, 60–61
Cogliati, Maria Grazia 263
Cohen, Hugo 132–33
Comba, Letizia 2–4
Common European Guidelines of the Transition from Institutions to Community Care 313
communism 228–33
community care/services 58, 71–75, 90, 98–99, 100, 104–5, 107, 108, 134, 157, 170, 176, 210, 328, 350
Congress on the Dialectics of Liberation 34, 35–36
Convention on the Rights of Persons with Disabilities (UN) 56, 61–62, 83–84
conversion model 308–9
Cooper, David 23–24, 24*f*, 26–27, 28, 29, 36, 38–39, 154–55, 214, 258, 281–82, 351
Cooperativa Lavoratori Uniti Franco Basaglia 133–34
cooperatives 133–34, 165, 169, 285
Corcés, Valentin 156
Costa, Filipe 339
criminalization 323–24, 326–27, 339
Crimini di Pace (Basaglia) 87
critical psychiatry 258–59
Crossley, Nick 215, 258, 261
Cuba 108
cultural issues 324–28, 338–39
Cunnold, Joan 28

Dabrowski, Stanislaw 249
Dal Bo, Agostino Zanon 7
Daumézon, Georges 276
Dedijer, Vladimir 6*f*
De Girolamo, Giovanni 196–97
deinstitutionalization 45, 46–48, 53, 58, 80–81, 89–90
Argentina 130–31, 132–35
Brazil 80, 104–5, 119
France 282–89
Greece 167, 170, 172
human rights 55, 61
institutional relationship 50–52
Italy 19, 58, 80–81, 89–90, 187, 354–55
meanings 89
Netherlands 269, 270–71
Sweden 334–39, 341–42
therapeutic relationship 52
UK 176, 186, 189
US 318–19
Yugoslavia 295, 301–7, 309–10
Delgado, Paulo 118–19
Del Giudice, Giovanna 140
Dell'Acqua, Giuseppe 263, 317
democratic psychiatry xiii–xiv, 50, 153, 218–20, 260–64
De Oliveira Marques, E.M. 122–23
diffusion of innovations 247–53
Divided Self, The (Laing) 24–26
Donzelot, Jacques 281–82
Doray, Bernard 280
Dörner, Klaus 239
double disease 44–46

electroconvulsive therapy 184–85
Elkaïm, Mony 280
El Salvador 97
empowerment 54–55, 62–63, 117, 307
England *see* United Kingdom
Escher, Sandra 214
Esterson, Aaron 23–24, 28, 29
everyday life 49
evidence-based practice 186
Ey, Henri 277, 278

Falconnet, Claude 279
family involvement 101, 103, 327
Faraone, Silvia 130

Farren, M. 34
Finzen, Asmus 227–28
Fischer, Andrea 227
Fo, Dario 57*f*
Foucault, Michel 45, 154–55
Foudraine, Jan 258–59
France 275
  Alternatives à la Psychiatrie 280–81
  Association pour l'Etude et la Promotion des Structures Intermédiaires (ASEPI) 281, 283
  Centre d'Entraînement aux Méthodes de Pédagogie Active 281
  deinstitutionalization 282–89
  Events 279
  Housing First 288
  involuntary commitment 287–88
  Le Cheval Bleu 280, 281
  psychothérapie institutionalle 276
  secteurs 276–77, 282, 283–85
  Syndicat de la Psychiatrie 281–82, 283
freedom
  freedom from/freedom to 184
  'freedom is therapeutic' 46*f*, 58–59, 91, 169
Freire, Paulo 121–22

Galende, Emiliano 131–32
Galli, Vincente 130–32
García, Ramón 149–50
gender issues 351
general hospitals 101, 103, 139–40
Gerais, Minas 119, 124
Germany 227
  after Law 180 237–40
  communists 228–33
  depiction of Italy 229
  German Society for Social Psychiatry (DGSP) 234, 236–37
  Informationszentrum Rote Volksuniversität 236
  left-wing terrorism 229
  Mannheimer Kreis 236–37
  Nazis 228–33, 245
  Psychiatrie-Enquête' silver jubilee 227
  Socialist Patients' Collective (Patientenfront) 234–37
Gillet, Michel 279
Gilli, G.A. 301–2
global mental health 89–91
Goffman, Erving 154–55, 182, 248–49
Goldenberg, Mauricio 134
Goldman, Lucien 279
Gorizia mental hospital 15–17, 33–34, 187
Goulart, Daniel Magalhães 222–23
Gramscian existentialism 88
grand theories 176, 183–85
Greece 161
  Chania Mental Hospital, Crete 171–72
  deinstitutionalization 167, 170, 172
  Dromokaiteion Mental Hospital 165
  Leros Colony of Mental Patients 165–71
  Psychiatric Hospital of Attica 164–65, 172
  Thessaloniki Mental Hospital 164
Greenwood, Mark 211–12, 216
guardianship 51
Guattari, Félix 214, 262, 280, 282

Haafkens, Joke 265
Haaster, Harrie 266
Häfner, Heinz 233
Hanaghan, Jonathan 195
Harrington, V. 212–13
Hartman, Mark 196
Havers, Joseph 35–36
Hayward, S.T. 26
healing 47–48, 49, 54
health, in everyday life 49
Hearing Voices movement 214
Heinrich, Kurt 239–40
Hervé, Edmond 284
Hippius, Hanns 233
holistic approach 62
homelessness 270–71, 320–21, 339
housing 288, 319–20, 339–40
Huber, Wolfgang 234–35
human rights 50–51, 55, 59–61, 98–99, 138, 139, 199

ideology 85–86, 126, 183, 355
illness
  in brackets 62, 117, 163, 325, 338, 351–52
  in everyday life 49
implementation 354
institutional double 44–46
institutionalism 44–46
In the Name of Reason 119
involuntary commitment and treatment 287–88, 322–23, 340
Ireland 191
  Great Famine 193
  lack of professional journals 196
  psychoanalysis 194–96
  Report of the Commission of Inquiry on Mental Illness 193–94
  Roman Catholic Church 194
  Scheper-Hughes book 197–98
Italy 69
  community mental health 71–75
  deinstitutionalization 19, 58, 80–81, 89–90, 187, 354–55
  Department of Mental Health 72, 74, 75–76
  Falucci Commission (integration of disabled school pupils) 70–71

Italy (*cont.*)
forensic psychiatric hospitals 74–75
German depiction of 229
Hot Autumn revolutionary movement 278
Law 180 (Basaglia's Law) xiii, 18–20, 55, 70–71, 161–62, 260, 282–83
Law 658 (addiction services) 71
National Health System 70, 72, 73–74, 75
Psichiatria Democratica xiii–xiv, 50, 153
Trieste experience xiii–xiv, 17–18, 56–59, 80–81, 89–90, 180–81, 187, 205, 210–16, 261–62

Jakubovicz, Albert 279
Janssen, Marc 264, 266
Jaroszewski, Zbigniew 246–47
Jaspers, Karl 229–30, 231–32
Jenner, Alec 206, 207–8, 210–11, 214, 216, 222
Jenner, Barbara 207–8
Jenz, Hans Werner 238
Jervis, Giovanni 2–4, 11, 12, 13, 17
Jones, Kathleen 177–82, 196–97
Jones, Maxwell 182, 185, 351–52

Kecmanovic, D. 299
Kendall, Tim 207–8, 211, 222
Kingsley Hall 28–31, 33–34, 35, 38–39
Korngold, Murray 38–39
Kos, Anica 301–2
Kotowicz, Zbigniew 31–32
Kouba, Anik 280
Kraepelin, Emil 25
Kulenkampf, Caspar 233

Lacey, Ron 177
Lainé, Tony 280
Laing, R.D. 23–26, 28, 29, 30, 32–33, 37–38, 83, 84, 181, 210, 215, 258
Latham, John 34
Law 180 (Basaglia's Law) xiii, 18–20, 55, 70–71, 161–62, 260, 282–83
Law 658 71
Leder, Stefan 251
Le Guillant, Louis 277–78
Levav, Itzhak 97
L'Istituzione Negata (Basaglia) 81, 114
lived citizenship 53
López Ibor, Juan José 151, 156
Louzoun, Claude 280
Lovell, Anne M. 197–98

McCann, Eamonn 35
McCarthy, Robert 199
McGrath, Tom 34
McLaughlin, Terence 216–18
McQuaid, John C. 195
Mad Movement 222
Mak, Geert 261
Mallet, Serge 279
Mamelet, Marie-Rose 282
Manuali, Carlo 265
map of the shame 150
Marco Cavallo (horse) 187, 261, 280
Martin, Jean-Pierre 280
Martins, Hélder xv–xvi
Marxism 297–98, 355–56
Matti da Slegare 262
medical model 321–22, 325
mental hospital, definitions 357–58
mental suffering 133, 138
Metge, Jean-Luc 280
Mezzina, Roberto 317
Milner, Marion 30
Minguzzi, Gian Franco 6*f*, 237
Minkowski, Eugeniusz 246
Minoletti, Alberto 106–7
Montejo, Javier 158*f*
Montgomery, Stuart 37
Mosher, Loren 177
Mozambique xv–xvi

Natella, Graciela 132–33
Nazis 228–33, 245
neo-institutionalization 105–6
Netherlands 257
'Amsterdam model' 264–67
'Amsterdam muddle' 270–71
Clients Union 260–61
critical psychiatry movement 258–59
deinstitutionalization 269, 270–71
enthusiasm for democratic psychiatry 260–64
homeless 270–71
Pandora Foundation 260–61
Runaway Shelters 257, 263–64
Santpoort Psychiatric Hospital 264, 267, 269
Social Psychiatric Service Centre 266–67, 269, 270
Nicaragua 97
normality, pathologizing 342–43
Nowlan, David 198
Nuttall, Jeff 34, 35

Odenbach, Erwin 238
Ongaro, Alberto 8–9
Ongaro, Franca 1, 4, 8–9, 14, 15–16, 114, 158*f*, 351
Oury, Jean 282

Palermo, George B. 197
Panama 103, 107

Pan American Health Organization (PAHO)
  Mental Health Unit 97–98
  psychiatric care in Latin America 99, 100–2
Parker, Ian 215–16
participation 52–55
Pascal, Jean-Charles 282
patients' protagonism 142
pedagogy of power 51
Pembroke, Louise 220–21
Penjeam, Alfredo 106–7
Permanent Conference for Psychiatric Reform of Southern European Regions 98
personal recovery 47, 60–61
person-centred approach 62
Peru 108
Petraglia, Sandro 262
Petry, Detlev 269–70
Philadelphia Association (Institute) 28–29, 30, 34, 35
Piel, Eric 285–86
Pirella, Agostino 16, 234, 260, 262, 283
Piro, Sergio 354
Plan of Action of Mental Health (PAHO/WHO) 101
Poland 245
  communication and diffusion of innovations 247–53
  Nazi extermination policy 245
  sectorization 249
Poletti, Alison 177–82, 196–97
power 50–52, 87, 307
pragmatism 176, 184–85, 186
primary care 98–99, 100, 105, 106, 107, 108, 349–50
Project Sigma 34
Prot-Klinger, Katarzyna 251, 252
Psichiatria Democratica xiii–xiv, 50, 153
Psychiatric Coordinator 148–55
psychoanalysis 131–32, 194–96

Querido, Arie 267

radicalism 125–26
Ralite, Jack 284
Ramon, Shulamit 196–97, 206
Ratton, Helvécio 119
Reali, Mario 236, 305–6
recognition 52–55
recovery 43–44, 171, 224, 325
  clinical 47, 60–61
  from the institution 44–46
  human rights 59–61
  personal 47, 60–61
  social factors 48
  subjectivity 46–48
reduction 117
reductionist view 43–44
rehabilitation 51, 186–87
Reich, Wilhelm 301
research programmes 102, 186
Roelandt, Jean-Luc 280, 285–86
Rogers, Everett M. 247–48
Romme, Marius 214, 268
Rotelli, Franco 73–74, 80, 81, 84–85, 97, 129, 135–36, 167, 283
Roth, Joseph 231
Roth, Martin 176

Salvini, Matteo 161
Saraceno, Benedetto 97
Sarkozy, Nicolas 287–88
Sartre, Jean-Paul 6*f*
Sassolas, Marcel 279
Schatzman, Morton 29
Scheper-Hughes, Nancy 197–98
Schmid, Sil 238, 260
Schmidt-Gante, Helmtraud 233
Schork, Werner 235
science, neutrality of 125
sectorization 249, 276–77, 282, 283–85, 336
Sedgwick, Peter 31–32, 33, 210
Sen, Amartya 83–84, 142
Sepulveda, Rafael 106–7
Serós, Ana 150
service users 101, 103, 211
Shenley Hospital 26–27
Sigal, Clancy 28
Simon, Hermann 232–33
Simons, Thomas 238–39
Sinclair, Simon 353
Sivadon, Paul 276
Slavich, Antonio 10
social body 47–48
social capital 354–55
social control 116–17
social engineering 333–34, 338, 339–40
social enterprise 134
social exchange 51–52, 169
social factors, recovery 48
social integration 54
socialist feminism 213
social psychiatry 297–301
societal change 216–18
societal engagement 187–88
Spain 79, 147
  Basaglia's influence 156–57
  conservative psychiatry 151
  General Health Law 157–59
  Mental Institute of the Holy Cross 149–50

Spain (*cont.*)
Ministry of Health 155
MIR Coordinator 153
Psychiatric Coordinator 148–55
Psychiatric Hospital of Salt 150
Socialist Party victory 157–59
Spanish Association of Neuropsychiatry 157
Spanish Society of Psychiatry 151
tardofranquismo 147
university student movements 147
specialist services 74, 186–87, 350
Strategy and Plan of Action on Mental Health (PAHO/WHO) 101
Stritih, Bernard 301–2
subjectivity 46–48, 87
substance abuse 323
substitution model 308–9
survivor movement 220–22
suspension 117
Sweden 333
civil rights 340–41
context 333–34
cultural issues 338–39
deinstitutionalization 334–39, 341–42
folkhemmet 333–34
involuntary treatment 340
National Board of Social Affairs reports 335–36
sectorized hospitals 336
social engineering 333–34, 338, 339–40
sterilization programme 334
Swift, Jonathan 194–95
Szafranski, Tomasz 252
Szasz, Thomas 218–19, 258

Tansella, Michele 73, 186, 196–97
technological paradigm 44
Terzian, Hryay 10, 13
therapeutic communities 26–29, 149, 157, 182, 185, 218, 260, 305, 356–57
therapeutic dimension 163–64
Tobino, Mario 13
Tomkiewicz, Stanislas 280
Tommasini, Mario 13, 262
Torrent, Luis 150
Tosquelles, François 276
training 102, 131
Tranchina, Paolo 30–31, 33, 283
transinstitutionalization 252, 298–99, 339
Trieste experience xiii–xiv, 17–18, 56–59, 80–81, 89–90, 180–81, 187, 205, 210–16, 261–62
Trimbos, Kees 259, 268
Trocchi, Alexander 34, 35

United Kingdom
Alpha Club 26
anti-psychiatrists 23
Anti-University of London 34, 36–37
Birmingham mental health service 81
Braziers Park conference 34–35
British Journal of Psychiatry articles 177–82, 196–97
Cochrane Collaboration 186
community care 176, 210
Congress on the Dialectics of Liberation 34, 35–36
deinstitutionalization 176, 186, 189
Dingleton Hospital 182–83, 185
evidence-based practice 186
Harpurhey resettlement team 211–13
Hearing Voices Network 214
Kingsley Hall 28–31, 33–34, 35, 38–39
Mental Health Act 1959 182
NICE 186
Philadelphia Association (Institute) 28–29, 30, 34, 35
pragmatism 176, 184–85, 186
Project Sigma 34
recruitment and morale in psychiatry 188
rejection of Basaglia 82, 175
research 186
service developments inspired by Trieste 210–14
Shenley Hospital 26–27
specialist rehabilitation services 186–87
Springfield Psychiatric Hospital 211–12, 213
suspicion of grand theories 176, 183–85
Team for the Assessment of Psychiatric Services (TAPS) 186
therapeutic communities 26–29, 182, 185
Villa 21 26–27, 33–34, 38–39
United Nations, Convention on the Rights of Persons with Disabilities 56, 61–62, 83–84
United States 317
criminalization 323–24, 326–27
cultural values 324–28
deinstitutionalization 318–19
Fountain House 328
Golden Gate Bridge suicides 326–27
involuntary commitment 322–23
mental health system 321–23
model treatment programmes 328–29
Program for Community Living 328
segregation 327–28
social and economic infrastructure 319–21
Soteria House 218
substance abuse 323
tax structure 326
transinstitutionalization 299
Village 328

Valdés Miyar, M 151
Van der Klinkenberg, Tineke 266–67
van der Poel, Egbert 264–65, 266, 268
van der Wilk, Hans 260–61, 268
van Weeghel, Jaap 270–71
Venezuela, Caracas Declaration 98–100, 134–35
Venturini, Ernesto xvi
Vermorel, Henri 278–79
Villa 21 26–27, 33–34, 38–39
Viney, Michael 198
Virden, Phil 207, 219

Wall, Oisin 352
Walsh, Dermot 196, 198–99
Wilkinson, R.K. 28
Winkler, Walter Theodor 233
Winnicott, D.W. 30
women's-only services 351
work participation 133–34, 165, 169, 215–16, 285
World Health Organization (WHO)
  World Health Day (2001) 100
  World Health Report (2001) 89, 100
Wulff, Erich 234, 237, 239–40

Yugoslavia 295
  Community Mental Health Studies 303–4
  deinstitutionalization 295, 301–7, 309–10
  Marxist psychiatry 297–98
  Occupy Movement 304
  social psychiatry 297–301
  South East Europe Mental Health Project 305–6
  Tempus programme 303–4, 305
  transinstitutionalization 298–99
  Walkout 304

Zavoli, Sergio 187